Quick Reference to

EAR, NOSE, AND THROAT DISORDERS

WILLIAM R. WILSON, M.D.

Associate Professor of Otolaryngology
Harvard Medical School
Associate Surgeon, Department of Otolaryngology
Massachusetts Eye and Ear Infirmary
Boston, Massachusetts

JOSEPH B. NADOL, JR., M.D.

Associate Professor of Otolaryngology
Harvard Medical School
Associate Surgeon, Department of Otolaryngology
Massachusetts Eye and Ear Infirmary
Boston, Massachusetts

with medical illustrations by ROBERT J. GALLA,
Massachusetts General Hospital

Quick Reference to

EAR, NOSE, AND THROAT DISORDERS

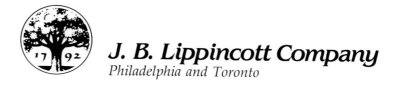

J. B. Lippincott Company
Philadelphia and Toronto

Sponsoring Editor: Richard Winters
Manuscript Editor: J. Bruce Martin
Indexer: Deana Fowler
Art Director: Maria S. Karkucinski
Designer: Ronald Dorfman
Production Supervisor: N. Carol Kerr
Production Coordinator: Charles W. Field
Compositor: Waldman Graphics, Inc.
Printer/Binder: Halliday Lithographic

The authors and publisher have exerted every effort to ensure that drug
selection and dosage set forth in this text are in accord with current rec-
ommendations and practice at the time of publication. However, in view
of ongoing research, changes in government regulations, and the constant
flow of information relating to drug therapy and drug reactions, the reader
is urged to check the package insert for each drug for any change in indications and dosage and for added warnings and precautions. This is particularly important when the recommended agent is a new or infrequently
employed drug.

1   3   5   6   4   2

Library of Congress Cataloging in Publication Data
Wilson, William R.
Quick reference to ear, nose, and throat disorders.
Bibliography
Includes index.
1. Otolaryngology—Handbooks, manuals, etc.
I. Nadol, Joseph B. II. Title. [DNLM:
1. Otolaryngology—Handbooks. WV 100 W754q]
RF56.W54   617'.51   82-15315
ISBN 0-397-50519-1   AACR2

CONTENTS

PREFACE *vii*

ACKNOWLEDGMENTS *ix*

1 Functional Anatomy, Physiology, and
Examination of the Ear
Joseph B. Nadol, Jr. *1*

2 Hearing Loss
Joseph B. Nadol, Jr. *25*

3 The Draining Ear
Joseph B. Nadol, Jr. *51*

4 The Dizzy Patient
William R. Wilson *71*

5 Ear Emergencies
Joseph B. Nadol, Jr. *97*

6 A Brief Review of Nasal Anatomy and Physiology
William R. Wilson *113*

7 Nasal and Sinus Congestion and Infection
William R. Wilson *127*

8 Nasal and Facial Emergencies
William R. Wilson   145

9 Pain Syndromes in the Head and Neck
Joseph B. Nadol, Jr.   175

10 Salivary-Gland Disorders
Joseph B. Nadol, Jr.   185

11 Sore Mouth and Throat and Hoarseness
William R. Wilson   197

12 Airway Emergencies
William R. Wilson   227

13 Evaluation of Neck Masses
Joseph B. Nadol, Jr.   237

14 Radiology of the Ears, Nose, and Throat
for the Primary-Care Physician
Alfred L. Weber and William R. Wilson   255

APPENDIX   315

INDEX   319

PREFACE

Quick Reference to Ear, Nose, and Throat Disorders evolved from a syllabus developed for a course for primary-care physicians given by the Department of Otolaryngology of the Harvard Medical School at the Massachusetts Eye and Ear Infirmary in Boston, Massachusetts. It is intended to help primary-care physicians improve their practice of office and emergency otolaryngology by providing practical information in a concise, quick-reference form. This is a symptom-oriented text that includes discussions not only of diagnosis and treatment but also of when to refer to, and what may be the expected treatment prescribed by, the consulting otolaryngologist. The Appendix describes instruments that are necessary for a well-stocked office.

It is our hope that this book will serve as a teacher and guide to our primary-care colleagues.

William R. Wilson, M.D.
Joseph B. Nadol, Jr., M.D.

ACKNOWLEDGMENTS

We wish to thank the following people for their assistance in the preparation of this book: Ms. Jean Dinon, Ms. Debra Kavesh, Harold F. Schuknecht, M.D., William W. Montgomery, M.D., Alfred Weber, M.D., Howard M. Ecker, M.D., and A. J. Gulya, M.D. We wish to thank members of the staff of the Massachusetts Eye and Ear Infirmary and Children's Hospital Medical Center who have helped us with lectures and clinical sessions: Elaine D. Carrol, M.D., Roland D. Eavey, M.D., Richard L. Fabian, M.D., Gerald B. Healy, M.D., Michael Joseph, M.D., Ely A. Kirschner, M.D., William G. Lavelle, M.D., Joseph A. Moretti, M.D., Thomas J. Mulvaney, M.D., Angelo J. Pappanikou, M.D., James T. Rhea, M.D., Stephen A. Smith, M.D., and Michael Zoller, M.D. We also wish to thank other members of the staff of the Massachusetts Eye and Ear Infirmary and our students.

In addition, we would like to acknowledge the support of the members of our families: Elizabeth, David, Anne, and Carolyn Wilson and Ruth, Joseph, and Benjamin Nadol.

Quick Reference to

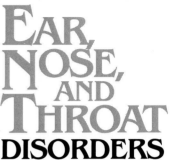

EAR, NOSE, AND THROAT

DISORDERS

1

FUNCTIONAL ANATOMY, PHYSIOLOGY, AND EXAMINATION OF THE EAR

Joseph B. Nadol, Jr.

Functional anatomy and physiology
  Auricle and external auditory canal
  Tympanic membrane
  Middle ear and mastoid cell system
  Ossicles
  Inner ear and internal auditory canal
  Facial nerve
Examination of the ear
  Inspection and cleaning
  Otoscopy
  Tests of auditory function
    Tuning-fork and whisper tests

    Behavioral audiometry (standard hearing tests)
    Special behavioral tests
    Auditory evoked-response testing
    Tympanometry
    Tests for functional hearing loss
  Vestibular testing
    Caloric tests
    Positional testing
    Fistula test
  Facial-nerve tests
    Site-of-lesion testing
    Neurophysiologic tests of neuronal viability

FUNCTIONAL ANATOMY AND PHYSIOLOGY

The ear is divided anatomically into external, middle, and inner portions (Fig. 1-1). The external ear consists of the auricle and the external auditory canal. The middle ear consists of the ossicular chain and air space continuous with the mastoid air-cell system; it is separated from the external ear by the tympanic membrane. The inner ear consists of the bony otic capsule, auditory and vestibular receptor organs, and the first portion of the eighth nerve.

AURICLE AND EXTERNAL AUDITORY CANAL

The auricle, with the exception of the lobule, contains a cartilaginous skeleton that develops from cartilaginous accumulations, or "hillocks," derived from the first (mandibular) and second (hyoid) branchial arches. Therefore, congenital malformations of these arches are commonly associated with auricular abnormalities. The intrinsic musculature of the auricle allows rotation of the external ear in animals, but this function is vestigial in the human.

The lateral one third of the external auditory canal is composed of cartilage extending from the auricle and is covered by skin with appendages specialized for cerumen production. The medial two thirds of the

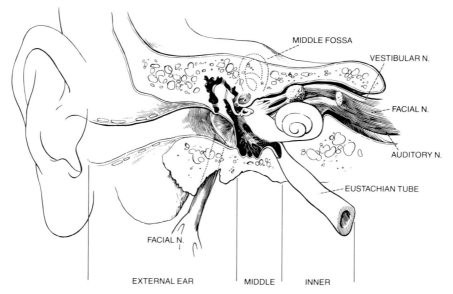

Fig. 1-1. Coronal section of the right ear and temporal bone.

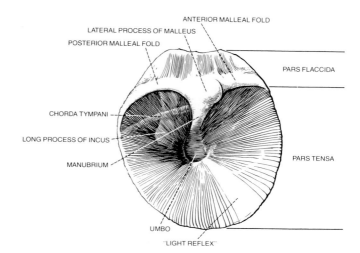

Fig. 1-2. Otoscopic view of tympanic membrane, which is divided into the pars flaccida and pars tensa by the anterior and posterior malleal folds.

external canal has a bony skeleton derived from the tympanic, mastoid, and squamous portions of the temporal bone. The skin here is thin and devoid of appendages. Therefore, disordered embryologic development in the first branchial groove may result in stenosis or atresia of the external canal.

TYMPANIC MEMBRANE

The eardrum, or tympanic membrane (Fig. 1-2), is divided into two distinct parts. The pars flaccida, or Shrapnell's membrane, lies above the anterior and posterior malleal folds. The pars tensa comprises the rest of the tympanic membrane. Landmarks visible on routine otoscopy include the lateral process of the malleus, which forms a bony prominence at the junction of Shrapnell's membrane and the pars tensa; the manubrium; and the umbo, where the pars tensa is attached to the end of the malleus. In the young, translucent tympanic membrane, the long process of the incus, the suprastructure of the stapes, and the chorda tympani nerve all may be visible. The "light reflex" is a wedge-shaped reflection of light seen with the otoscope as originating at the umbo and extending anteroinferiorly to the edge of the tympanic membrane. Although often present, the light reflex does not ensure the absence of disease, nor does its absence signify pathology.

It is important that the examiner visualize both parts of the drum. The pars flaccida is the most commonly overlooked, and it is in this area that the most serious disease processes, such as cholesteatoma, may be located.

The tympanic membrane serves several important functions. First, it closes the middle-ear space from the external ear canal. Second, it collects and transmits sound selectively to the oval window of the inner ear. Third, it protects the round window—the second opening between middle and inner ear—from sound waves, thus providing an important phase difference between the oval and round windows.

MIDDLE EAR AND MASTOID CELL SYSTEM

The middle ear and eustachian tube are derived from the dorsal end of the first pharyngeal pouch. The pneumatization of the mastoid is limited at birth to the antrum, the cell area closest to the middle ear. There is a wide range of normal variability in the extent of pneumatization, which progresses during the first 2 decades of life.

The medial two thirds of the eustachian tube is cartilaginous and ends in the nasopharynx. It is normally closed and opens during swallowing owing to the muscular activity of the tensor veli palatini.

OSSICLES

The ossicular chain consists of the malleus, incus, and stapes. Their function is to transmit mechanical energy from the tympanic membrane across the air-filled middle ear to the fluid-filled inner ear. The malleus is the longest ossicle, but only the manubrium and a portion of the neck are visible by otoscopy. The head of the malleus lies above the level of the tympanic membrane in the epitympanum. There it articulates with the body of the incus, which in turn articulates with the head, or capitulum, of the stapes. The ossicles are suspended within the middle ear by the suspensory, anterior, and lateral ligaments of the malleus and the posterior ligament of the incus.

The relative lengths of the malleus and incus and their axis of rotation produce a mechanical advantage, a lever mechanism, which results in a gain of approximately 2.5 db as sound is transmitted through the middle ear. An additional mechanical advantage is achieved through a hydraulic effect that results from the ratio between the effective surface areas of the tympanic membrane (approximately 55 sq mm) and the stapes footplate (approximately 3.2 sq mm). This ratio provides an additional gain of 25 db.

The ossicular chain, with the exception of the stapes footplate, is derived from first and second branchial arches. Middle-ear abnormalities and conductive hearing loss are commonly associated with first and second branchial arch syndromes such as Crouzon's disease and Treacher-Collins syndrome.

There are two middle-ear muscles: the stapedius and tensor tympani. The stapedius originates in the bony facial canal, inserts on the capitulum or neck of the stapes, and is innervated by the seventh cranial nerve. The tensor tympani originates in a semicanal superior to the eustachian tube, inserts at the neck of the malleus, and is innervated by the fifth cranial nerve. It is thought that these muscles decrease the compliance of the ossicular chain and tympanic membrane and may serve a protective role in the presence of intense auditory stimulation.

INNER EAR AND INTERNAL AUDITORY CANAL

The inner ear is contained in the bony otic capsule. The membranous labyrinth is divided anatomically into two parts: the auditory portion, or cochlea, and the vestibular labyrinth, consisting of the three semicircular canals, the utricle, and the saccule (Fig. 1-3). The entire membranous labyrinth, both auditory and vestibular, is suspended in perilymphatic fluid that is contained by the surrounding bony otic capsule. Perilymph is similar chemically to extracellular fluid and cerebrospinal fluid. The perilymphatic space completely surrounds the entire

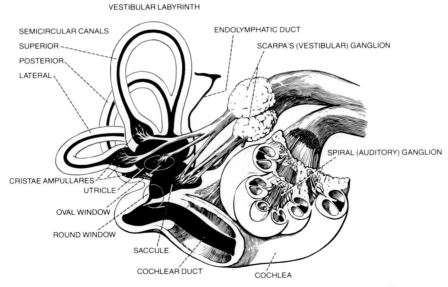

Fig. 1-3. Inner ear. The cochlea has been sectioned along the modiolus. The endolymphatic space is shown in black.

membranous labyrinth and is continuous with the subarachnoid space around the nerves of the internal auditory canal and the cochlear aqueduct. It is thought that perilymph is produced not only by simple diffusion of cerebrospinal fluid into the inner ear but also as an ultrafiltrate of plasma.

The membranous labyrinth, which is suspended like a complex balloon within the perilymph, contains endolymph. This fluid is most similar to extracellular fluid and has a very high potassium level (150 ± 10 mEq). The endolymphatic fluid space of the cochlear system is connected to that of the vestibular system by a narrow duct, the ductus reuniens (Fig. 1-4). It is thought that the stria vascularis of the cochlear portion of the membranous labyrinth and the dark cell area of the vestibular portion are responsible for the production of endolymph. The endolymphatic sac, which extends from the utricle and saccule into the posterior fossa, is thought to be at least partly responsible for resorption of endolymph. The exact mechanism for maintenance of the ionic gradients between perilymph and endolymph is not known.

The neuroepithelium of both the auditory and vestibular systems lies at an interface between perilymph and endolymph. The internal and external hair cells lying in a spiral array on the basilar membrane are the auditory receptor cells of the organ of Corti (Fig. 1-5). It is thought that the mechanical properties of the basilar membrane produce a max-

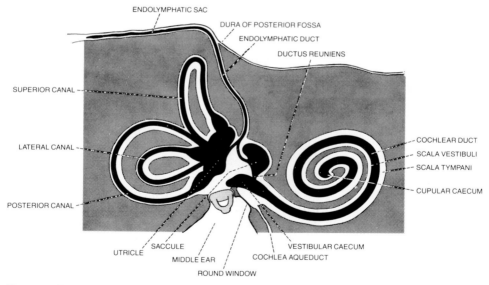

Fig. 1-4. Schematic drawing of the fluid spaces of the inner ear. The endolymphatic space is shown in black. The perilymphatic space is shown in white.

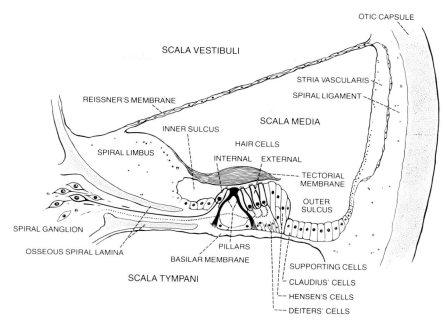

Fig. 1-5. Radial section of the organ of Corti.

imal point of vibration at a different site along it for each frequency in the physiologic range of the organism. Displacement of the basilar membrane leads to stimulation of the hair cells, which in turn causes depolarization of the first-order cochlear neuron and the conduction of an action potential. Thus, the basilar membrane serves as a first-order frequency analyzer. High-frequency sounds are detected at the basal end of the cochlea; low-frequency sounds are detected at the apical end. The afferent signals from each ear are distributed to both cerebral hemispheres by way of several brain-stem nuclei.

The semicircular canals of the vestibular apparatus lie in the three planes of space (Fig. 1-3). The sense organs, or cristae ampullares, are sensitive to angular acceleration in the plane of each canal. Two additional sense organs, the maculae, are contained in the utricle and saccule. The overlying otolithic membrane allows the macula to be sensitive to linear acceleration, or gravitational pull. As in the cochlea, displacement of the inner-ear fluid results in stimulation of hair cells, which in turn causes depolarization of the first-order vestibular neuron. The afferent impulse is then transmitted to the vestibular nuclei in the brain stem. Both auditory and vestibular nerves pass from the inner ear through the internal auditory canal and the subarachnoid space to brain-stem nuclei.

FACIAL NERVE

Because of its anatomical relationships with other structures of the inner ear, disorders of the facial nerve are often treated by the otolaryngologist. The motor root of the facial nerve originates in the facial nucleus of the pontine brain stem (Fig. 1-6). The nerve then passes through the anterosuperior aspect of the internal auditory canal, adjacent to auditory and vestibular nerves. Next the nerve passes through the geniculate ganglion, which contains the cell bodies of sensory fibers that also travel in the trunk of the nerve. The course of the nerve bends sharply posteriorly at the first genu and then sharply inferiorly at the second genu near the stapes footplate. It then descends in the bony fallopian canal in the most anterior part of the mastoid and exits at the skull base through the stylomastoid foramen. The nerve trifurcates at the pes an-

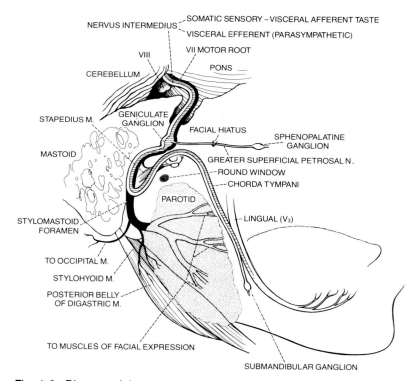

Fig. 1-6. Diagram of the course of the facial nerve. The facial nerve has both motor (black) and sensory fibers. The sensory fibers have their cell bodies in the geniculate ganglion and together with the visceral efferent fibers are called the nervus intermedius. The visceral afferent fibers are shown in white, the visceral efferent fibers as striped.

serinus shortly after exit from the stylomastoid foramen and innervates the muscles of facial expression. The motor root of the facial nerve innervates the muscles of facial expression, the stapedius, the occipitalis, the buccinator, the platysma, the stylohyoid, and the posterior belly of the digastric.

The nervus intermedius portion of the facial nerve contains somatic sensory, visceral afferent, taste, and general visceral efferent fibers. The somatic sensory fibers carry sensation from the posterior aspect of the external auditory canal and synapse in the spinal tract of cranial nerve V. The visceral afferents carry sensation from the pharynx, nose, and palate to the tractus solitarius by way of the greater superficial petrosal nerve. Taste from the anterior two thirds of the tongue is transmitted to the nucleus of the tractus solitarius by way of the chorda tympani branch of the facial nerve. General visceral efferent fibers pass through the nervus intermedius portion of the facial nerve from the superior salivatory nucleus as preganglionic parasympathetic fibers. These fibers pass peripherally either through the greater superficial petrosal nerve to the lacrimal gland and the glands of the nose and palatine mucosa or through the chorda tympani nerve and submandibular ganglion to the submandibular and sublingual glands.

EXAMINATION OF THE EAR

INSPECTION AND CLEANING

Cerumen, which is produced in specialized apocrine glands located in the lateral one third of the external auditory canal, often accumulates in sufficient quantities to interfere with examination of the canal and drum. Wax may be removed by irrigation with water at body temperature or with either a loop or ring curette, a handheld speculum, and a headlight or mirror. Ninety-five percent of whites and blacks have dark, oily wax. Most orientals have dry, light, flaky wax.

OTOSCOPY

By positioning the seated patient with his head tilted backward approximately 30 degrees, the examiner has a clear view without resorting to contortions of his own head and neck. The examiner should hold the otoscope in his nondominant hand to free his dominant hand for manipulation or suctioning of the external canal. In a child or a combative adult the examiner should place the fifth finger of the hand holding the otoscope against the squamous portion of the patient's skull to prevent injury to the skin of the external canal during head movements.

Examination of the ear canal and tympanic membrane should be done in an orderly fashion starting with a circumferential inspection of the bony external canal. The most constant landmark in the diseased tympanic membrane is the lateral process of the malleus. The examiner should identify this first because it will automatically orient him as to the location of the pars flaccida and the pars tensa. The pneumatic otoscopic head allows the examiner to induce movements of the drum and therefore to determine the presence of fluid or masses behind the tympanic membrane. In addition, moving the tympanic membrane may make healed perforations of the tympanic membrane that are almost transparent more visible. Additional magnification may be achieved by using the operating microscope. With his dominant hand the examiner straightens the external canal by pulling on the auricle posterosuperiorly in the adult and posteriorly in the child. Once the speculum is inserted, the auricle may be released, and the examiners dominant hand is freed for other manipulation.

The otoscopic findings can be summarized by diagraming the tympanic membrane as a circle and the malleus as an obtuse angle formed at the lateral process of the malleus (Fig. 1-7). Perforations may be illustrated simply by outlining the location in red. Pathology visualized in the middle ear may be the result of more significant disease in the nasopharynx. Hence, nasopharyngoscopy should be performed routinely in cases of serous otitis media in adults to rule out a neoplastic process.

Eustachian-tube function may be evaluated by examining the movement of the tympanic membrane while the patient performs a modified Valsalva maneuver. This is done by filling the patient's oropharynx with air and having him blow out against closed lips and nose or by having the patient blow up a balloon. If there is a perforation, the

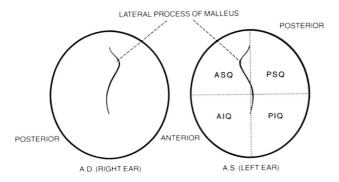

Fig. 1-7. Schematic representation of both ear drums used to diagram pathology. The principal anatomical landmark is the malleus and its lateral process. The drum may be divided into four quadrants as shown in the diagram of the left ear. (ASQ) anterosuperior quadrant; (PSQ) posterosuperior quadrant; (AIQ) anteroinferior quadrant; (PIQ) posteroinferior quadrant.

function of the tube may be evaluated by listening through a small rubber catheter or Toynbee tube placed in the external auditory canal while the patient swallows or performs a modified Valsalva maneuver. With good tubal function, either a click or a hiss of air will be heard. If these techniques fail, more forceful insufflation of air into the patient's middle ear may be achieved by politzerization. This consists of forcing air through one nares of the nose with the other nares occluded while the patient swallows or says "kick" or "Coca-Cola" to lift the soft palate and close the nasopharynx. The air source may be a Politzer bag or low-pressure compressed air.

TESTS OF AUDITORY FUNCTION

TUNING-FORK AND WHISPER TESTS

It is advisable to perform tuning-fork and whisper tests on all patients even though audiology may be obtained subsequently. The Rinne test is based on a comparison of sound conduction by bone and sound transmission through the air of the external auditory canal. A 512-cps fork is best for this purpose. The fork is struck against the examiner's knee or base of the thumb and held firmly against the patient's mastoid bone where the skin is thinnest. The examiner's opposite hand must be used for counterpressure to ensure firm apposition of tuning fork to bone. The tuning fork is then held at the external auditory canal with the two blades of the tuning fork aligned with the axis of the external canal. In most adults and some young children, a modified Rinne test is performed by asking the patient to compare the loudness of the stimulus transmitted by bone and air. If this is confusing to the patient, the classical Rinne test may be performed by holding the base of the fork against the patient's mastoid process until its tone is no longer heard. The fork is then held at the external auditory canal, and the patient is asked if the tone is still audible. The Rinne is recorded as positive if air conduction is superior to bone conduction or negative is the converse is true. When the Rinne is positive, the hearing may be normal or a sensorineural hearing loss may be present. A negative Rinne usually implies a conductive hearing loss. However, a false-negative Rinne may be produced by ipsilateral profound sensorineural deafness and transmission of sound by bone conduction to the opposite ear.

The Weber test is a test of lateralization of sound and is performed with the same tuning fork. The fork is placed on a midline structure such as the patient's forehead or the vertex of his skull. The patient is asked in which ear, if either, the sound is heard to be louder. In a sensorineural hearing loss the sound will be heard in the midline or will lateralize to the better-hearing ear; in a conductive hearing loss it will lateralize to the poorer-hearing ear. This test is most sensitive if the fork is placed on the central incisors of the maxilla.

Hearing acuity can be estimated by using voice tests. A series of spondaic words, such as "baseball," "hot dog," "earthquake," "sidewalk," "mousetrap," and "greyhound" is spoken at graded intensities at the external canal, and an approximation of threshold is made. A whisper lies in the range of 0 db to 30 db HL, normal conversational speech between 40 db to 60 db HL, and a shout between 60 db to 90 db HL. Masking of the opposite ear must be done and is best achieved using the Barany noisemaker, which can achieve masking levels of approximately 80 db (see Appendix).

BEHAVIORAL AUDIOMETRY (STANDARD HEARING TESTS)

The best test of auditory function in a cooperative child or adult is behavioral audiometry. Thresholds of frequencies between 250 cps and 8000 cps are measured in db HL (a scale of loudness with 0 db HL being the threshold of normal controls at each frequency). Air conduction and bone conduction are measured separately in each ear. If there is a hearing loss, masking may be necessary in the contralateral ear because sounds 40 db and greater will be transmitted by bone conduction across the skull to the opposite ear. The various symbols for masked and unmasked air conduction and bone conduction are illustrated in Figure 1-8.

With normal hearing, both air conduction and bone conduction will be superimposed at each test frequency between 0 db and 10 db. It is important to realize that 0 db HL is the threshold for both bone conduction and air conduction and that the normal superiority of air conduction over bone conduction is taken into account by the normalization of testing. If air conduction is inferior to bone conduction, a conductive hearing loss is present. A conductive hearing loss is due to a disorder in the external auditory canal, tympanic membrane, or middle ear. A sensorineural hearing loss is indicated by a bone curve lying below the 0-db to 10-db threshold at any frequency tested. This implies pathology in the inner ear or auditory neural pathways.

After pure-tone audiometry is performed, the *speech-reception threshold* (SRT) is determined for each ear. Beginning at a level approximately 20 db above the average of the three midfrequencies, two-syllable words of equal stress (spondees) are presented in 2-db decrements. The SRT is defined as the faintest level at which the patient can correctly identify approximately 50% of the words. The purpose of speech-reception testing is twofold. First, it serves to confirm the patient's midfrequency pure-tone responses, and second, it determines the intensity at which subsequent speech-discrimination tasks are to be presented. The following Spondaic Words for Determination of SRT are useful for office whisper testing.

Spondaic Words for Determination of SRT

Greyhound	Hot dog
Schoolboy	Padlock
Inkwell	Mushroom
Whitewash	Hardware
Pancake	Workshop
Eardrum	Horseshoe
Headlight	Armchair
Birthday	Baseball
Duck pond	Stairway
Sidewalk	Cowboy

Pure-tone levels are not a complete indication of how well the patient hears because comprehension also depends on discrimination ability. The *word-discrimination test* is performed at a level 40 db above the previously determined SRT for each ear in order to approximate a comfortable level for the comprehension of speech. Masking is used in the contralateral ear, and a list of 50 phonetically balanced, monosyllabic words such as "yes," "church," and "boy" is read to and repeated by the patient. The patient's discrimination score is reported as the percentage of words identified correctly. Discrimination testing also provides diagnostic information as to the site of a lesion. In the instance of a conductive hearing loss or a sensorineural loss with pathology at the cochlear hair-cell level, the speech-discrimination score will be above 80%. On the other hand, when the primary site of hearing loss is neuronal (retrocochlear), very low discrimination scores are the rule.

Flat hearing losses are usually associated with good discrimination scores. Individuals with flat hearing losses are good candidates for satisfactory hearing-aid usage. In general, the more steeply a hearing loss slopes, particularly into the high frequencies, the worse the discrimination scores. Patients with steep hearing loss, usually the elderly, complain that they hear but do not understand. Although amplification is useful, it does not solve this problem.

SPECIAL BEHAVIORAL TESTS

Recruitment signifies an abnormally rapid growth of sensation of loudness in a diseased ear. In the clinic, the patient will complain that loud noises are "too loud" or that they "irritate" his affected ear. The presence of recruitment is an indication of a cochlear, rather than retrocochlear, lesion.

(Text continues on p. 16)

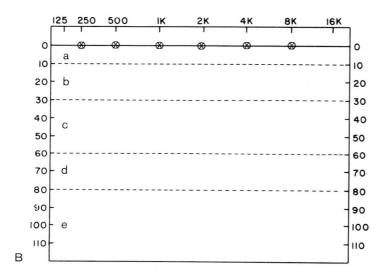

Fig. 1-8. (*A*) Symbols used in behavioral audiometry. (*B*) A normal audiogram. The hearing threshold for both ears is 0 db HL at each frequency tested. (*a*) Normal hearing (0 db to 20 db—if both ears hear equally): A small hearing loss relative to the other ear can be detected and still be within the normal range. Perfectly normal hearing should be in the 0 db to 10 db range. Most speech, except for fricatives, falls within the 750 Hz to 2000 Hz frequency range. (*b*) Mild hearing loss (20 db to 35 db): Patient is aware of hearing difficulty when there is background noise or when in groups. He must concentrate in school and at meetings. Preferential seating is beneficial. (*c*) Moderate hearing loss (35 db to 50 db): Impaired communication. Patient hears a loud conversational voice in a one-to-one situation but is confused by background noise. He has difficulty hearing on the telephone. Hearing aid(s) are advisable when discrimination scores are good. Most patients begin to lip-read. (*d*) Severe hearing loss (50 db to 80 db): Amplification (hearing aids) is mandatory. The value of the hearing aid depends in large part on the patient's ability to understand. Hearing aid use is much better if discrimination scores are greater than 80%. (*e*) Profound hearing loss (80 db or greater): Hearing aids are of adjunctive value only. Many patients cannot hear their own voice and therefore speech may be affected. Powerful body hearing aids are usually employed. Profound hearing losses are usually accompanied by poor discrimination.

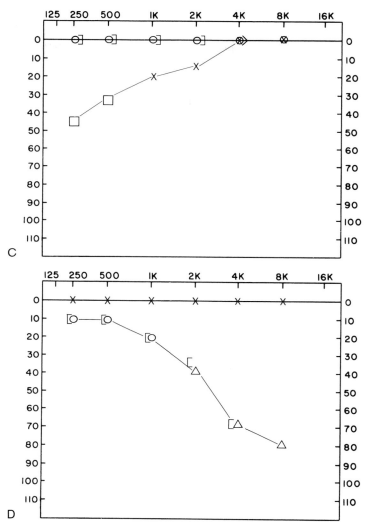

Fig 1-8. *Continued* (C) Normal hearing in the right ear and a low-frequency conductive hearing loss in the left ear. Masking of the right ear with white noise during testing of the left ear is required because of the large difference in hearing between right and left. The masked bone conduction is normal in the left ear, but air conduction hearing is reduced for the low frequencies, indicating a conductive hearing loss (for explanation of symbols see Figure 1-8A). (D) Normal hearing in the left ear and a descending sensorineural hearing loss in the right ear. The masked bone conduction is the same as the air conduction in the right ear, indicating a sensorineural hearing loss. Masking for bone-conduction testing is almost always required. Masking for air conduction is required if a differential of greater than 40 db exists between the ears. Because of the slope of this audiogram, one would expect the discrimination score to be affected as well (for explanation of symbols see Figure 1-8A).

A 512-Hz tuning fork can be used to assess recruitment. First, the fork is struck softly, and the patient compares the sound level heard in one ear to the sound level heard in the other. Then the fork is struck sharply, and the process is repeated. In the second instance, if recruitment is present, the sound should be perceived in the diseased ear as equal to or louder than in the normal ear.

One specific audiologic test for the measurement of recruitment is the alternate binaural loudness balance test (ABLB). The patient is asked to compare the loudness of two tones of the same frequency that are presented alternately to the unimpaired and impaired ear until the tones are perceived as being of equal relative loudness.

The *tone-decay* test detects abnormal function of the auditory nerve. In this instance, a constant sound will be perceived as fading out over a 60-second period in the patient's affected ear(s). An objective measure of tone decay is made by presenting a barely perceptible pure tone and recording the increment in decibels necessary for the patient to sustain perception of the tone for 60 seconds. A positive test (30 db or greater of added sound energy) suggests that the primary site of hearing loss is neuronal and is often interpreted as an indication of retrocochlear (auditory nerve) pathology.

Special Behavioral Audiometry Tests to Determine Site of Lesion

Discrimination score: Low score indicates retrocochlear (i.e., auditory) nerve pathology.

Recruitment: Positive recruitment test indicates cochlear injury.

Tone decay: Positive test indicates auditory nerve pathology.

Békésy audiometry is an automated audiometric test that compares the test subject's threshold for a continuously presented tone with his threshold for an interrupted tone. Five types of tracings are described. This testing has provided no additional useful information in my experience.

AUDITORY EVOKED-RESPONSE TESTING

Behavioral audiometry may be difficult or impossible to perform in patients under the age of 2½ years or in adults with emotional or neurologic disorders. In such patients, auditory evoked-response techniques may be useful in approximating a threshold. This technique is based on computer summation of evoked response from the cochlea, auditory nerve, and brain-stem pathways in response to an acoustic stimulus (click).

Depending on the electrode placement and the time window after the stimulation, one may selectively examine electrical activity at the cochlear, eighth-nerve, brain-stem, or cortical levels. When the parameters of the recording are set up to best detect activity in the cochlea and eighth nerve, the testing is called *electrocochleography*. When set up for waves generated from the auditory pathway within the brain stem, the recording is called a *brain-stem evoked response (BSER)*. When set up for the auditory portion of the electroencephalogram (EEG), the recording is called a *cortical evoked response*. Unlike electrocochleography and BSER, cortical evoked responses are drastically altered by various drugs or varying levels of attention.

BSER is the most popular of these three techniques because it can be performed with surface electrodes rather than canal or middle-ear electrodes, which are required in electrocochleography. (Electrocochleography requires a local anesthetic in the adult and a general anesthetic in the child.) Furthermore, BSER provides information not only at the eighth-nerve level but also at brain-stem levels. The findings of this test are unchanged by state of awareness, pharmacologic levels of drugs, or general anesthesia. In addition to approximation of hearing (pure tone) threshold, the BSER has also proved useful in evaluating patients for retrocochlear pathology. BSER requires no anesthesia in an adult, and in a child it may be done during natural sleep or under mild sedation.

By means of a summing computer, the BSER measures the electrical response of the auditory system to a series of rapid clicks that can be presented to the ear at different intensities. Once the sounds have exceeded hearing threshold, a series of wave forms numbered 1 through 7 can be detected within the first 10 milliseconds. The first wave represents the action potential from the eighth nerve, the second is probably generated at the cochlear nucleus, and the others have complex origins from progressively higher centers in the brain stem. Each wave peak has an expected latency. The fifth peak is the largest and most predictable and is therefore used as an indicator of hearing threshold level by BSER (Fig. 1-9A and B).

Conductive hearing losses and cochlear injuries will raise waveform thresholds but in general will not change the wave forms or interwave latencies. Eighth-nerve and brain-stem injuries such as tumors or multiple sclerosis do cause wave-form distortions and increased interwave latencies, thus making the test a very sensitive indicator of pathology in these regions (Figure 1-9C).

TYMPANOMETRY

For impedance audiometry, the ear canal is sealed, and the pressure within the external auditory canal may be varied. With the use of a probe tone, the impedance or, conversely, the compliance of the eardrum and attached ossicular chain may be measured. This technique

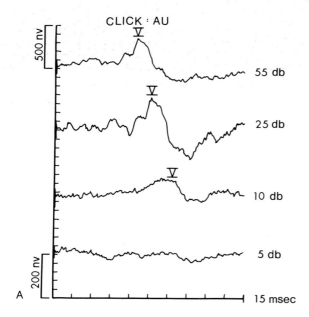

Fig. 1-9. (*A*) Hearing threshold determination using brain-stem evoked-response (BSER) audiometry. Wave *V* is detectable at a threshold below 10 db.

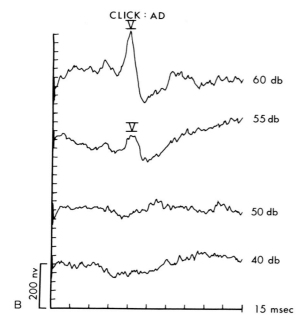

(*B*) Hearing threshold determination using brain-stem evoked-response (BSER) audiometry. The threshold for wave *V* is approximately 50 db, suggesting approximately 40 db of hearing loss in the right ear.

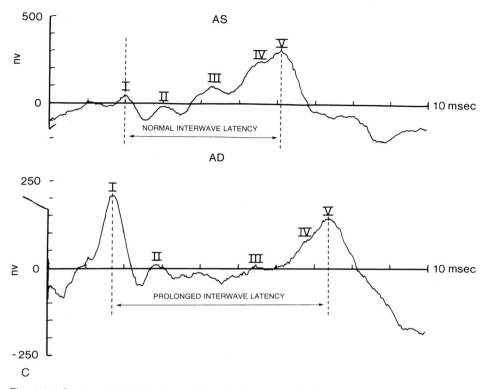

Fig. 1-9. *Continued* (C) Waveforms from brain-stem evoked-response (BSER) audiometry. Documented case of vestibular schwannoma in the right ear. The absolute latency of wave *V* and the interwave latency (*I* through *V*) are prolonged in the right ear, suggesting retrocochlear pathology.

may be helpful in the diagnosis of middle-ear disorders and is frequently used as an adjunct to audiometry in the screening of schoolchildren because they have a high incidence of otitis media.

Five types of tympanograms have been identified (Fig. 1-10). Type A demonstrates a normal middle-ear compliance. Type AS demonstrates decreased compliance at each pressure tested, which is consistent with stiffness of the ossicular chain. Type AD shows infinite compliance and is consistent with ossicular discontinuity. Type B shows no point of maximum compliance and very little change in compliance over the range −200 to +200 mm H_2O and is consistent with middle-ear effusion. Type C is similar to type A except that the maximum point of compliance is found by applying negative pressure to the external

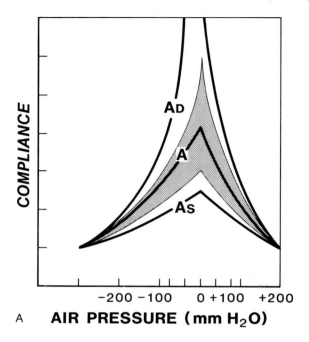

A   **AIR PRESSURE (mm H₂O)**

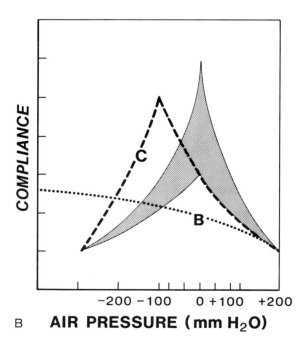

B   **AIR PRESSURE (mm H₂O)**

Fig. 1-10. Tympanometry patterns. The normal range is indicated by the shaded area. *A.* (*A*) Normal tympanogram. (*AS*) A "stiffness" lesion. Stiffness of the ossicular chain will demonstrate a peak at normal pressures but decreased compliance. This pattern may be seen in otosclerosis. (*AD*) A "discontinuity pattern." There is infinite compliance and an extrapolated peak at normal pressure. This is due to a disruption of the ossicular chain or an extremely flaccid tympanic membrane. *B.* (*B*) No peak compliance—consistent with middle-ear effusion (such as serous otitis or acute otitis media). (*C*) Compliance is in the normal range, but a peak at −150 mm H₂O is consistent with negative middle-ear pressure. This is a sign of early eustachian-tube blockage or otitis media.

auditory canal, and this is consistent with partial eustachian-tube dysfunction and middle-ear atelectasis.

Because the contraction of the stapedius muscle results in measurable changes in the impedance of the tympanic membrane, the same equipment may be used for measuring the acoustic reflex threshold (ART) and acoustic reflex decay (ARD). The ART has been used as a somewhat rough but objective measurement of hearing in neonates and in difficult-to-test patients and as a means of corroborating behavior threshold. In addition, the ART and ARD may be used in conjunction with ipsilateral and contralateral stimuli as a means of evaluating the site of lesion in a sensorineural hearing loss.

TESTS FOR FUNCTIONAL HEARING LOSS

In patients suspected of malingering or of having psychogenic deafness, special behavior tests, such as the Stenger, Lombard, and delayed-feedback tests, may be used by the audiologist. Recently, BSER has been used with totally uncooperative patients.

VESTIBULAR TESTING

CALORIC TESTS

The function of the vestibular system is best examined by caloric testing. This may be done in an office setting, using Frenzel's lenses to prevent ocular fixation. First, the eyes are examined for spontaneous nystagmus. Next, the ear canal and drum are checked for obstruction or perforation. Then the minimal caloric test, or Kobrak test, is determined by the instillation of 5 ml of water at 80°F with the patient in a sitting position and the head inclined backward 60 degrees. The time of onset and time of termination of nystagmus are noted. After 10 minutes, the opposite ear is tested. If no response is achieved with water at 80°F, 5 ml of iced water is used. The range of normal response to thermal calorics is great; hence, this test is best applied to a unilateral lesion by comparison with the opposite normal side. Nystagmus is more accurately measured with the use of electronystagmography (ENG) (see Chap. 4). When there is a perforation of the tympanic membrane, thermal stimulation can be performed by using 2 ml of iced sterile saline or otic drops.

POSITIONAL TESTING

If a patient complains of vertigo that occurs in one position only, positional testing should be done. The patient is placed on an examining table so that his head may hang over the end of the table. The following positions are assumed by the patient with the examiner controlling the patient's head: head hanging; head hanging with left ear down; head hanging with right ear down. Between each position the patient is brought to the fully erect position. The examiner records whether vestibular symptoms are present, whether nystagmus is present, whether the onset of nystagmus is immediate or delayed, and whether the nystagmus fatigues by maintaining the provocative position or by repeating the provocative position. The most common form of positional nystagmus is benign positional nystagmus, or vertigo, also called *cupulolithiasis*. In this disorder the nystagmus is rotatory, demonstrates a latency of several seconds, and fatigues, and there is an intense feeling of vertigo with the affected ear downward. The Aschan classification of positional nystagmus is commonly used.

Aschan Classification of Positional Nystagmus

Type I: Nystagmus is nonfatigable, and direction changes with head position.

Type II: Nystagmus is nonfatigable, but direction remains fixed despite change of head position.

Type III: There is positional nystagmus in any direction but it demonstrates definite latency and fatigue.

Patients with type I findings almost always have a central disorder. Those with type II may have a peripheral vestibular disorder, but again most patients with type II findings have central disorders. Type III findings are almost always peripheral in origin.

FISTULA TEST

In the fistula test, objective nystagmus and a subjective sensation of unsteadiness or shift in body position may be induced by changing the pressure in the external auditory canal. This is most conveniently done with a Politzer bag with an olive tip while the examiner observes the patient's eyes with Frenzel's lenses. In the presence of chronic otitis media, a positive test usually implies a labyrinthine fistula due to cholesteatoma. With an intact eardrum, a positive test has been described in congenital syphilis (Hennebert's sign) and Meniere's disease.

FACIAL-NERVE TESTS

It is often valuable in cases of facial paralysis to determine (1) the sites of involvement of the facial nerve in its anatomical course from brain stem to the periphery and (2) whether the lesion is caused by degeneration of the nerve fibers (neurotmesis) or simply a physiologic block (neuropraxia).

SITE-OF-LESION TESTING

Because of the mixed nature of the facial nerve, with motor, somato-sensory, viscerosensory, taste, and visceral efferent components, the site of lesion may be evaluated in several ways:

1. Salivary flow test (chorda tympani): The submaxillary ducts are anesthetized and cannulated with No.-60 polyethylene tubing. Lemon juice is used to stimulate salivary flow, and the number of drops secreted per minute on each side is compared. A difference of 70% or more between the two sides is considered significant.

2. Taste (chorda tympani): Taste can be compared on the two sides either with physiologic stimuli, such as concentrated salt and sugar solutions, or with an electrogustometer.

3. Stapedial reflex: The function of the stapedial branch (motor division) is tested with impedance audiometry techniques.

4. Lacrimation (greater superficial petrosal nerve at the level of geniculate ganglion): This is evaluated by the Schirmer's test.

NEUROPHYSIOLOGIC TESTS OF NEURONAL VIABILITY

There are a number of tests, each with limitations, that over time will differentiate between neuropraxia and nerve degeneration. These include the nerve excitability test, electromyography, and electroneurography. All of these require special equipment. The major limitation of the neurophysiologic tests is that, even in the case of total transection of a nerve, transmission as tested distal to the site of the lesion will be little affected for approximately 3 days.

2
HEARING LOSS

Joseph B. Nadol, Jr.

Definitions and history taking
Specific diagnoses
  Conductive hearing loss
    Conductive hearing loss secondary to obstruction of the external canal
    Cerumen
    Foreign body
    External otitis
    Developmental defects
    Exostoses
    Conductive hearing loss secondary to disorders of the tympanic membrane
    Hyalinization and tympanosclerosis
    Perforation
    Conductive hearing loss due to disorders of the middle ear
    Effusions
      Serous otitis media
      Other effusions
    Mass lesions within the middle ear
    Malleus fixation
    Incus resorption
    Stapes fixation
  Sensorineural hearing loss
    Bilateral sensorineural hearing loss

Presbycusis
  Treatment: Hearing aids
Genetically determined sensorineural hearing loss
Congenital, nonhereditary deafness
Ototoxicity
Unilateral, or asymmetrical, sensorineural hearing loss
Otitis media
Bacterial meningitis
Direct trauma
Acoustic trauma
Syphilis
Neurologic disorders
Neoplasms
Cerebellopontine-angle tumors
Hearing loss associated with other metabolic or systemic disorders
  Arterial disease
  Other metabolic disorders
Disorders of unknown cause
  Meniere's disease
  Collagen vascular diseases
  Sudden idiopathic sensorineural deafness

DEFINITIONS AND HISTORY TAKING

To evaluate hearing loss the examiner must devise a diagnostic strategy in order to establish whether or not the hearing loss requires urgent treatment and which additional diagnostic tests are necessary to determine its cause. Several aspects on the clinical history are critical in this evaluation.

1. Is the hearing loss unilateral or bilateral? Generally speaking, a unilateral loss, especially sensorineural loss, will require more diagnostic work-up.
2. Is the hearing loss slowly progressive or was the onset sudden? A sudden hearing loss may require emergency treatment.
3. Are there any associated symptoms that will help differentiate various forms of hearing loss?
   a. Is there tinnitus? Subjective tinnitus, or head noise, is a sound, apparently produced in the hearing centers of the midbrain, that may accompany both sensorineural and conductive hearing loss. Although it is an annoying symptom, it is rarely debilitating, and most patients are not disturbed by it when they are active and busy. However, patients may be kept awake by it at night, in which case a radio playing or a mild sedative may help the patient to sleep. Tinnitus may disappear if the hearing loss is corrected. The efficacy of "tinnitus maskers" is not proven. Objective tinnitus can be heard by the examiner as well as by the patient by using a Toynbee tube. Pulsative tinnitus may be due to an arterial venous malformation, a partial arterial occlusion and bruit, or a vascular tumor, such as a glomus tumor, in or about the ear. Repeated clicking sounds, the same as those heard on swallowing, can be the result of myoclonic spasms of the palate. Breath sounds can be heard in the ear as the result of a patulous eustachian tube. This condition occurs following alteration of fat deposits around the tube, such as following a marked weight loss or during pregnancy.
   b. Are there vestibular symptoms? Here, the terminology used in questioning a patient is important. Patients often do not understand the meaning of the term *vertigo* but do understand "unsteadiness," "imbalance," or "spinning dizziness."
   c. Is the hearing loss associated with pain in either ear?
   d. Is there any history of drainage from the ear canal at the onset of the hearing loss or preceding it?
   e. Is there history of trauma preceding the hearing loss? This

is particularly important in sudden sensorineural loss. Trauma may occur as a result of direct injury, such as a blow to the head, skull fracture, slap injury to the external canal, and insertion of a foreign body into the external canal, or as a result of barotrauma. Barotrauma implies a sudden change in ambient pressure such as may occur during aircraft descent and scuba diving or because of an explosion.

f. What is the history of drug administration? This would pertain to a patient with a bilateral sensorineural hearing loss and may be associated with progressive or sudden deterioration in hearing.

g. Are there other associated medical illnesses, such as neurologic disturbances, either central or peripheral; blood dyscrasias; diseases of bone; a history of neoplasm that might result in metastasis to the temporal bone; or collagen vascular disease?

h. Particularly, but not exclusively, in children, a brief inquiry should be made into the family history of auditory or vestibular disturbances. In addition, are there any familial deformities or abnormalities?

The brief history should be followed by examination of the ear, including the auricle, external canal, and tympanic membrane. The tuning fork test and clinical approximation of speech-reception threshold should be performed. An audiogram or other tests can then be ordered on an emergent basis or can be planned as part of a future evaluation by the primary physician, or the patient may be referred to an otologist for these tests.

SPECIFIC DIAGNOSES

A final or working diagnosis should be made after the preliminary evaluation. In the following sections, brief descriptions of several specific disorders as well as the criteria for their diagnosis are given. The usual treatment is outlined, including possible surgical remedies. When surgery is a therapeutic alternative, a brief description of the surgery is given as well as nonsurgical alternatives.

CONDUCTIVE HEARING LOSS

By definition conductive hearing loss implies that the site of dysfunction is in the external canal, tympanic membrane, or middle-ear space.

CONDUCTIVE HEARING LOSS SECONDARY TO OBSTRUCTION OF THE EXTERNAL CANAL

Obstruction may be the result of simple cerumen accumulation, a foreign body, edema, or neoplastic or congenital obstruction of the external canal.

Cerumen

Cerumen may be removed by irrigation, suction, or curettage. Irrigation may be the easiest treatment for both patient and physician, but it should not be used if a perforation of the drum is known or suspected. An additional disadvantage of irrigation is that irritation of the tympanic membrane may occur and make any further diagnosis difficult at that time. When irrigation is done, it should be performed with water maintained at body temperature to avoid a caloric response. This is best achieved with a cerumen syringe (see Appendix). The stream of water is directed toward the posterior canal wall so that a plane of cleavage is created between skin and wax and the full force of the water does not strike the tympanic membrane. Care should be taken so that a tight seal in the external canal, with resulting damage to the drum, does not occur. Automatic ear-irrigation devices are available for office use.

If there is soft wax or mucopurulent debris in the external canal, suction is essential. Depending on the consistency of the obstructing material, a No.-5 or No.-20 French suction tip is used (see Appendix). Suction is performed using a handheld speculum with headlight and mirror or through an otoscope.

For practiced hands, simple curettage is done with a ring or wire curette, Hartmann's forceps (see Appendix), handheld speculum, and headlight and mirror. The forceps may also be used through an otoscope. Hard or particularly deep wax impactions may be removed by first softening them with a glycerin and hydrogen peroxide mixture (Debrox) t.i.d. for several days prior to irrigation or aspiration.

Foreign Body

Foreign bodies in the ear canal are common in children and occasionally may be seen in adults. Several guidelines of therapy are in order. First and foremost, a nonemergency situation should not be made into an emergency by pushing a foreign body further into the canal and possibly damaging the drum or middle-ear structures. Local or general anesthesia should be used if necessary. Nonspherical objects may be simply grasped with alligator forceps and lifted straight out of the external canal. For spherical objects, a hook placed behind the object or a suction tip may be useful. Living insects should be drowned in mineral oil to prevent unpleasant footfalls on the tympanic membrane and then are removed *in toto* or piecemeal with ear forceps (Hartmann's or alligator) or suction. After the foreign body has been removed, the tympanic membrane is carefully inspected to ensure that no perforation of the drum has occurred. Vestibular symptoms and signs should be sought, and the patient's hearing should be tested clinically.

External Otitis

External otitis is an inflammatory process involving the skin and occasionally the cartilages of the external canal. This is often accompanied by cerumen impaction within the canal. The treatment of external otitis will be outlined in Chapter 3.

Developmental Defects

Atresia or dysplastic stenosis of the external auditory canal may occur alone or in association with other abnormalities of first and second branchial arches or auricular deformities. This is commonly associated with middle- and inner-ear abnormalities. Surgical correction is possible in selected cases, based on assessment of inner-ear function and the severity of malformation. In general, a patient with unilateral atresia of the external canal with a contralateral normal ear is not an ideal surgical candidate because surgery usually does not result in total correction of the hearing loss. In cases of total atresia, surgical risks include damage to inner-ear function and to the facial nerve because it often runs an aberrant course. Consultation with an otologist should answer the following questions: What are the risks in this particular case? What is the expected gain in hearing? Is a hearing aid a reasonable option?

When auricular deformities are present and reconstruction is planned, this should be carefully integrated with the external canal surgery.

Exostoses

Exostoses in the bony external canal usually appear as two to three bony white excrescences covered by skin. These are asymptomatic unless progressive stenosis of the bony canal results in entrapment of water or other material between the exostoses and the tympanic membrane. Surgery, usually performed either through the ear canal or through an incision behind the ear, involves removal of the exostoses with a drill or curette, followed by skin grafting of the external canal. General anesthesia is usually required, and the major risks include possible damage to the tympanic membrane or ossicular chain during the course of the surgery.

CONDUCTIVE HEARING LOSS SECONDARY TO DISORDERS OF THE TYMPANIC MEMBRANE

Hyalinization and Tympanosclerosis

As a result of repeated infections of the middle-ear space, hyaline may be deposited within the drum and middle ear. It appears as white plaques on the tympanic membrane and may result in a hearing loss due to ossicular fixation. Isolated hyalin deposits within the drum rarely produce significant hearing loss unless associated with ossicular fixation. Some patients with this form of conductive hearing loss are surgical candidates. The suitability for surgery as determined by an otologist is based on a number of considerations, including hearing on the contralateral side, age of the patient, and eustachian-tube function.

Perforation

Perforations may be either marginal or central. A marginal perforation implies that the perforation extends to the tympanic annulus. A central perforation is one that is surrounded by a remnant of normal tympanic membrane. An acute central perforation is likely to heal without intervention; a marginal perforation is less likely to do so. Furthermore, squamous epithelial ingrowth into the middle ear with cholesteatoma formation is much more common with a marginal perforation (see Chap. 3). A posterior perforation, either central or marginal, especially over the round window area, may result in a conductive hearing loss of up to 40 db.

Acute perforation of the drum may result from direct trauma or barotrauma and constitutes an otologic emergency if there is evidence of injury to the ossicular chain or to the inner ear (see Chap. 5). Chronic perforations may be the result of a large, unhealed traumatic perforation or, more commonly, of chronic otitis media.

Treatment. The treatment of a chronic, dry perforation consists of myringoplasty or tympanoplasty, type I. Repair of a perforation of the tympanic membrane may be done to correct the conductive hearing loss and because the patient desires to avoid the annoyance of water precautions for hairwashing and showering. Even so, surgical repair of an uncomplicated perforation, with or without conductive hearing loss, must be considered elective. Nonoperative treatment of an uncomplicated perforation by an otologist might include chemical cauterization of the perforation margins and application of a small cigarette-paper patch. With this method, a perforation might be waxed to close over a period of a week to several months. All patients with a perforated tympanic membrane should take precautions against recurrent middle-ear infections due to water entering the middle ear. Ear plugs (which can be purchased in a pharmacy) are generally satisfactory for showering, but most will leak to some degree if put under the stress of swimming. In addition, perforations, especially of the marginal type, should be observed by an otologist to ensure that there is no ingrowth of squamous epithelium into the middle-ear space (*e.g.,* cholesteatoma formation).

Surgical correction of a small perforation (up to 2 mm) may be done as an outpatient procedure under local anesthesia, using a fat graft. Surgical correction of an anterior perforation behind an anterior canal-wall bulge, a perforation associated with large conductive loss, or a perforation in which squamous epithelial ingrowth is possible is performed as an inpatient procedure. Small posterior perforations with or without a hearing loss are usually corrected by a transcanal technique similar to the approach used for stapes surgery under local anesthesia. Temporal fascia is the most common graft material used to patch the drum. Larger perforations or anterior perforations require endaural incisions that open the canal wide and permit the surgeon to visualize the entire drum.

The overall success rate of tympanoplasty is approximately 85%. Thus, the greatest risk of this surgery is a 15% chance of failure. Other complications include those from anesthesia and a very small risk of damage to the ossicular chain, facial nerve, or inner ear. The usual hospital stay for such procedures is 2 to 3 days. Treatment of perforation with drainage is discussed in Chapter 3. The treatment of an acute perforation is discussed in Chapter 5.

CONDUCTIVE HEARING LOSS DUE TO DISORDERS OF THE MIDDLE EAR

Hearing loss resulting from disorders of the middle ear may be caused by middle-ear effusions, stiffness lesions, or discontinuity of the ossicular chain.

Effusions

Serous Otitis Media. Serous otitis media is recognized by the presence of an air–fluid level in the middle ear or of a golden-to-bluish discoloration of the drum and lack of compliance of the drum as tested by pneumo-otoscopy. Serous otitis media is the most common cause of conductive hearing loss in children. It is much less common in adults, but may be seen as a complication of upper respiratory infection or allergy. In an adult, the presence of serous otitis media must initiate a search for neoplastic obstruction of the nasopharyngeal end of the eustachian tube. This is done by indirect or direct nasopharyngoscopy, soft-tissue radiography of the nasopharynx, basal-skull tomography in selected cases, and nasopharyngeal biopsy if indicated. There is a relatively higher incidence of nasopharyngeal carcinoma in Chinese men.

In children, the treatment of serous otitis media involves a preliminary search for a medically treatable cause of eustachian-tube dysfunction. For example, questions concerning allergic symptoms may lead to a formal allergic evaluation. Examination of the nasopharynx either by mirror examination or with a lateral x-ray view may demonstrate adenoid hypertrophy sufficient to cause stasis within the nasopharynx and eustachian-tube dysfunction. Craniofacial abnormalities, either gross or relatively subtle, particularly those involving the mandible and occlusion, are associated with a relatively high incidence of ear disease secondary to eustachian-tube dysplasia or dysfunction. And certain family groups will have ear disease in each generation apparently related to physiognomy.

Palatal abnormalities, particularly cleft palate, may be associated with serous otitis media. The eustachian tubes are opened during swallowing and yawning by the contraction of the right and left tensor veli palatini muscles. These muscle pairs meet at the median palatal raphe and pull against one another. In the child with a cleft palate the eustachian tubes have a greatly compromised mechanism for opening. Hence, most of these children require long-term otologic care for recurrent serous otitis media.

There is evidence that the intermittent mild-to-moderate impaired hearing associated with serous otitis media, which can range up to 45 db, will result in a deficit in language development among preschool and school-aged children. School hearing-screening programs as well as the increased awareness of hearing problems by physicians and parents have helped reduce this problem.

If the preliminary search for an identifiable cause of eustachian-tube dysfunction is unrewarding, a trial of decongestants and antihistamines is usually tried. Self-inflation through the use of a modified Valsalva maneuver, the blowing up of balloons by the patient, or the use of a Politzer bag may also help. If the fluid is persistent and is causing a significant hearing loss, a myringotomy and the insertion of a ventilating tube constitute a reasonable temporizing maneuver. In an adult, this can be performed under local anesthesia, and in a child, under general anesthesia. Occasionally, iontophoretic anesthesia is employed. This involves the use of a small electric current to painlessly draw molecules of the anesthetic, lidocaine 4%, into the tympanic membrane over a 10- to 20-minute period. A myringotomy is made in the anterior drum, the fluid is aspirated, and a ventilating tube is inserted. The tube does not serve as a drain but as an alternate means for air to pass to the middle ear; drainage from a ventilating tube usually means there is an infection in the middle ear or mastoid. Risks of myringotomy are minimal but include possible production of a permanent perforation or surgical damage to the ossicular chain. The patient with tubes in place must not allow water to enter the external canal from showering or swimming, and the patient or parent should understand that drainage from the ear may be the only indication of acute infection because the usual pain associated with acute suppurative otitis media may not occur with a tube in place. For children with recurrent serous otitis media and adenoid hypertrophy, myringotomy may be combined with adenoidectomy (placement of a tube is a temporizing maneuver). In addition to reduced inflammation from proper middle-ear ventilation, improved eustachian-tube function will result from growth, allergic treatment, and, if indicated, adenoidectomy. A ventilating tube usually remains in place for 8 to 12 months. However, in ears in which tubes have been place so many times that the fibrous layer of the drum that holds the tube in place has been compromised, the tube may be lost within a few weeks.

Other Effusions. Blood or cerebrospinal fluid within the middle ear may also produce a conductive hearing loss. Hemotympanum in the presence of significant head injury implies a basal skull fracture despite negative radiologic evaluation, including tomography. The hemotympanum need not be treated because the blood will resorb spontaneously within several days. A hemotympanum may also result from barotrauma during airplane descent or scuba diving.

Mass Lesions Within the Middle Ear

Variants in anatomy, such as high-riding and dehiscent jugular bulb, aberrant internal carotid artery, aneurysm of the carotid artery, or neoplastic growths, such as glomus tumors, may present as a conductive loss but are usually visible as a mass behind the tympanic membrane. For such lesions, otologic and radiographic consultation is needed.

Malleus Fixation

The malleus may be fixed to the bone of the epitympanum by new bone or fibrous tissue as a result of inflammatory changes or bone dysplasias. Fixation of the malleus may be detected by pneumo-otoscopy or ma nipulation of the malleus handle.

Incus Resorption

As a result of trauma or septic or aseptic necrosis, the incudostapedial articulation may be disrupted. The long process of the incus is most commonly affected because of the relatively poor blood supply to this portion of the ossicle. Total discontinuity in the presence of an intact drum will produce a characteristic hearing loss of 60 db and a characteristic discontinuity pattern on tympanometry. Lesser degrees of disruption, such as subluxation of the incus or a fibrous union between the incus remnant and the capitulum of the stapes, will result in lesser degrees of loss. If the drum becomes retracted against the stapes head in the face of resorption of the incus—a situation called *myringostapediopexy*—very little if any hearing loss may be detectable. Disorders of the malleus, the incus, and the ossicular articulations can usually be corrected by transcanal ossiculoplasty (Fig. 2-1). In an adult, this is done under local anesthesia. Rearrangement of ossicles or substitution with alloplastic materials may result in elimination of the conductive hearing loss. The risks of these procedures are minimal and consist of those attendant to anesthesia and surgical trauma.

Stapes Fixation

Stapes fixation may occur as the result of congenital fixation in association with a branchial arch syndrome, or it may occur as an isolated congenital abnormality. Fixation of the stapes may also occur as a result of bone dysplasias and hyaline or fibrous deposition at the stapediovestibular joint due to recurrent, acute, or chronic middle-ear infection. The most common cause of stapes fixation, though, is otosclerosis. Otosclerosis is a disorder inherited as an autosomal dominant with variable penetrance. It occurs only in the human and only in the temporal bone. The prevalence of conductive hearing loss due to otosclerosis ("clinical otosclerosis") is approximately 1 in 100 among whites and 1 in 1000 among blacks and those of Oriental extraction. Hearing loss results from disordered bone growth at the stapediovestibular joint causing fixation. Conductive loss occasionally may be caused by bony closure of the round-window niche. The disorder is usually bilateral, but the stage of progression is different in each ear, and otosclerosis may present as a unilateral conductive loss. The natural history of otosclerosis is slow progression, but it is rare that a conductive hearing loss will exceed 50 db. Some authorities believe that otosclerosis may also cause a sensorineural loss.

Diagnosis. The diagnosis is presumptive, based on normal ear canal and tympanic membrane, normal motion of the malleus, and the presence of a conductive loss. Some radiologists believe that polytomography may be used to diagnose otosclerosis, although this opinion is not universally held. The ultimate diagnosis is made during surgical exploration of the middle ear.

Treatment. When the hearing loss becomes handicapping, usually when the threshold reaches 30 db or worse in the better-hearing ear, treatment may consist of either amplification with a hearing aid or surgical correction. Amplification is reserved for individuals with an only hearing ear and for those who cannot or will not take the risks involved in surgical correction.

A stapedectomy usually is performed under local anesthesia and requires approximately 1 hour (Fig. 2-1D). The posterior drum is turned back, and the stapes is either partially or totally removed. Most often, a prosthesis made of Teflon or steel and shaped like a miniature piston is fitted into an opening in the footplate and fixed to the long process of the incus, thus replacing the stapes. The success rate as measured by closure of the air–bone gap to within 10 db is approximately 96%. The risks of surgery include a 2% incidence of sensorineural hearing loss that may be profound and preclude the subsequent use of a hearing aid. In such cases, a vertigo, usually temporary, may also occur. The most common complication is impaired taste on the ipsilateral anterior tongue due to an injury to the chorda tympani. Perforations of the drum or damage to the facial nerve are rare complications. Relative contraindications include a mixed hearing loss in which the degree of sensorineural hearing loss will still require amplifications despite a successful stapedectomy. With severe mixed cases, stapedectomy may permit successful amplification by elevating the air-conduction threshold. Surgery for otosclerosis should never be performed in an only hearing ear. Age is not a contraindication.

SENSORINEURAL HEARING LOSS

A presumptive diagnosis of the cause of a sensorineural hearing loss is made largely on the basis of history and audiometric pattern. Usually, a unilateral hearing loss requires further evaluation in the form of vestibular or radiographic evaluation and will be treated separately.

BILATERAL SENSORINEURAL HEARING LOSS

Presbycusis

Approximately 30% of the adult population over 70 years of age has a handicapping sensorineural hearing loss ascribable to no other cause than the cumulative effects of the aging process. Diagnosis is made by history and audiometric pattern.

Diagnosis. The hearing loss caused by presbycusis is slowly progressive and bilaterally symmetrical. Four patterns of presbycusis have been described by Schuknecht (Fig. 2-2):

(Text continues on p. 40)

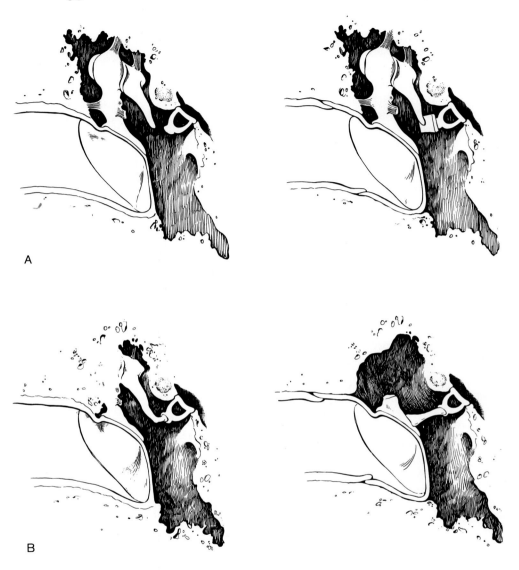

Fig. 2-1. (*A*) Ossiculoplasty, type II. A conductive loss caused by discontinuity of the incudostapedial joint (*left*). This is corrected by a bone interposition (*right*). (*B*) Ossiculoplasty, type IIIa (minor columella). The conductive hearing loss is caused by fixation of the head of the malleus and the body of incus (*left*). This is corrected by interposition between the malleus handle and stapes capitulum (*right*).

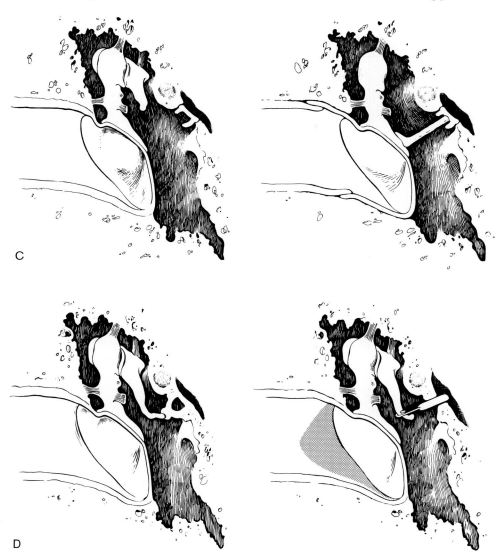

C

D

Fig. 2-1 *Continued* (*C*) Ossiculoplasty, type IIIb (major columella). A conductive hearing loss is caused by loss of the suprastructure of the stapes and the long process of incus (*left*). This is corrected by an interposition between the malleus handle and the stapes footplate (*right*). (*D*) Stapedectomy. The conductive hearing loss is caused by ankylosis of the stapes footplate (*left*). This is corrected by fenestration of the footplate and replacement of the stapes suprastructure with a teflon wire prosthesis from the incus to the oval window (*right*).

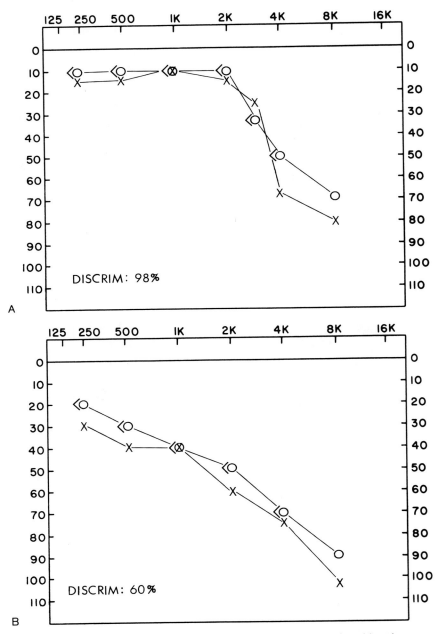

Fig. 2-2. (*A*) Patterns of presbycusis, sensory: bilateral sensorineural hearing loss with sharp onset and good discrimination; consistent with loss of hair cells in the basal turn. Discrimination remains good because hearing is preserved at normal levels in the speech frequencies, 125 Hz to 2000 Hz. (*B*) Patterns of presbycusis, neural: bilateral, downsloping sensorineural hearing loss with poor discrimination; consistent with degeneration of first-order cochlear neurons of the auditory nerve.

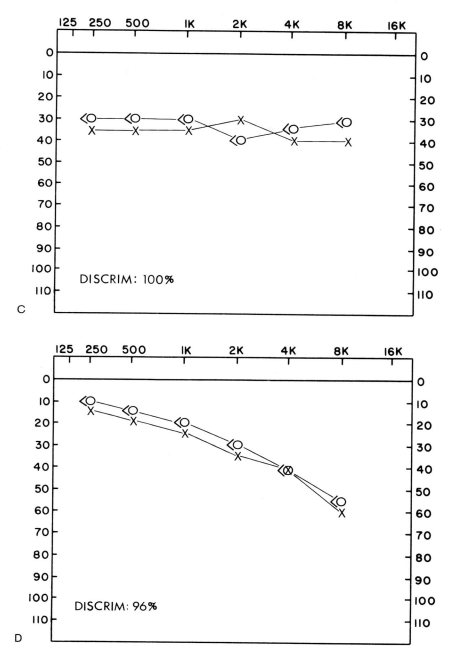

Fig. 2-2. *Continued* (C)Patterns of presbycusis, metabolic: bilateral, flat sensorineural hearing loss with good discrimination; consistent with atrophy of the stria vascularis. (*D*) Patterns of presbycusis, mechanical: bilateral, downsloping sensorineural hearing loss with good discrimination; consistent with an inner ear "stiffness lesion."

1. Sensory presbycusis: The usual audiometric pattern in this form of degeneration is a bilateral high-frequency hearing loss starting at 2 kHz to 3 kHz. Discrimination scores are good, and recruitment may be present. The histopathologic correlate is loss of hair cells in the basal turn of the cochlea.
2. Neural presbycusis: The typical audiometric pattern in this form of degeneration is a slowly descending threshold curve with reduced discrimination scores. The histopathologic correlate is primary degeneration of nerve elements of the inner ear and probably higher auditory pathways.
3. Metabolic presbycusis: The audiometric pattern is bilateral "flat" thresholds (*i.e.*, with equal decrement of threshold at all frequencies). The discrimination score is usually good except in severe hearing losses. The histopathologic correlate is degeneration of the stria vascularis, an epithelial component in the inner ear thought to be involved in inner-ear fluid homeostasis.
4. Mechanical presbycusis: The usual clinical finding is a symmetrical, descending audiometric pattern but with good discrimination, unlike in the neural group. Histologically, there is no loss of hair cells, neurons, or stria to correlate with the hearing loss, and disorders of mechanical elements of the inner ear have been postulated.

Slow progression is common in all forms of presbycusis. Patients may be told that the average rate of deterioration is approximately 5 db of speech-reception threshold in 3 to 5 years. However, this rate varies considerably from patient to patient. In a patient with the usual onset of hearing loss in the third to fifth decade of life, a typical audiometric pattern, bilateral symmetry, and no complicating medical factors, no further investigation is needed to make this diagnosis.

Certain families have a strong tendency for progressive hearing loss beginning in the fifth and sixth decades. Early in the course of presbycusis many older persons deny or fail to recognize this hearing loss, attributing their difficulties to mumbling or background noise, until it is pointed out by others. As with other forms of hearing loss, the first symptom of presbycusis is often tinnitus. Another complaint is increased inability to hear at meetings or difficulty hearing someone in the next room. Very commonly, poor discrimination accompanies hearing loss, and for such patients loud sounds and voices are irritating, yet comprehension is poor. As the hearing loss progresses, the patient has increased difficulty hearing the telephone and doorbell ring. In order to communicate with the patient, others may have to begin speaking loudly, a source of irritation to both the patient and his family. Most patients acquire some self-taught lip-reading skills; many become frustrated and tend to withdraw, not wishing to suffer the embarrassment of not hearing well in social situations. Patients with presbycusis, like all hearing-impaired persons, hear better when spoken to directly in quiet surroundings. Speaking slowly and clearly is more helpful than shouting. For patients with presbycusis the act of listening requires concentration, but many have slowed cognitive functions as well, compounding their difficulties.

Treatment: hearing aids. One or two hearing aids are usually prescribed when the speech-reception threshold exceeds 30 db to 35 db in the better-hearing ear. It is a common misconception that a hearing aid is not useful in sensorineural hearing loss. Nothing could be further from the truth in most cases, although several factors will influence the success of amplification. For instance, patients with low discrimination scores will have more difficulty using their hearing aid than will those with normal scores, but even patients with discrimination scores of under 10% may obtain useful information with amplification. Also, the presence of recruitment and a sharply downsloping audiometric pattern may make amplification difficult. Patients with a flat sensorineural hearing loss with good discrimination, that is, those with the metabolic type of presbycusis, almost always do extremely well with the aid of amplification.

There are several types of hearing aids. In air-conducting aids the amplification system may be contained in a mold within the ear or it may be suspended behind the auricle or worn in a pocket or harness at the chest level. This last type of hearing aid is usually reserved for severe-to-profound hearing loss where a high gain is necessary, such as in children with large congenital hearing losses or in adults with severe presbycusis. The amplification system may be incorporated into eyeglass frames; however, this combination may prove inconvenient if either hearing aid or lenses become nonfunctional. A more sophisticated hearing aid is the contralateral-routing-of-signals (CROS) aid, designed for individuals with a unilateral deafness. A microphone in the deafened ear reroutes sound to a receiver in the hearing ear. A further variant is the bicross aid for individuals with bilateral hearing loss in which only one ear is able to process amplified sound. In this situation, microphones are placed at each ear, and both signals are routed to the ear with usable hearing. The *bone-conduction hearing aid* transmits sound to the skull rather than through the external canal. This may be necessary in cases of atresia of the external canal or cases in which chronic ear discharge cannot be controlled.

With the burgeoning variety of design and gain characteristics, a hearing-aid fitting should be done with the guidance of an audiologist in a hearing and speech center. Optimal use of a hearing aid requires training, and courses for patients to learn to use their instrument should be provided at such centers. Inadequate training and motivation, rather than the impracticability of amplification, is the most common cause of failure to use a hearing aid. The principal drawback of a hearing aid is that it will not return hearing to a normal state like eyeglasses will restore normal vision in cases of myopia. It helps but does not overcome the problem of poor speech discrimination. Hearing aids amplify ambient noise (wind, traffic, kitchen noises) as well as more useful sounds and require frequent adjustment because of changing sound levels. Another drawback is the initial cost and the cost of replacement batteries. Also, small hearing aids are difficult to use by the elderly with arthritic fingers or severe tremor.

Genetically Determined Sensorineural Hearing Loss

Diagnosis. Dominant forms of inheritance constitute approximately 25% of genetically determined sensorineural hearing loss. The onset is typically after birth and is rapidly progressive. Recessive forms constitute 75% of the total, are typically present at birth, and are nonprogressive. Hearing loss of both the dominant and recessive types may be associated with defects in other systems that may be used as markers to identify the hearing loss as genetically determined. A partial listing of known genetically determined syndromes involving a hearing loss is presented under Hereditary Nerve Deafness, below, and the reader is referred to the Selected Readings at the end of the chapter for further description of the clinical presentation, progression, and diagnosis of individual entities. Fifty percent of all hereditary deafness is unassociated with other defects.

Hereditary Nerve Deafness

I. Dominant (25% of total); onset of hearing loss typically after birth and progressive)
  A. Without associated defects
    1. Congenital severe deafness
    2. High-tone deafness
  B. Inborn errors of metabolism and deafness
    1. Amino acids
      a. Tyrosine
        (1) Tietze's syndrome (albinism and deafness)
        (2) Waardenburg's syndrome: 1% of total hereditary deafness; 20% of dominant types
      b. Proline
        (1) Hereditary mental retardation, prolinemia, and deafness

    c. Methionine

       (1) Hereditary mental retardation, homocystinemia, deafness, dislocated lenses, fatty degeneration of liver

C. Nephropathies and deafness

  1. Alport's syndrome (1% of hereditary deafness)

    a. Hereditary nephritis and deafness

  2. Hereditary nephritis, urticaria, amyloidosis, and dominant nerve deafness

    a. Progressive sensorineural hearing loss from youth

  3. Hereditary nephritis, mental retardation, epilepsy, diabetes, and dominant nerve deafness (Hermann's syndrome)

D. Ectodermal defects and deafness

  1. Ectodermal dysplasia, anhidrotic type, and deafness

  2. Bilateral acoustic tumors and deafness

E. Degenerative disease of nervous system and deafness

  1. Huntington's chorea

F. Skeletal defects and deafness

  1. Craniofacial dysostosis (Crouzon's disease)

  2. Cleidocranial dysostosis

  3. Mandibulofacial dysostosis

II. Recessive (75% of total; typically congenital and nonprogressive)

A. Without associated defects (50% of hereditary deafness)

  1. Recessive congenital deafness

  2. High-tone deafness

  3. Mid-tone deafness

B. Inborn errors of metabolism

  1. Amino acids

    a. Tyrosine

       (1) Albinism and deafness

       (2) Photophobia and nystagmus

       (3) Deafness (congenital)

  2. Carbohydrates

    a. Mucopolysaccharides

       (1) Gargoylism (Hurler's syndrome)

       (2) Morquio's disease (osteochondrodystrophy)

       (3) Onychodystrophy

  3. Lipids

    a. Ganglioside lipidoses

       (1) Amaurotic familial idiocy (Tay-Sachs disease)

    4. Minerals

        a. Copper

            (1) Wilson's disease (hepatolenticular degeneration)

  C. Degenerative diseases of the nervous system

    1. Friedreich's ataxia

    2. Schilder's disease

    3. Unverricht's epilepsy

  D. Skeletal defects

    1. Generalized defects

        a. Osteopetrosis (Albers-Schönberg disease)

    2. Defects of vertebrae

        a. Klippel-Feil syndrome

  E. Congenital heart disease and deafness

    1. ECG abnormalities (Jervell and Lange-Nielsen syndrome)

  F. Endocrine abnormalities

    1. Thyroid

        a. Nonendemic goiter and deafness (Pendred's syndrome) (10% of hereditary deafness)

  G. Eye abnormalities

    1. Retinitis pigmentosa (Usher's syndrome; 10% of hereditary deafness)

    2. Retinitis pigmentosa, mental retardation, dwarfism (Cockayne's syndrome)

III. Trisomies

  A. Trisomy 13

  B. Trisomy 18

The estimated incidence of profound hereditary deafness is approximately 1 in every 2000 live births in the United States. The genes involved in the development of the ear number in the thousands, and either single or multiple gene dysfunction may result in abnormalities. The diagnosis of a genetically determined hearing loss is presumptive and based on the pattern of onset and progression, the exclusion of other causes of hearing loss, and a family history consistent with the diagnosis. Further laboratory investigation may include tomography of the temporal bone to diagnose forms of dysplasia involving the bony otic capsule. This carries little therapeutic significance, however. Chromosomal studies are not useful except in severe and multiple associated congenital defects.

Treatment. In cases of partial hearing loss an attempt should be made to place the disorder into the known varieties of genetically determined loss so that a probable natural history may be determined. A hearing aid is usually prescribed when the hearing threshold in the better ear is greater than 30 db. In congenitally severe-to-profoundly deaf children, habilitation is usually best coordinated at a school for the deaf.

Congenital, Nonhereditary Deafness

Not all congenital deafness is genetically determined. Known cases include those resulting from rubella, ototoxic drugs, anoxia, and birth injury. Early onset of deafness may be secondary to bacterial meningitis, and presumed inner-ear damage may be due to measles and mumps.

Ototoxicity

The list of drugs known or thought to be ototoxic continues to grow. The most common include the aminoglycoside antibiotics, loop diuretics, quinine and its derivatives, salicylates, and chemotherapeutic agents. The hearing loss caused by ototoxicity is usually bilateral and symmetrical. Ototoxicity may be increased by concurrent renal disease. The vestibular system may be selectively affected before the auditory system by some drugs, such as streptomycin and gentamicin.

UNILATERAL, OR ASYMMETRICAL, SENSORINEURAL HEARING LOSS

Otitis Media

Chronic and, rarely, acute otitis media may be complicated by suppurative labyrinthitis with resultant destruction of the inner ear. The diagnosis is based on associated signs of infection. Hearing can rarely, if ever, be saved once suppurative labyrinthitis has occurred.

Bacterial Meningitis

Partial or complete bilateral or unilateral hearing loss occurs as a sequela in approximately 21% of cases of bacterial meningitis. This is due to damage to the cochlear nerve in the infected subarachnoid space or to spread of the suppurative process into the perilymphatic space by way of the cochlear aqueduct. In addition, transient hearing loss may occur as a result of metabolic dysfunction in the inner ear. Predisposing factors to the development of a hearing loss include a delay between the onset of meningitis and treatment, the presence of meningococcus as the infective organism, and the development of other neurologic sequelae.

Direct Trauma

Temporal-bone fractures, particularly transverse fractures, may result in total profound hearing loss and are commonly associated with vestibular and facial-nerve injury. Hearing loss may occur without fracture as a result of transmission of acoustic energy to the inner ear from a blow to the head. This usually results in an abrupt high-tone hearing loss that is worse in the ear closest to the site of injury. Penetrating wounds, such as those resulting from putting a pencil or cotton-tip applicator through the drum, may result in perilymphatic leakage and sensorineural hearing loss (see Chap. 5).

Acoustic Trauma

Exposure to loud noise may result in a unilateral or bilateral sensorineural hearing loss. This may result from one exposure to intense noise, or it may be cumulative over years of exposure to high-intensity industrial noise. The audiometric pattern demonstrates abrupt loss in the 3-kHz to 4-kHz area in cases of single exposures to high-intensity sound and a gradually downsloping pattern with long-term exposure to loud but less intense noise. The diagnosis is made by the typical audiometric pattern and a consistent history of noise exposure. For an example of hearing loss from acute noise trauma, see Chapter 5.

Syphilis

Syphilis, either congenital or acquired, may produce a sensorineural hearing loss. This may be symmetrical, but usually one ear is more affected than the other. Routine serology or Venereal Disease Research Laboratory (VDRL) and rapid plasma reagin (RPR) card tests may not be positive in late latent syphilis, and hence a fluorescent treponemal antibody-absorption (FTA-ABS) test should be performed in suspected cases. Cerebrospinal fluid serology usually is not positive. The hearing loss may be sudden in onset, rapidly progressive, or fluctuating (similar to the hearing loss in Meniere's disease). Discrimination scores are characteristically low, and severe vestibular hypofunction as determined by caloric testing and vestibular symptoms are usually present.

Treatment with oral corticosteroids and intramuscular antibiotics over a several-month period has proved effective in some patients (see Chap. 4).

Neurologic Disorders

Loss of hearing or vestibular function may be a presenting symptom of a demyelinating disease such as multiple sclerosis. The usual pattern of hearing loss is a progressive, high-frequency type, although it may be sudden and unilateral and may recover to a degree. Speech discrimination is usually decreased.

Neoplasms

Rarely, primary tumors of the temporal bone may invade the inner ear and cause a sensorineural hearing loss. Metastatic lesions may demonstrate no local manifestation with the exception of hearing and vestibular dysfunction. The most common sources of metastatic lesions of the temporal bone in order of frequency are carcinomas of the breast, kidney, lung, stomach, larynx, prostate, and thyroid. Temporal-bone x-ray films or bone scan in suspected cases are diagnostic.

Cerebellopontine-Angle Tumors

Vestibular schwannoma (acoustic neuroma) and other tumors of the cerebellopontine angle, such as meningiomas, may cause a unilateral dysfunction or auditory and vestibular dysfunction.

Diagnosis. The hearing loss may be slowly to rapidly progressive, although cases of sudden hearing loss have been described. Audiometric criteria that raise the suspicion of a cerebellopontine-angle tumor include poor discrimination, positive-tone decay, and acoustic-reflex decay. Severe ipsilateral vestibular hypofunction is seen in the majority of cases.

When no other cause of a unilateral sensorineural loss is found by history or examination, further investigation is indicated to rule out this class of tumors. For instance, caloric testing with or without electronystagmography (ENG) will detect vestibular hypofunction. (Often these patients have little or no vestibular symptoms despite marked loss of caloric function.) Also, brain-stem evoked-response audiometry has proved to be a sensitive test for the presence of cerebellopontine-angle tumors. Interwave latency prolongation, either I–III or I–V, suggests the diagnosis. Radiographic techniques, in order of sensitivity, include plain views of the interal auditory canal, tomography of the internal auditory canal, enhanced computed tomography (CT) scanning of the posterior fossa, and contrast myelography of the posterior fossa and internal auditory canal using Pantopaque or metrizimide. Bilateral vestibular schwannomas may occur in von Recklinghausen's disease.

Treatment. Most tumors of the cerebellopontine angles are benign and slowly progressive. No treatment may be indicated in the aged or debilitated individual. For patients who are surgical candidates, it is usually best to remove the tumor when first discovered because the morbidity and mortality of surgery correspond directly to tumor size. The surgical approach depends on the size of the tumor, the presence of usable hearing, and the necessity of preserving this hearing. A tumor under 2 cm in diameter, in a patient with no usable hearing, is probably best removed through a transmastoid–translabyrinthine approach, which requires little retraction of intracranial structures. For larger tumors or in cases in which the decision has been made to attempt to preserve hearing, a combined neurosurgical and otologic procedure by way of the suboccipital route is most popular.

Complications of tumor removal are significant. Temporary or permanent facial paresis or paralysis occurs in at least 30% of cases. Severe neurologic deficits or death may result from bleeding or interruption of brain-stem arterial supply. In aged and debilitated patients who require surgery because of the progression of symptoms, intracapsular subtotal removal is often indicated to limit the morbidity.

Hearing Loss Associated With Other Metabolic or Systemic Disorders

Arterial Disease.   Although the concept of hearing loss due to involvement of the blood supply of the inner ear by arteriosclerotic cardiovascular disease is intuitively attractive, there is little evidence to support such a hypothesis. Hemorrhage into the inner ear or certain well-described vascular insufficiencies of the posterior circulation are rare but do occur. These include occlusion of the anterior inferior cerebellar artery and the lateral medullary syndrome. Lateral medullary syndrome, or Wallenberg's syndrome, is caused by occlusion of the vertebral or posterior inferior cerebellar artery. Symptoms consist of headache, vertigo, vomiting, diplopia, and dysphagia. Findings include ipsilateral facial analgesia, ipsilateral ptosis and miosis, contralateral trunk analgesia and thermanesthesia, and ipsilateral paralysis of the soft palate, pharynx and larynx. The occlusion of the anterior inferior cerebellar artery may be suspected with the sudden onset of vertigo, hearing loss, facial paralysis, and cerebellar and sensory signs including ipsilateral loss of pain and temperature sensation on the face, including corneal hypesthesia. Partial loss of pain and temperature sensation on the contralateral side may occur.

The syndrome of vertebrobasilar ischemia is probably invoked more often than it occurs. The diagnosis is not warranted unless the hearing loss and vertigo are associated with other sensory and motor disturbances such as diplopia, blurred vision, transient hemianopsia, dysarthria, and hemiparesis.

Other Metabolic Disorders.   A number of authors have associated sensorineural hearing loss with diabetes mellitus, although convincing evidence is lacking. The same is true of thyroid disease with the exception of Pendred's syndrome, a coincidently inherited syndrome of thyroid and auditory dysfunction.

Disorders of Unknown Cause

Meniere's Disease. In Meniere's disease, the hearing loss is usually unilateral, although it may be bilateral in 20% of cases. A characteristic low-frequency sensorineural loss is present. Hearing loss is commonly fluctuant and is associated with acute attacks of prostrating vertigo and tinnitus and a feeling of fullness within the affected ear. Variant forms are recognized. For example, the cochlear variant of Meniere's disease consists of fluctuating low-tone sensorineural hearing loss, tinnitus, and aural fullness, without vestibular symptomatology. In uncomplicated cases the diagnosis is made by history and audiometric patterns. In cases of severe sensorineural loss, exclusion of a cerebellopontine angle tumor may be necessary (see above, Cerebellopontine-Angle Tumors).

Collagen Vascular Diseases. Unilateral or bilateral sensorineural loss and vestibular symptoms have been described as complicating Wegner's granulomatosis, periarteritis nodosa, temporal arteritis, Cogan's syndrome, and a relapsing polychondritis.

Sudden Idiopathic Sensorineural Deafness. Sudden idiopathic sensorineural deafness is diagnosed after other causes of sudden sensorineural hearing loss have been excluded. The disorder is most commonly unilateral but in rare cases may be bilateral or sequential. Vestibular complaints may accompany the hearing loss. The precise etiology is uncertain, though many authors believe it is related to viral disease. Although a number of treatments have been recommended, to date only steroid therapy in selected patients has proved to be efficacious. This disorder is more fully discussed in Chapter 5.

SELECTED READINGS

KONIGSMARK BW, GORLIN RJ: Genetic and Metabolic Deafness. Philadelphia, WB Saunders, 1976

NADOL JB JR: Hearing loss as a sequela of meningitis. Laryngoscope 88:739–755, 1978

NADOL JB JR: Pathoembryology of the middle ear. In Gorlin RJ (ed): Fifth International Conference on Morphogenesis and Malformation of the Ear, pp 181–209. New York, Alan R. Liss, 1980

WILSON WR, BYL FM, LAIRD N: The efficacy of steroids in the treatment of idiopathic sudden hearing loss. Arch Otolaryngol 106:772–776, 1980

3

THE DRAINING EAR

Joseph B. Nadol, Jr.

External otitis (swimmer's ear)
  Diagnosis
  Treatment
    Systemic antibiotics
    Topical antibiotics
    Analgesia
  Malignant external otitis
    Diagnosis
    Treatment
  Chondritis of the auricle
  Bullous myringitis
  *Herpes zoster oticus (Ramsay
      Hunt syndrome)*
  Chronic fibrosing external otitis
Acute suppurative otitis media
  Diagnosis
  Role of paracentesis
  Treatment
  Follow-up
  Complications
    Rupture of eardrum
    Acute mastoiditis
      Bezold's abscess
      Facial paresis
      Role of mastoidectomy

Chronic otitis media
  *Chronic active otitis media
              without cholesteatoma*
    Diagnosis
    Treatment
  *Chronic active otitis media with
      cholesteatoma*
    Diagnosis
    Treatment
  *Complications of chronic active
      otitis media*
    Labyrinthine fistula
    Facial-nerve paresis
    Petrositis
    Brain abscess and meningitis
    *Phlebitis and thrombosis of
        the lateral venous sinus*
      Diagnosis
      Treatment
Surgery of the infected ear
  Risks of surgery
  Expectations of surgery

Drainage from the external auditory canal in the absence of trauma implies infection in the external canal or middle ear and mastoid. There are basically three entities, and variations of them, that need to be considered: external otitis, acute suppurative otitis media, and chronic otitis media.

EXTERNAL OTITIS (SWIMMER'S EAR)

Dermatologic conditions that affect the rest of the body, including eczema, may also affect the squamous epithelium of the external auditory canal, and the treatment for a dermatologic condition involving the ear is similar to the treatment for the condition in general. These conditions rarely cause drainage, but they may cause itching, flaking, and the accumulation of desquamated epithelial debris, which requires periodic cleaning.

Infectious external otitis causes drainage, intense pain, tenderness, and hearing loss owing to obstruction of the external canal.

DIAGNOSIS

The usual clinical setting includes precedent maceration of the external canal resulting from water retained from swimming or showering or resulting from trauma caused by an attempt to clean the external canal. Often the accumulation of cerumen or debris in the canal may result in infection by causing retention of water in the canal and by prompting the patient to manipulate the ear.

It is important to differentiate external otitis from otitis media. Both cause pain, and both may cause drainage from the canal. Although the external auditory canal is usually normal in cases of otitis media, it may be somewhat macerated, especially if perforation of the drum has occurred and the ear is draining. The attribute that best distinguishes external otitis from otitis media is tenderness. External otitis causes intense tenderness over the tragus and pain when the auricle is displaced, whereas uncomplicated otitis media does not.

External otitis and otitis media may coexist. For example, untreated acute suppurative otitis media with perforation and drainage may cause secondary inflammatory changes in the external canal for a few days. In such cases both disorders should be treated; oral antibiotics should be administered for otitis media and topical antibiotics for otitis externa.

TREATMENT

The ear must be cleaned in order to properly diagnose external otitis and exclude middle-ear pathology and to initiate proper treatment for external otitis. When the debris within the canal is loose or liquid, cleaning is best accomplished with a No.-5 Barron or No.-70 Pilling suction tip (see Appendix). Suction aspiration of the ear canal is done with a headlight and handheld speculum or through an otoscope. The drum is examined for perforation and evidence of middle-ear pathology. In external otitis, the squamous epithelium of the lateral surface of the drum may be macerated and inflamed in the absence of middle-ear pathology. Once the canal is cleaned, a screening hearing evaluation should be performed with a tuning fork and whisper tests. In general, tuning-fork tests are normal in otitis externa. Evidence of a conductive hearing loss is strongly suggestive of concomitant middle-ear disease.

SYSTEMIC ANTIBIOTICS

Oral antibiotics are generally not useful in the treatment of external otitis and are not used unless there is evidence of early cellulitis at the meatus or of significant adenopathy in preauricular or infra-auricular areas. Culture of the drainage is usually not performed in uncomplicated cases. The usual causative organisms are *Staphylococcus aureus* or *Pseudomonas aeruginosa,* but external otitis also may be caused by fungi. Fungal otitis is usually recognized by the appearance of spores or mycelia in the external canal.

TOPICAL ANTIBIOTICS

Commercially available antibiotics or acidic eardrops combined with hydrocortisone are essential in the treatment of external otitis. These include Cortisporin, Pyocidin, and Vosol HC. Cortisporin is available as a suspension or solution. The suspension is said to be less likely to cause pain in an inflamed ear, but it has the disadvantage of causing accumulation of suspended ingredients in the ear canal. There is little reason to differentiate between these drugs, although Vosol has the advantage of not containing an antibiotic. Any of these solutions may be used in the presence of a perforation, but some otologists prefer not to use an ototoxic antibiotic, such as neomycin, with an open middle ear. Also, neomycin may cause a contact dermatitis in sensitive individuals.

If the ear canal is swollen shut, it may be necessary to insert an ear wick to act as a conduit for topical drops. Wicks may be obtained commercially or may be made from a neurosurgical patty or simply a segment of 4 × 4 sponge. The wick is inserted into the ear canal using Hartmann's or bayonet forceps. It is usually premoistened with otic drops, and the patient continues to apply 3 drops to the lateral aspect of the wick three times a day. The patient is usually asked to remove the wick in 2 days. Drops should be continued for a minimum of 1 week at the same dosage. Follow-up for uncomplicated external otitis is usually not necessary, but patients are instructed to return if the symptoms do not resolve after this course of treatment. Also, if it was impossible to examine the eardrum, follow-up after edema has subsided is necessary to assess the drum, middle ear, and hearing.

ANALGESIA

Otitis externa causes intense pain, and narcotic analgesics are usually required for the first 2 to 3 days.

MALIGNANT EXTERNAL OTITIS

Simple external otitis in diabetics may progress to a life-threatening disorder known as malignant external otitis. The infective organism is always *P. aeruginosa,* and the usual clinical situation involves an elderly diabetic. It is thought that the diabetic angiopathy seen elsewhere in the body also occurs in the skin of the external auditory canal and allows a superficial infection to become invasive. Once the epithelial barrier is broken, the infectious process spreads rapidly anteriorly into the parotid space or, more often, inferiorly into the retromandibular fossa. From there the cellulitis may then spread to the stylomastoid foramen, causing facial paresis and paralysis, and to the jugular foramen, causing lower-cranial-nerve paresis and thrombosis of the sigmoid sinus. This may lead to the spread of the process along vascular and fascial planes across the skull base. Late in the course of this disease, osteomyelitis of the mastoid tip, skull base, and petrous apex may occur.

DIAGNOSIS

External otitis in an elderly diabetic should always raise the question of malignant external otitis. If the usual course of treated external otitis does not occur (*i.e.,* gradual improvement of symptoms starting at the second or third day, resulting in complete resolution within 7 to 10 days), malignant external otitis should be considered. The earliest presenting sign is breach of the epithelial barrier, usually on the floor of the cartilaginous external canal, with granulation tissue replacing lost epithelium. Later, there may be exposed cartilage or tympanic bone in the ear canal. Facial and lower-cranial-nerve paresis must be considered late signs, and morbidity and mortality are directly related to the stage reached prior to treatment. Plain mastoid films or tomography of the temporal bone are negative until late in the disease when osteomyelitis has occurred. Furthermore, radiographs may lag several weeks behind the stage of disease.

TREATMENT

Long-term intravenous antibiotic treatment is essential in malignant external otitis. The usual regimen is a combination of carbenicillin and tobramycin, the drug selection being based on culture and sensitivities. Surgical intervention is necessary if the canal is occluded by granulation, and simple office curettage may be all that is necessary. Late in the disorder when osteomyelitis or abscess formation at the skull base has occurred, extensive transmastoid surgery may be necessary for salvage. Antibiotic therapy at our institution is maintained for 4 weeks when there is no evidence of osteomyelitis and for 6 weeks when there is evidence of bone involvement.

CHONDRITIS OF THE AURICLE

Cellulitis of the auricle and subsequent chondritis of the auricular cartilage may occur as a sequela of external otitis or as a complication of an injury to the auricle.

The most common causative organisms of cellulitis and chondritis are *S. aureus* and *P. aeruginosa*. Intravenous antibiotics are usually required and are selected by culture if drainage is present. Empirical treatment should include coverage for both organisms. If a hematoma is present, it must be drained. If the cellulitis responds poorly to antibiotics, debridement of sequestered cartilage may be necessary.

BULLOUS MYRINGITIS

Bullous myringitis may be confused with external otitis. In this disorder, thought to be caused by a virus, the ear canal is normal. However, the layers of the drum are separated by bullae that contain serosanguineous fluid. This is usually extremely painful but does not produce systemic signs. Puncture of the blebs with a myringotomy knife may be necessary for control of pain.

HERPES ZOSTER OTICUS (RAMSAY HUNT SYNDROME)

Herpes zoster oticus is a herpetic disorder that is often heralded by intense pain in the ear before the herpetic vesicles appear. Hearing loss, vertigo, and facial paralysis also may occur.

Treatment consists of supportive measures, including analgesics. Because the herpetic vesicles may become superinfected, prophylactic antibiotics are often used. *S. aureus* is a frequent offender.

CHRONIC FIBROSING EXTERNAL OTITIS

Chronic fibrosing external otitis, which is relatively rare, is due to chronic or repeated episodes of external otitis in which subepithelial fibrosis causes stenosis of the external canal, thickening of the drum, and eventually a conductive hearing loss. Surgical treatment is required. The skin of the external canal and lateral aspect of the drum is removed, the bony ear canal and meatus are enlarged, and the lateral surface of the drum and ear canal are covered with split-thickness skin grafts.

ACUTE SUPPURATIVE OTITIS MEDIA

Acute suppurative otitis media, an infection of the middle-ear space, is a common complication of serous otitis media in children and may be a sequela of an upper respiratory infection in children or adults. The most common organisms include pneumococcus, *Streptococcus*, and *Hemophilus influenzae*. The incidence of *H. influenzae* is higher in children under 5 years of age. *Staphylococcus aureus* also may occasionally cause otitis media. Virus and microplasma organisms have been implicated in a minority of cases of otitis media, based on the clinical finding that a percentage of cultured middle-ear exudates show no growth.

DIAGNOSIS

Although the tympanic membrane is usually intact early in the course of otitis media, it may rupture very early with streptococcal infections or if it contained a thin neomembrane from a previous perforation. Within the first few hours of infection, the only physical finding may be some erythema in the posterosuperior quadrant. Shortly thereafter, bulging and widespread erythema of the tympanic membrane occur. A slight conductive hearing loss may be produced, and adults may complain of a slight sense of unsteadiness. There should be no tenderness of the external canal or auricle or over the mastoid cortex. In the absence of signs of complication, no x-ray films are necessary. Culture may be done if perforation has occurred.

ROLE OF PARACENTESIS

Paracentesis for the release and culture of purulent material is usually not indicated except in extenuating circumstances, such as in an immunosuppressed individual or in a patient with concurrent meningitis, mastoiditis, or facial-nerve paresis. Paracentesis can be accomplished with a local anesthetic in the posterior canal wall, using 1% Xylocaine with 1:100,000 epinephrine or with the use of iontophoresis. Needle aspiration or myringotomy should be performed in the anterior inferior quadrant of the drum to avoid damage to the facial nerve or ossicular chain.

TREATMENT

In the adult the drug of choice is penicillin. The usual dosage is 250 mg by mouth, four times a day for 10 days. A decongestant–antihistamine may be used, especially if the patient has congestion from an upper respiratory infection. Erythromycin is a reasonable alternative to penicillin in the presence of penicillin allergy. Treatment of acute otitis media in children up to 7 years of age requires an antibiotic effective for both pneumococcus and *H. influenzae*. The choice for an effective therapy might be amoxicillin (20 mg/kg/day) divided into three doses or ampicillin (50 mg/kg/day) in four doses for 10 days. If the child is allergic to penicillin, erythromycin (40 mg/kg/day) plus sulfisoxazole (100 mg/kg/day) divided into four doses can be used. Decongestants (*e.g.,* Actifed and Dimetapp) probably have little direct effect upon otitis media, but they may be useful in patients with an associated blocked nose and rhinorrhea. Pediatric nose drops, such as xylometazoline (Otrivin), are also useful in this regard.

FOLLOW-UP

All patients with acute otitis media should be reexamined in approximately 2 to 3 weeks. They should be told that pain associated with otitis media should resolve within hours of the initiation of antibiotic treatment. If persistent pain or drainage occurs, the patient should return for further examination. Especially in children, serous otitis media may persist for some weeks after an acute episode of suppurative otitis media and should be treated in the same fashion as uncomplicated serous otitis media (see Chap. 2).

Occasionally, a child will develop recurrent otitis media of one or both ears despite apparently proper antibiotic therapy. A typical history might be right acute otitis media (RAOM) in a 5-year-old child, treated with ampicillin for 10 days with apparent resolution of infection, followed in 2 weeks by another RAOM, treated properly with a good response, but followed 2 weeks later by a third infection and so on throughout the winter. It is likely that this is the same infection, which is suppressed but not eliminated by the course of antibiotics and continues to recur. Following a 10-day course of ampicillin or erythromycin and sulfisoxazole, the patient should be placed on prophylactic antibiotics, such as ampicillin (125 mg) or sulfisoxazole (500 mg), each morning for 3 to 6 months. This long-term therapy is very effective for this problem, rarely leads to the growth of resistant bacteria or antibiotic sensitivities, and avoids the hazards of recurrent infections and fevers.

If prophylactic antibiotics fail to prevent recurrent acute otitis media, the placement of a ventilating tube, even without evidence of persistent serous otitis, may be effective.

Adults often complain of a strange feeling or a slight ache in the ear even in the absence of serous otitis for 3 to 6 weeks after a bout of acute otitis media. A follow-up clinical evaluation of hearing should be done, and if an abnormality is suspected, audiometry should be performed. Persistent serous otitis media in an adult should result in a search for a cause of eustachian-tube dysfunction, such as nasopharyngeal carcinoma.

COMPLICATIONS

RUPTURE OF EARDRUM

An eardrum may rupture rapidly with streptococcal infections or in the presence of an organism, often *Staphylococcus aureus,* not sensitive to the prescribed antibiotic. If rupture has occurred, the drainage should be cultured, and topical antibiotics should be used in addition to oral antibiotics. Some otologists hesitate to use otic drops containing neomycin in the presence of a perforation. Rupture of the tympanic membrane due to an otherwise uncomplicated suppurative otitis media usually heals spontaneously within a few weeks after the drainage has subsided. Occasionally a perforation will persist and may require tympanoplasty.

ACUTE MASTOIDITIS

Acute mastoiditis was common in the preantibiotic era and still occurs today occasionally, usually because of delay in treatment of acute suppurative otitis media. Pathognomonic signs of mastoiditis include persistent pain after initiation of antibiotic treatment, tenderness or periosteal elevation over the mastoid cortex, displacement of the auricle anteriorly caused by periosteal elevation, and sagging of the posterosuperior external canal wall. The diagnosis is confirmed by plain x-ray films of the mastoid. These will show loss of the normal bony trabecular pattern of the mastoid cells in addition to fluid density. The treatment of acute mastoiditis includes intravenous antibiotics and a myringotomy for culture, drainage of purulent material, and, usually, the placement of a ventilating tube. Intravenous antibiotics are continued for 7 to 10 days based on gram stain and culture.

Bezold's Abscess

If the treatment of mastoiditis is delayed, or if a loculation of pus develops in the mastoid tip, an abscess may occur below the mastoid tip in the neck owing to breakdown of the lateral mastoid cortex. Because the sternocleidomastoid muscle originates on the lateral surface of the mastoid cortex, this abscess is medial to it, and hence fluctuance may not be palpated. A Bezold's abscess requires immediate drainage and a simple mastoidectomy for drainage of the loculated purulence within the central mastoid tract in order to prevent spread of the infectious process to the carotid space and beyond.

Facial Paresis

Facial paresis may occur in the presence of mastoiditis; it does not require additional treatment unless the paresis progresses despite antibiotic treatment and paracentesis. If total paralysis and evidence of neuronal degeneration occur, exploration of the mastoid and facial nerve may be necessary.

Role of Mastoidectomy

Simple mastoidectomy for treatment of acute mastoiditis was the most common otolaryngologic procedure in the preantibiotic era. It is now rarely performed. It is necessary when the infection has resulted in the resorption of the bony mastoid cells, as in coalescent mastoiditis, or in the face of complications such as facial paralysis and Bezold's abscess.

CHRONIC OTITIS MEDIA

Chronic otitis media applies to ears that are actively draining and those that have drained chronically in the past. *Chronic inactive otitis media* implies a perforation of the eardrum and scarring in the middle ear but no active drainage. *Chronic active otitis media* implies chronic drainage through a perforation in the drum and may exist with or without *cholesteatoma*.

CHRONIC ACTIVE OTITIS MEDIA WITHOUT CHOLESTEATOMA

A variety of bacterial species have been cultured from chronically draining ears. Gram-negative organisms predominate. The most common pathogens are *P. aeruginosa, Streptococcus, Escherichia coli,* and *Staphylococcus aureus.* Often multiple organisms are cultured.

Rarely, *Mycobacterium tuberculosis* may cause chronic drainage from the ear. The rapid progression and presence of abundant granulation tissue helps to differentiate tuberculosis from other forms of chronic otitis media. The facial nerve and inner ear may be involved and demonstrate dysfunction relatively early compared to chronic bacterial otitis media. Also, multiple perforations of the drum are thought to be pathognomonic of tuberculous otitis media. Wegener's granulomatosis must be differentiated from this disorder.

DIAGNOSIS

The diagnosis is based largely on the history and otologic findings. Roentgenograms may be useful if cholesteatoma is suspected. In chronic active otitis media, the usual radiographic report includes mention of "underdeveloped or under pneumatized mastoid with sclerosis." This usually does not help in guiding treatment and is not needed to make the diagnosis.

TREATMENT

The first consideration in treatment is to determine whether chronic active otitis media can be transformed into chronic inactive otitis media with medical treatment only. Medical treatment includes the use of topical drops, which has been previously discussed in connection with otitis externa; periodic cleaning of the ear to remove keratin debris; and instruction to the patient not to allow water to enter the ear canal. Oral antibiotics play little role in the treatment of chronic active otitis media.

Occasionally, parenteral antibiotics may be beneficial for treating particularly active purulent drainage.

If the ear becomes dry with this treatment, further treatment becomes elective. The patient may become a candidate for tympanoplasty or ossiculoplasty to repair the drum and ossicular chain, or he may choose to live with the perforation and hearing loss. If the ear fails to become dry with this therapeutic trial, surgery is recommended in the form of a mastoid tympanoplasty to remove chronic infection from mastoid air cells.

CHRONIC ACTIVE OTITIS MEDIA WITH CHOLESTEATOMA

DIAGNOSIS

A history of perforation, usually with chronic, foul-smelling drainage, and the finding of keratin debris within the middle ear—most often in the pars flaccida area—is sufficient for the otologist to make a diagnosis of cholesteatoma. Pathologic verification is seldom necessary at this stage. Roentgenograms may be useful in special situations to define the limits of the cholesteatoma or to provide evidence of destruction of ossicles or thinning of the otic capsule.

TREATMENT

Cholesteatoma requires surgical treatment unless there are extenuating circumstances in the medical history. The surgical procedure is tailored to the extent of the cholesteatoma. For example, a small cholesteatoma may be removed by the transcanal route; a larger one in the attic may be removed by atticotomy, but usually mastoid tympanoplasty is required. A description of mastoid surgery is found later in this chapter under "Surgery of the Infected Ear."

COMPLICATIONS OF CHRONIC ACTIVE OTITIS MEDIA

Longstanding suppuration within the mastoid air-cell system, especially with concurrent cholesteatoma, may produce a number of complications.

LABYRINTHINE FISTULA

A labyrinthine fistula is caused by resorption of bone of the otic capsule by the action of enzymes associated with cholesteatoma or chronic active suppurative osteitis. The most common site for a fistula is the lateral semicircular canal in the mastoid antrum. However, any of the canals may be involved, and a cochlear fistula may occur in the middle ear or epitympanum. Untreated, fistulae may progress to bacterial labyrinthitis with destruction of auditory and vestibular end-organs and may cause a bacterial meningitis. The presence of a fistula is indicated by subjective episodes of unsteadiness and a positive fistula test, in which a nystagmus is elicited by the application of positive or negative pressure to the external canal. The presence of a fistula with chronic active otitis media constitutes an urgent indication for surgery.

FACIAL-NERVE PARESIS

Bone resorption and chronic active infection may uncover the facial nerve, usually in its descending portion. This may result in facial paresis and destruction of a segment of the facial nerve if untreated. Paresis in the presence of chronic active otitis media is an urgent indication for surgery.

PETROSITIS

Petrositis implies an extension of the suppurative process to the apex of the petrous bone. With acute suppurative otitis media, this occurs as a rare complication called Gradenigo's syndrome. More commonly, it occurs in the clinical situation of chronic active otitis media in the face of an immune deficiency or debilitation.

The diagnosis is suggested by deep head pain, perceived as temporal or retro-orbital, secondary to trigeminal-nerve inflammation. Also, there is often a loss of ipsilateral lateral gaze due to a sixth-nerve paresis, meningismus, and white blood cells in the cerebrospinal fluid on spinal tap. Profound sensorineural hearing loss and vertigo can occur with inner-ear involvement. Temporal-bone tomography may indicate the osteomyelitis process or abscess formation at the petrous apex. If surgery is possible, it should be done immediately, before septic involvement of the temporal portion of the carotid artery or contamination of the subarachnoid space has occurred.

BRAIN ABSCESS AND MENINGITIS

Bone erosion from chronic infection or cholesteatoma may eventually produce dehiscences in the tegmen of the mastoid and middle ear. In addition, a dehiscence in this area may be an occasional variant of normal anatomy. The suppurative process in these instances is then free to extend to the dura and subarachnoid space. Infection may also spread from the central mastoid tract to the posterior fossa and cerebellum.

Intracranial complication occurs in less than 1% of cases of chronic otitis media. A subdural empyema or brain abscess is usually in direct continuity with the point of entry from the temporal bone. It is rare that the abscess will occur with intervening normal brain tissue between it and the diseased temporal bone. Symptoms suggesting the development of an intracranial abscess include headache, nausea, vomiting, drowsiness, and fever—none of which are seen in uncomplicated chronic otitis media. More advanced disease may result in seizures, neck rigidity, aphasia, papilledema, and coma. Cerebellar abscess may be accompanied by ataxia and nystagmus. The most common bacteria found in cerebral abscesses are *Staphylococcus aureus, Streptococcus pyogenes, Diplococcus pneumoniae, E. coli, Proteus,* and *Pseudomonas.* Mixed infections are not uncommon.

Computed tomography (CT) is currently the most valuable diagnostic maneuver to demonstrate an abscess. Lumbar puncture is done if there is no evidence of marked elevation of intracranial pressure. Management usually involves a high dose of antibiotics followed by drainage of the brain abscess either before or concurrently with mastoidectomy. The mortality rate, despite antibiotic treatment and surgical drainage approaches, is 20%.

PHLEBITIS AND THROMBOSIS OF THE LATERAL VENOUS SINUS

Sequestrated suppuration with or without cholesteatoma may progress posteriorly to involve the lateral venous sinus within the folds of the posterior fossa dura and cause phlebitis or septic thrombosis. The presence of high, spiking fevers, with chills, septicemia, sweating, and tachycardia in the presence of either acute or chronic ear infection, should raise the suspicion of lateral venous sinus thrombosis. The fever course has been described as similar to a picket fence, in that the patient's temperature may go up to 105°F and then drop to normal, presumably corresponding to showers of septic emboli and intervals between them.

Diagnosis

The clinical signs are most important in diagnosis. The white blood count is usually elevated. Lumbar puncture in the absence of otitic hydrocephalus is usually normal. The Tobey-Ayer test will be positive only if thrombosis has already occurred. With extensive thrombosis, otitic hydrocephalus and papilledema may occur. Roentgenograms are not specific; a CT scan demonstrates ipsilateral cerebral edema.

(*Text continues on p. 68*)

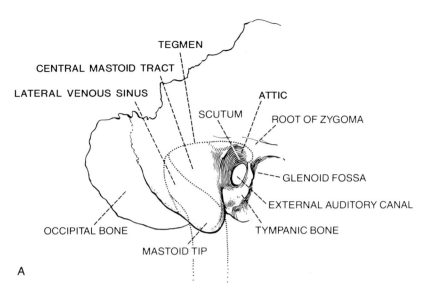

A

Fig. 3-1. (*A*) Surface anatomy of the lateral aspect of the temporal bone. The approximate locations of pertinent internal structures are also indicated. (*B*) The dotted line indicates the area of bone removal for an antrotomy, used to investigate the possibility of a cholesteatoma or granulations in the mastoid antrum. This procedure is done following an exploratory examination of the middle ear if disease is found that could extend into the mastoid antrum. (*C*) The dotted line indicates the area of bone removed to open the attic and antrum (atticoantrotomy), used to remove a cholesteatoma or granulations limited to these areas. Once the disease and affected ossicles are removed, the ear is reconstructed according to one of the methods illustrated in Figure 3-2. (*D*) The dotted line indicates the area of bone removal for a simple mastoidectomy, used to explore the mastoid in such cases as antibiotic-resistant mastoiditis. The middle ear and hearing are usually unaffected by this surgery. (*E*) The dotted line indicates bone removal for a "canal-wall-up mastoidectomy," used to remove chronic disease from the mastoid and middle ear space. The posterior wall of the external auditory canal is preserved. (*F*) The dotted line indicates bone removal for a "canal-wall-down," or standard radical mastoidectomy. This procedure includes removal of the posterior wall of the external auditory canal to gain wider exposure and to exteriorize the mastoid into the external canal.

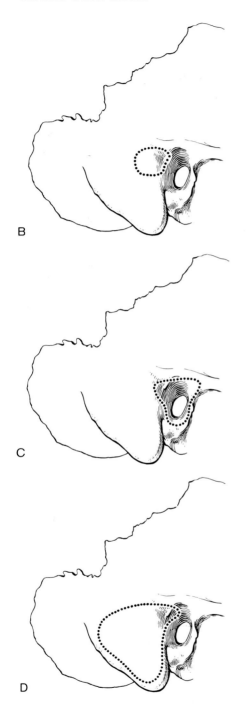

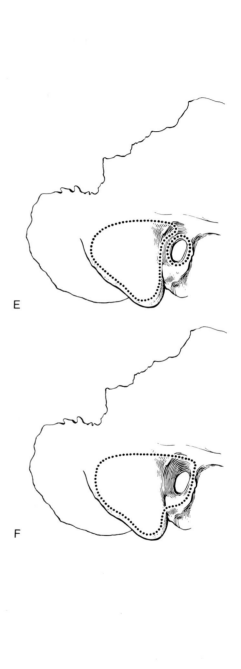

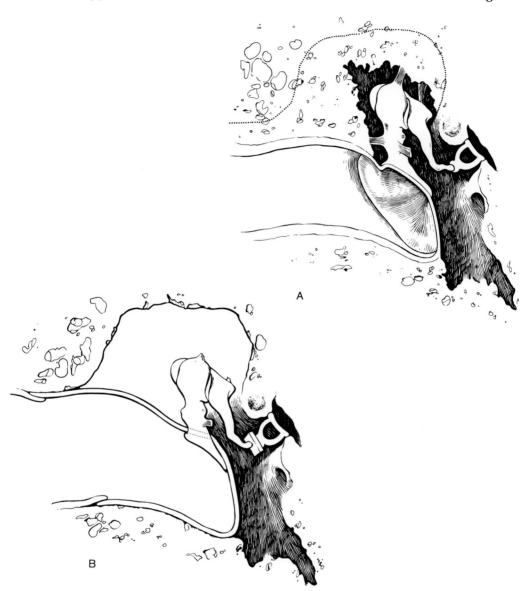

Fig. 3-2. (*A*) The dotted line indicates the area of bone removal in atticotomy or mastoidectomy. (*B*) Type II tympanoplasty. The mastoid air cell system has been removed, a fascial graft replaces the drum, and a bone chip reestablishes continuity between the incus and stapes. (*C*) Type III tympanoplasty. A fascial graft has been laid down on the capitulum of the stapes. (*D*) Type IV tympanoplasty. The drum has been replaced by fascia temporalis, and a split-thickness skin graft has been placed on the footplate. No other ossicles remain. (*E*) Type Va tympanoplasty. No ossicles, including the stapes footplate, remain. The temporalis fascial graft is laid over a fat graft placed on the oval window.

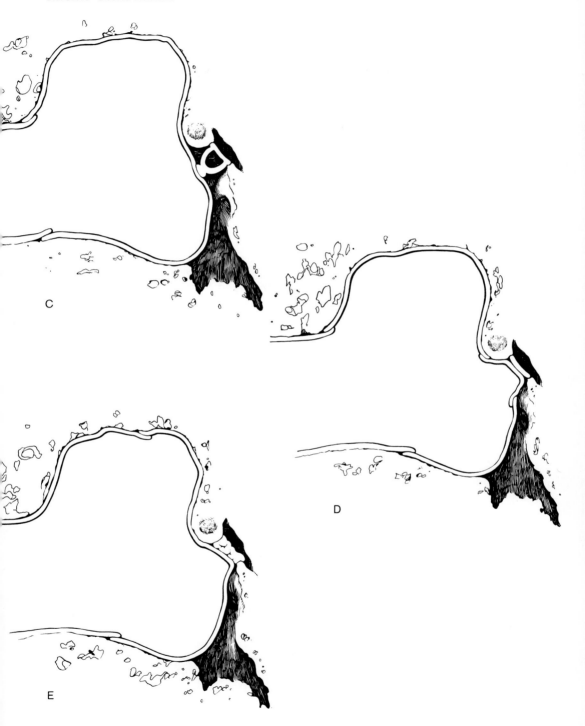

C

D

E

Treatment

Broad-spectrum antibiotics are used intravenously until the specific organism is identified, based on blood cultures, ear-canal drainage, or
purulence obtained at mastoid surgery. With adequate blood levels of
antibiotics, the mastoid should be explored on an emergent basis. Necrotic bone and purulence are removed, and if indicated the dura and
lateral venous sinus are explored with a needle. If thrombosis has occurred, removal of the septic thrombus is performed. If the internal
jugular vein has been thrombosed, this is explored as well.

SURGERY OF THE INFECTED EAR

Several surgical procedures are employed depending on the findings.
A *simple mastoidectomy* implies removal of the pneumatized air cells of
the central mastoid tract without entering the middle-ear space. This is
done most often for acute mastoiditis that does not respond rapidly to
parenteral antibiotics or when the bony cells of the mastoid are seen by
radiography to have broken down.

For chronic otitis media, various forms of *tympanomastoidectomy* are
currently used (Fig. 3-1). The goals of mastoid surgery in order of importance should be (1) the elimination of disease and the establishment
of a safe ear; (2) the rearrangement of anatomy to discourage recurrent
disease; and (3) the reconstruction of the ear to allow useful hearing if
possible. Preservation or removal of the posterior canal wall that sepa-
rates the ear canal from the mastoid determines whether the procedure
will be a "canal-wall-up" or "canal-wall-down" mastoidectomy. In the
presence of cholesteatoma, most surgeons at this time prefer canal-wall-
down mastoidectomy to achieve better exposure. Once the air cells and
cholesteatoma that are present are removed, a graft is put in place to
protect the middle ear. The usual grafting material is fascia taken from
the lateral surface of the temporalis muscle.

Depending upon which ossicles remain, various forms of tympanoplasty are possible. For example, type I tympanoplasty implies preservation of all ossicles. When combined with a canal-wall-down
mastoidectomy, this would be called a Bondy-modified mastoidectomy.
The forms of tympanoplasty most often combined with mastoidectomy
are types III, IV, and V (Fig. 3-2). The type III tympanoplasty, combined
with canal-wall-down mastoidectomy, implies placement of a graft directly on the stapes capitulum. Type IV implies that the graft has been

placed on the stapes footplate. Type V tympanoplasty implies that the footplate has been removed and replaced with fat underlying the fascial graft.

RISKS OF SURGERY

The usual risks that should be explained to the patient include an anesthesia of 1 to 4 hours, risks to auditory and vestibular function, and the risks to the facial nerve. These are all relatively low in incidence. In essence, surgery involves the same types of risks inherent in an unsafe ear left unoperated, but the incidence of these complications is much lower with surgery.

EXPECTATIONS OF SURGERY

The vast majority of chronic draining ears should be rendered dry, and all should be rendered safe. This implies the altering of anatomy or the exteriorization of pathology to the point that complications are no longer likely. With modern techniques, the patient with mastoidectomy usually can swim and shower without protection, and hearing results are often in the 30-db range if there is reasonable eustachian-tube function. The hospital stay is usually 4 days. Postoperative care involves removal of sutures, outer mastoid dressing, and packing after 1 week, removal of inner packing after 2 weeks, and follow-up cleaning and perhaps delayed skin grafting in the next 4 to 6 weeks. Thereafter in an asymptomatic ear all that is required is semi-annual cleaning of the ear canal and mastoid bowl to prevent accumulation of wax and keratin debris.

4

THE DIZZY PATIENT

William R. Wilson

Evaluation of vertigo
  History
  Examination
    Ear canal and tympanic membrane
    Spontaneous nystagmus
    Positional tests
    Caloric test
    Electronystagmography
Treatment of vertigo
  Mild to moderate (V1-V2) vestibular attacks
  Marked vertigo (V3) associated with nausea and vomiting
  Chronic positional imbalance and mild to moderate vertigo (V1-V2)
Vertiginous disorders involving the inner ear and vestibular nerve
  Meniere's disease
    Treatment
      Surgery
      Streptomycin and gentamicin therapy
  Acute viral labyrinthitis
    Epidemic vertigo
    Ramsay Hunt syndrome
    Inner-ear membrane rupture
Vertiginous disorders involving the inner ear and vestibular nerve—no hearing loss

Cupulolithiasis
Viral vestibular neuritis
Vertiginous disorders involving the inner ear and vestibular nerve as part of a larger syndrome
Vestibular toxicity
Acoustic neurinoma
Dysequilibrium as a result of aging
Multiple sclerosis
Syphilis: Congenital and tertiary
Rare disorders
  Waldenström's macroglobulinemia
  Relapsing polychondritis
  Cogan's syndrome
Vertigo resulting from neck injury
Vertigo of brain-stem origin
  Vascular disease
  Transient basilar-artery ischemia
  Wallenberg's syndrome
  Anterior inferior cerebellar-artery syndrome
  Subclavian steal syndrome
  Neoplastic disorders

EVALUATION OF VERTIGO

HISTORY

The history is a very important part of the evaluation of dizziness, and it must be taken in a manner that is succinct and useful to the physician. To the layman, dizziness is a general term that encompasses not only vertigo but also the various forms of lightheadedness, and at times syncope as well. The physician, therefore, must establish that the patient does indeed have vertigo. The patient should have the sensation that the world is spinning (eyes open) or that he is spinning (eyes closed). A sense of imbalance, such that the floor is moving like a rocking deck, is also a form of vertigo. Vestibular disturbances are associated with a visceral response of pallor and, at times, nausea and vomiting. Occasionally a patient will become frightened and may hyperventilate as well, sometimes to the point of tingling and muscular cramping. Hyperventilation serves to enhance vestibular symptoms. Patients with vestibular disorders do not suffer a loss of consciousness, nor do they experience an aura such as that associated with epilepsy or migraine.

Other forms of dizziness may be due to postural hypotension, hypoglycemia, medications, and neurological and cardiac disorders, and should be separated by the history and physical examination and the appropriate laboratory work. During the history, it is helpful to establish the date of the first attack, the date of the last attack, and the frequency with which attacks occur within the following intervals: daily, weekly, or monthly. Next, the patient should describe the first attack. The history should obtain pertinent information, such as (1) the patient's activity at onset, (2) the intensity of the vertigo, (3) the duration of the attack, (4) the presence or absence of associated symptoms or hearing loss, and (5) the presence of other physical symptoms.

An assessment of the patient's activity at onset is important because *positional vertigo* may not be recognized as such by the patient. Complaints may include vertigo that occurs only during head movements, for instance, when washing dishes, hanging clothes, or rolling over in bed. Positional vertigo is most commonly associated with cupulolithiasis, postconcussion syndrome, whiplash injury, and, rarely, posterior-fossa tumors.

The intensity of vertigo can best be measured in terms to which the patient easily relates. Mild vertigo (V1) can be defined as an attack of spinning or imbalance that is not sufficiently severe to cause the patient to discontinue what he is doing. Moderate vertigo (V2) requires the patient to stop his current activities and sit quietly until it clears, usually in less than half an hour. Severe vertigo (V3) is characterized by a marked, spinning sensation with nausea and vomiting that requires the patient to take to bed.

Vestibular falling attacks, or the drop attacks of Tumarkin, come without warning and last a few seconds. They represent an unusual form of vestibular symptomatology and are distinguished from a faint or seizure by the fact that there is no loss of consciousness and by the onset of vertigo as soon as the patient is on the ground.

Patients suffering from vertigo may be incapacitated for varying periods of time. Attacks of vertigo can last for a few seconds or for several days. They may recur daily or, more commonly, at irregular intervals. The frequency of the subsequent attacks should be noted, and the intensity of the first should be compared to the intensity of the last. This information provides a guide for the physician as to the progress of the disorder.

Hearing changes are the most frequent symptom associated with vertigo. Even when there is no hearing loss present, patients may be able to determine the involved ear because of the sensation of pressure or discomfort. In other patients, hearing loss may have been present unilaterally or bilaterally for many years prior to the first episode of

---

Evaluation of Vertigo

History
Age: Sex: Weight:
Description of Vertigo: Hyperventilation?:
Review of Symptoms:
     Alcohol, cigarettes, caffeine, others:
     Other illnesses:
     Medications used regularly:
     Symptoms other than vertigo or hearing loss:
Detailed Description of First Attack: Date:
     Type of vertigo: imbalance, mild (V1), moderate (V2), severe (V3):
     Duration:
     Associated ear symptoms and hearing loss:
     Other symptoms:
     Treatment:
Subsequent Attacks: Date of last attack:
     Frequency of attacks:
     Usual type of vertigo:
     Ear symptoms and hearing loss:
     Treatments tried and effects:
     Estimated degree of disability:

vertigo. Hearing loss is often associated with tinnitus and a blocked sensation of the ear. Not uncommonly, vertigo is associated with sudden hearing loss.

Vertigo associated with fluctuating hearing suggests increased pressure of the endolymphatic fluid of the inner ear (cochlear hydrops). For example, the hearing in one ear may decrease for several days and then return, only to decrease again, and so on. These fluctuations most often occur in the low frequencies that are important for the understanding of speech. In addition, patients complain of noise recruitment, a characteristic finding if hearing losses are due to cochlear injury. In this condition, loud noises are perceived in the affected ear as being irritatingly loud. Cochlear hydrops is associated with Meniere's disease and chronic syphilitic otitis.

Most vestibular disorders are short-lived and amount to a minor medical problem. However, occasionally they result in a significant alteration of lifestyle or, in unusual cases, total disability. Treatment, medical or surgical, should be carefully selected to be appropriate for the symptoms.

EXAMINATION

EAR CANAL AND TYMPANIC MEMBRANE

In almost every vestibular disorder, the tympanic membrane is normal. The exceptions are vertigo associated with a painful vesicular eruption involving the pinna, canal, or drum, suggestive of herpes zoster oticus, or vertigo associated with tympanic-membrane perforation, with or without drainage.

The fistula test should be used on all patients with vertigo. In patients with chronic ear disease, a positive test is a suggestion of a fistulous tract between the middle ear and inner ear. When a positive fistula test is present in patients with an intact tympanic membrane, it suggests the presence of adhesions in the inner ear, most commonly secondary to chronic luetic otitis.

One method of performing the fistula test is to face the patient and ask him to look directly ahead. Press the tragus firmly into the ear canal to create a positive pressure, and release. If the patient feels a sense of turning with this maneuver, it is a positive test. There may be a few beats of nystagmus, best seen if the patient is wearing magnifying (Frenzel's) glasses. An alternate method of performing the fistula test is presented in Chapter 1.

Vestibular nystagmus is known as "jerk nystagmus" because there is a slow deviation of the eye in the horizontal plane and then a very rapid, or jerklike, recovery. When rapid, this nystagmus appears to be beating in the direction of the fast phase (jerk). For instance, if it were to the right, the nystagmus would be named right-beating horizontal nystagmus. However, it is the slow phase of nystagmus that is controlled by the vestibular system; the fast phase, called a saccade, is a recovery movement of the eye controlled by the central nervous system. A disorder producing jerk nystagmus may be located at any point in the vestibular system: the end-organ, nuclei, or central vestibular tracts.

A second, less common form of vestibular nystagmus is rotatory nystagmus. In this form the eye moves in the horizontal plane and rotates relative to the vertical axis as well. This form is usually induced by positional testing.

On the other hand, jerk nystagmus in a vertical plane is indicative of a central vestibular dysfunction and requires thorough neurological evaluation. Other varieties of nystagmus, such as pendular nystagmus, congenital nystagmus, and searching nystagmus, are associated with the neuro-ocular system.

SPONTANEOUS NYSTAGMUS

Most often, vestibular nystagmus will be suppressed by visual fixation when the eyes are open. There are several maneuvers used to elicit it.

Jerk nystagmus, characteristic of vestibular dysfunction, will be enhanced when the eyes are turned in the direction of the fast phase. In other words, if the rapid phase of the nystagmus is beating to the right, the nystagmus will be strongest, and in some cases only present, when the eyes are turned right. First-degree nystagmus is present only with the eyes turned in the direction of the nystagmus; second-degree nystagmus is present in midgaze as well; third-degree nystagmus is present in all fields of gaze.

The patient is asked to watch the examiner's finger at a distance of 2 to 3 feet. The finger is moved a short distance to the right or left in order to avoid end-position nystagmus, which is normally present near the limits of gaze. *Frenzel's glasses,* goggles with +20 diopter lenses and small lights within, are useful for vestibular-system diagnostics. In a darkened room, the patient is unable to see out, but the examiner has an excellent view of the patient's eyes and nystagmus (see Appendix).

Nystagmus that is not present in the light will often be noticeable in the absolute dark during examination of the fundus with an ophthalmoscope. This is an excellent way of determining the presence of spontaneous nystagmus that otherwise would be suppressed by visual fixation. During examination of the retina, the direction of the fast phase will be opposite that noted by direct observation of the eyes.

POSITIONAL TESTS

Vertigo and nystagmus can often be elicited by placing patients through positional changes. In the first positional test the patient is asked to sit on the examining table with his eyes open, preferably wearing Frenzel's glasses, and facing the examiner. The head is turned as far as it will go to the right and left. If this stimulus elicits vertigo or nystagmus, a proprioceptive muscular disorder of the neck—as might be seen after whiplash injury—is suspected. Also, transitory vascular compromise can be induced when pathology of the carotid or vertebral arteries is present.

The *Hallpike maneuvers* are illustrated in Figure 4-1. The patient sits on the examining table so that when lying supine his head will extend over the table edge. The examiner should support the patient's head between his hands and observe the eyes for nystagmus throughout. If

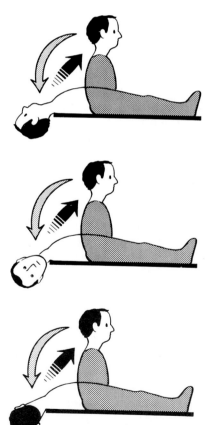

Fig. 4-1. The positional testing (Hallpike) maneuvers. The patient is seated so that his head will hang over the end of the examining table. Whichever maneuver—to the right or to the left—is indicated by the history to cause symptoms should be used first. The patient's head is held in the examiner's hands, brought quickly into position, and held for approximately 10 seconds before being returned to the upright position. The patient must be instructed to look straight ahead at all times and to keep his eyes open.

the patient has a history of vertigo when lying on one side, the examiner should begin by bringing the patient's head back to that side. Each head-hanging position should be held for about 10 seconds before the patient begins to sit upright again. Right, left, and straight head-hanging positions should all be tested. The type, direction, and duration of the nystagmus should be noted.

There are several responses that the examiner might expect from this test. *Direction-fixed positional nystagmus* is directed to one side only throughout all the position changes. It often fatigues after a few moments and most often represents a vestibular end-organ disorder. *Direction-changing positional nystagmus* takes several forms. The first type consists of a rotatory nystagmus that begins after a 1 to 2 second delay upon assuming the head-hanging position and is directed towards the lowermost ear. Upon sitting upright, the rotary nystagmus reverses direction for a few seconds and ceases. Subjectively, the patient has a frightening sense of whirling vertigo and is certain that he will roll off the table. These findings are pathognomonic of benign paroxysmal vertigo. This condition is the result of loose otoconia that are free to tumble about in the inner ear (cupulolithiasis).

The second type of direction-changing nystagmus is jerk nystagmus that changes direction with different head-hanging positions. For example, with the right ear down, left-beating nystagmus may be visible. This nystagmus changes to right beating in the head-hanging and left head-hanging positions. Direction-changing nystagmus of this type is seen with unilateral or bilateral vestibular end-organ disorders, but it occasionally may indicate central vestibular dysfunction.

A third form of direction-changing nystagmus is jerk nystagmus that changes direction randomly during a single positioning. For example, the patient might have left-beating nystagmus, then right-beating, followed by left-beating nystagmus over a 30-second period, all while maintaining the right head-hanging position. This nystagmus may be coarse and irregular and is not associated with vestibular symptoms. This type of response is most suggestive of a central vestibular disorder involving the brain stem.

CALORIC TEST

The horizontal semicircular canal can be stimulated by placing warm or cool water against the tympanic membrane. With the patient's head in the supine position, so that there is a vertical axis between the lateral canthus and external auditory canal, the horizontal semicircular canal is placed in a vertical plane. The temperature changes following irrigation of the external canal result in convection currents in the fluids of the horizontal semicircular canal that stimulate the end-organ. After

(Text continues on p. 80)

Office Examination for Vertigo

General
BP: sitting   standing
Pulse:
Respiration:
Heart: Lungs:
Otolaryngology Exam
  Tuning-Fork and Voice Testing
    AD:
    AS:
          256 Hz   *512 Hz*
    Rinne AD:
    Rinne AS:
    Weber Test: R   Midline   L
    Fistula Test: AD: AS:
  Neck Exam (for masses, bruits):
Vestibular-System Testing
1. Ask the patient to perform any maneuver that in his experience elicits vertigo.
2. Head shaking: With the patient's eyes closed, move his head briskly from side to side for 1 second.
3. Ask the patient to walk and turn 180 degrees rapidly, making repeated turns.
4. Head turning maneuver: Turn the patient's head to the far right and left, and extend it upwards for 20 seconds in each position.
5. *Hallpike positional tests* (in the light, with the patient's eyes open)
   upright (U): Straight down: U: AD down: U: AS down:
6. *Minimal Caloric test:*
  Water temperature and amount:
  Response: (duration, speed, amplitude)

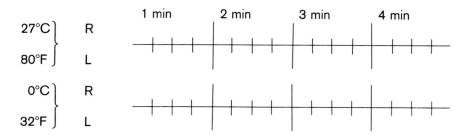

7. Hyperventilate (up to 3 minutes)
8. Neurological and funduscopic examination

    I:

    II:

    III, IV, VI: EOMs, pupil

    VII:

    IX, X:

    XI:

    XII:

    Cerebellar tests: Romberg:

                        Rapid movements:

                        Past pointing:

  Gait:

  Muscle strength:

  Tendon reflexes:

Audiological Studies

    Pure-tone audiometry with air- and bone-conduction levels. This involves speech discrimination scores and tests for recruitment (ABLB, alternate binaural loudness balance test or SISI, short increment stimulus intensity) and tone decay.

    Brain-stem evoked-response audiometry:

    Electronystagmography (ENG):

Blood Tests

CBC, VDRL or FTA-ABS, glucose and 5-hr GTT, and thyroid-function studies

X-ray Studies

Transorbital view of internal auditory meati, cervical-spine films, skull series, CT scan

EEG

ECG

Summary of impressions:

the use of cold water, the nystagmus beats towards the opposite ear, after warm water towards the same ear. This fact can be remembered as "COWS": cold, opposite; warm, same.

The office caloric test is a rough measure of vestibular function, but even so it is very useful. The most important parameter is the speed of the slow phase, which is hard to judge. Normally, both ears have a similar response. If there is a large difference in amplitude or duration of nystagmus between the two ears, the less responsive one is the affected ear.

The technique for office caloric testing requires Frenzel's glasses, a stop watch, and a syringe. Make certain that the tympanic membrane is intact and the canal is clear of wax. Using 5 ml of tap water at room temperature, irrigate the patient's ear over a 10- to 20-second period. The nystagmus should be observed for direction of the fast phase, amplitude, and duration. Another technique is to use a tuberculin syringe with a 1½-inch 20-gauge needle filled with 0.4 ml of iced water. After positioning, the iced water is injected through the speculum of an otoscope against the tympanic membrane. This method elicits approximately the same vestibular response as the first. If there is no response to the above tests in one or both ears, the exam is repeated using 5 ml of iced water, the maximum stimulus employed.

ELECTRONYSTAGMOGRAPHY

Electronystagmography (ENG) is vital to a thorough evaluation of vertigo. The test is used to separate nystagmus of central origin from that of peripheral origin, as well as to determine in cases of peripheral dysfunction which ear is impaired. It provides a permanent record of the signs of vestibular dysfunction.

An ENG is performed in a specially equipped laboratory and requires approximately 1 hour. The equipment permits recording with the patient's eyes closed, thereby eliminating unwanted visual suppression of the diagnostic eye movements. Electrodes are placed about the patient's eyes to record eye movements by the measurement of changes in the corneal-retinal potentials. Then the examiner establishes the presence or absence of horizontal or vertical spontaneous nystagmus and any deficiencies in eye-tracking ability. Next, attempts are made to induce nystagmus by means of head shaking, hyperventilation, and positional testing. Last, the Hallpike caloric tests are used. Warm and cool water, 7°C above and below body temperature, in a prescribed amount and flow rate (approximately 250 ml over a 30- to 40-second period), is used to irrigate the external canals. The recorded response (nystagmogram) is used to measure the vestibular function of each ear. In the event there is no response, the test is repeated with 5 ml of iced water.

Measurement of the slow phase of the nystagmus permits an accurate assessment of lateral semicircular canal function.

TREATMENT OF VERTIGO

The treatment of vertigo requires a blend of art and science. The symptoms are frightening and troublesome to patients, though they are usually representative of a benign disorder involving the inner ear. This fact should be used to reassure patients.

One of the most useful devices for treating vertigo is a daily record sheet of symptoms and treatment (Fig. 4-2). The form serves several purposes. For one, the patient is reassured of the continuous concern of the physician even though he may be seen at infrequent intervals, such as every 3 to 4 months. Also, when presented at the next office visit, the daily record establishes at a glance the clinical course of the disorder and the use or misuse of prescribed medications and exercises. And, finally, this method incorporates the patient as a partner in his medical care.

MILD TO MODERATE (V1 TO V2) VESTIBULAR ATTACKS

There are many medications suggested for the treatment of vertigo. Those that are effective are capable of suppressing mild to moderate vestibular activity. The dosage should be titrated against symptoms, adjusted upward or downward as necessary to keep side-effects—usually sleepiness and mild incoordination—to a minimum. Two medications that are effective are meclizine and diazepam. Frequencies of administration are shown below.

A similar sliding scale can be used for proprietary drugs, such as Dramamine and Bonine. Some physicians use promethazine HCl (Phenergan) 6.25 mg to 12.5 mg in a similar manner.

Mecilzine 12.5 mg (Antivert) or Diazepam 2 mg (Valium)

Beginning dosage	b.i.d.
If no response in 24 hours	t.i.d.
If no response in 24 hours	q.i.d.

When vertigo is controlled, reduce the number of pills by one every 5 days.

DAILY PATIENT RECORD
VERTIGO AND HEARING LOSS
MARK SYMPTOMS WITH AN X

NAME _____

UNIT # _____

PATIENT # _____

DAY NUMBER	DATE	NO SYMPTOMS	PRESSURE IN EAR	INCREASED EAR NOISE	HEARING CHANGE ⇄	IMBALANCE C CONTINUOUS I INTERMITTENT	VERTIGO* MILD (V1)	VERTIGO* MODERATE (V2)	VERTIGO* SEVERE (V3)	DROP ATTACK	TIME OF VERTIGO C CONTINUOUS OTHERWISE: HR, MIN, SEC	ACTIVITY AT ONSET	MEDICATION AND NUMBER OF PILLS	CAWTHORNE EXERCISE SCORE
1														
2														
3														
4														
5														
6														
7														
8														
9														
10														
11														
12														
13														
14														
15														
16														
17														
18														
19														
20														
21														
22														
23														
24														
25														
26														
27														
28														
29														
30														

*VERTIGO   MILD: PATIENT MAY CONTINUE ACTIVITIES
MODERATE: CLEARS AFTER PATIENT TAKES A SHORT REST
SEVERE: PATIENT MUST TAKE TO BED; HE EXPERIENCES NAUSEA AND SOMETIMES VOMITING

Fig. 4-2. Sample of daily record sheet of symptoms and treatment. The form is quite simple and takes only a few seconds to complete each day. If the patient is symptom-free, "no symptoms" is checked, and nothing further is marked for that day. An "x" is placed in the appropriate space if the patient experiences pressure or noise in the ear. Hearing changes and the sensation of imbalance are similarly indicated. Mild (V1), moderate (V2), and severe (V3) vertigo are noted when present, as well as any drop attacks. The duration of the vertigo, any activity that may have precipitated it, and the medications and exercises used for treatment are all recorded.

MARKED VERTIGO (V3) ASSOCIATED WITH NAUSEA AND VOMITING

For treatment of marked vertigo (V3) associated with nausea and vomiting, Tigan is administered 200 mg IM or suppository q. 8 hr PM along with IV fluids if necessary. An alternative to Tigan is Compazine, 10 mg IM or suppository.

CHRONIC POSITIONAL IMBALANCE AND MILD TO MODERATE VERTIGO (V1 TO V2)

The vestibular response in the injured system as well as in the intact system can be suppressed by repeated stimulation. This vestibular function, called *habituation,* is the mechanism that permits a figure skater to spin in a manner that a nonhabituated person could not tolerate. The tolerance of the injured system for motion can be improved by the Cawthorne-Cooksey exercise program:

Cawthorn-Cooksey Vestibular Exercise Program to Overcome Dizziness

    I. In order to derive the most benefit, exercises must be done diligently three times a day for at least 5 minutes.

    II. At each of these times, always start with number 1 in the schedule and proceed to the point at which the exercises cause discomfort from dizziness.

    III. As soon as dizziness occurs, stop and wait for the next exercise period.

    IV. All exercises are started in exaggerated slow time, then progress gradually to more rapid time. The rate of progression—from bed, to sitting, to standing—varies from patient to patient.

    V. A period of 2 months is needed to give the program a fair chance.

Exercises

    A. In bed, supine (only if you cannot sit up); otherwise in sitting position without arm rest.

        1. Head immobile, eye movements (at first slow, then quick)

            a. Up and down

            b. Side to side

            c. Repeat *a* and *b*, focusing on finger.

            d. Focus on finger moving back and forth from about 3 feet to 2 inches away from face.

2. Head mobile, head movements (at first slow, then quick).
   Later with eyes closed.
   a. Bend forward and backward.
   b. Turn from side to side.

B. Sitting position, *without arm rests.*
   Repeat as in 1 and 2.
   3. Shrug shoulders and rotate upper body.
   4. Bend forward and pick up objects from the ground.
   5. Rotate head and shoulders slowly, then quickly.
      a. Rotate head with eyes open, then closed.
   6. Rotate head, shoulders, and trunk with eyes open, then
      closed.

C. Standing
   7. Repeat number 1.
   8. Repeat number 2.
   9. Repeat number 5.
   10. Change from a sitting to a standing position with eyes
       open, and then with them shut.
   11. Throw ball from hand to hand (at eye level).
   12. Throw ball from hand to hand (above eye level).
   13. Change from sitting to standing and turn around in be-
       tween.
   14. Repeat number 6.

D. Walking
   15. Walk across the room with eyes open, then closed.
   16. Walk up and down slope with eyes open, then closed.
   17. Do any games involving stooping or stretching and aim-
       ing, such as bowling and shuffleboard.
   18. Stand on one foot with eyes opened, then closed.
   19. Walk with one foot in front of the other with eyes opened,
       then closed.

VERTIGINOUS DISORDERS INVOLVING THE INNER EAR AND VESTIBULAR NERVE

MENIERE'S DISEASE

Meniere's disease might better be called a disorder of the peripheral
vestibular system. It is due to a failure of the endolymphatic resorptive
system to keep pace with fluid production, resulting in increased fluid
volume in the endolymphatic compartments of the inner ear (cochlear

hydrops). Whether this failure occurs spontaneously or is secondary to an injury, such as a previous viral cochleitis, is not certain. However, several facts are known. With a few exceptions, Meniere's disease is not inherited. Endolymphatic hydrops can be created in animals by surgical injury to the endolymphatic sac, the site of resorption. Also, the onset of increased inner-ear volume may require many years. Chronic inflammatory conditions, such as long-standing luetic otitis, will produce cochlear hydrops as an end stage.

The term Meniere's disease should not be used interchangeably with labyrinthitis. The disorder has a clear pattern of symptomatology. As described in 1848 by Prosper Meniere, it consists of vertiginous spells associated with hearing loss, tinnitus, nausea, and vomiting. The spells of vertigo or hearing loss may precede one another by a matter of years, but they generally present simultaneously. The condition is unusual in children; the incidence climbs until the third and fourth decades, then declines. In 80% to 90% of the patients, Meniere's disease remains unilateral, but the opposite ear may become affected even many years after the first.

The episodes of spinning vertigo associated with Meniere's disease begin abruptly with little or no warning, reaching maximum intensity—often accompanied by nausea and vomiting—within a few moments. The marked vertigo usually lasts several hours, but occasionally may persist for 12 to 24 hours. Residual imbalance can continue for several days more. The recurrence rate of attacks is highly variable and sporadic. They may occur weekly, monthly, occasionally, after many years, or not at all. It is unusual for a patient with Meniere's disease to find it necessary to permanently alter his life-style or to become partially or fully disabled.

In practice, the hearing loss associated with Meniere's disease often begins with a sensation of pressure in one ear associated with some tinnitus. The tinnitus may represent the first symptom of hearing loss perceived by the patient. In early Meniere's disease, hearing loss occurs in the lower frequencies, which are important in the perception of speech. There are two features that characterize it further. First, the hearing loss will fluctuate, such that the hearing will be depressed for a few days and then improve, usually with a concomitant reduction in tinnitus. The fluctuation may be a single occurrence; however, some cases continue to fluctuate over many years, resulting in a gradually progressive sensorineural hearing loss. Second, patients note that the affected ear has an increased sensitivity to loud sounds, and they often find them disturbing. This phenomenon—known as recruitment—is characteristic of cochlear, rather than neural, auditory dysfunction. To test for recruitment in the office, strike a 512-Hz tuning fork softly, and have the patient listen to it alternately with the right and the left ear and determine in which ear it is louder. Then strike the fork sharply and ask the patient to compare his ability to perceive this loud sound with each ear. If the hearing loss in the affected ear is not too great, the loud sound will be perceived as equal between the ears or as greater in the ear with diminished hearing.

Lermoyez's syndrome is a variant of Meniere's disease in which the hearing loss improves subsequent to the episodes of vertigo, nausea, and vomiting.

In the office examination of patients with Meniere's disease, the middle ears are normal. There is usually no positional nystagmus. Examination of the eyes, particularly with Frenzel's glasses or in the dark with an ophthalmoscope, will often reveal direction-fixed horizontal nystagmus, most often directed away from the involved ear. Head shaking or hyperventilation can help elicit nystagmus. The whisper and tuning-fork tests will usually elicit a hearing loss and recruitment. A minimal cool caloric test will often demonstrate a unilateral reduced response. The neurological evaluation will be negative except for a disturbance of balance and gait that should be appropriate for the degree of vestibular upset.

Further laboratory studies should include an audiogram consisting of pure tones, discrimination scores, and tests for recruitment (ABLB, or SISI) and auditory-nerve function (tone decay). Also, electronystagmography should be done following the attack to determine the extent of injury to vestibular function and to assess residual spontaneous nystagmus. A fluorescent treponemal antibody-absorption (FTA-ABS) test is necessary to eliminate the possibility of congenital syphilis or latent tertiary syphilis (luetic otitis).

TREATMENT

The medical treatment of vertigo and imbalance associated with Meniere's disease is no different from the regimen described above for vestibular upset. Because something is known of the pathophysiology of this disorder, a variety of theoretical but unproven treatments abound. Most should be avoided because they are ineffective and potentially harmful. These include low-salt diets, all types of vasodilators, and all types of diuretics. The Cawthorne-Cooksey exercises may be of benefit in stabilized Meniere's disease with residual imbalance or slight vertigo.

Surgery

Surgical treatments for Meniere's disease abound as well, a testimony to their relative ineffectiveness and general lack of acceptance. They are listed below so that the referring physician will be familiar with the recommended procedures and the relative merits or drawbacks. Surgery or further medical therapy must be considered only when the patient is truly incapacitated by vertigo. Because of the highly unpredictable frequency of attacks and propensity for long, spontaneous remissions, the assessment of any treatment for Meniere's disease is difficult. This is doubly true for surgical therapy that is not easily controlled.

In the *Fick operation*, a needle is passed through the footplate to create a fistula between the endolymphatic and perilymphatic spaces. There are frequent relapses and a high risk to hearing. Not recommended.

The *tack operation* is a procedure similar to a Fick operation that implants a tack permanently through the footplate. This operation has only limited success and a high hearing risk. It is not recommended.

The *sac operation* uses a simple mastoidectomy to expose the endolymphatic sac and drain it into the subarachnoid space or mastoid. Whether drainage occurs has not been established. One series of twelve patients suggests an 83% success rate without hearing loss in the speech frequencies. The experience nationwide is not this good. This operation is recommended with reservations.

Vestibular nerve section is an intracranial procedure that is occasionally performed for unremitting unilateral vestibular upset. Except in very unusual situations, the risks to the seventh and cochlear nerves, as well as those of any intracranial procedure, seem unwarranted.

Ultrasound ablation of vestibular end-organs requires a simple mastoidectomy and application of the ultrasound probe against the horizontal semicircular canal. The success rate is approximately 70%. There are some problems with sensorineural hearing loss and occasional temporary facial paralysis.

Labyrinthectomy is a transtympanic destructive procedure that has a very high success rate for the control of vertigo. Because this procedure results in a total loss of hearing, it should be reserved for patients with no usable hearing in the affected ear and unilateral involvement. Postoperative imbalance persists for several weeks.

Labyrinthotomy (endocochlear shunt) is an experimental procedure similar to the Fick operation, except that the fistulization of the endolymphatic and perilymphatic spaces is performed through the round-window membrane. No conclusions about its effectiveness can as yet be drawn.

Streptomycin and Gentamicin Therapy

Use of streptomycin and gentamicin for the treatment of Meniere's disease takes advantage of the fact that the vestibular portions of the inner ear are more sensitive than the cochlea to ototoxic effects.

Transtympanic injection of gentamicin is associated with a relatively high recurrence rate of vertigo. About 25% of patients incur further sensorineural hearing loss.

Intramuscular streptomycin ablation is reserved for patients with bilateral progressive Meniere's disease with marked hearing loss and vertigo. It requires the administration of ototoxic levels of streptomycin for 2 to 4 weeks until there is no further vestibular response to an iced water caloric. Vestibular function and hearing are carefully monitored in a hospital setting. Ataxia persists for 2 or more months. Hearing is stabilized. This procedure is recommended for patients younger than 55 years of age.

ACUTE VIRAL LABYRINTHITIS

EPIDEMIC VERTIGO

Occasionally, an increased incidence of labyrinthitis involving all age groups will be seen in a community. Hearing loss may or may not be associated. When hearing loss is associated, these cases are categorized as sudden hearing loss with vertigo, rather than as epidemic vertigo. Nonetheless, it is likely the pathogenesis is the same, except that the expression of the disorder is altered by the viral infections according to the relative degree of involvement of the cochlea or vestibular end-organ.

This disorder is characterized by a single, marked vestibular upset. Nystagmus is usually present. Vertigo, nausea, and vomiting resolve in a few days, but imbalance may persist for several weeks. The tympanic membrane and middle ear are normal. The caloric response is usually reduced or absent in the affected ear. Hearing loss may be temporary or permanent.

Routine therapy for vertigo is employed. Sudden sensorineural hearing loss, if seen within 10 days of onset, should be treated by corticosteroid therapy (see Chap. 5).

RAMSAY HUNT SYNDROME

Ramsay Hunt syndrome is characterized by deep ear pain and a vesicular eruption of the ear canal and auricle. Frequently, there is an associated facial paralysis, hearing loss, and vertigo, all of which may be mild or severe. The disorder is due to a regional herpes zoster polyneuritis.

The symptoms are unmistakable. Recovery is dependent upon the magnitude of the original injury. There is evidence that improvement in facial function and hearing is enhanced by corticosteroid therapy.

INNER-EAR MEMBRANE RUPTURE

Membrane ruptures involving the round window and the annular ligament about the stapes are known to occur during abrupt changes in atmospheric pressure or cerebrospinal fluid (CSF) pressure. A typical history might involve a scuba diver who noted a "pop" in his ear followed by tinnitus and dysequilibrium during an ascent or descent. Or a weightlifter might notice similar symptoms from increased CSF pressure. The hearing loss, if not complete initially, will usually progress over the next few hours and may fluctuate, improving in the morning but worsening during the day. Dysequilibrium is present, and positional vertigo often can be elicited with the injured ear down. It is theorized that purely intracochlear ruptures of Reissner's membrane can occur as well.

Examination will demonstrate an abnormal ear or the effects of barotrauma upon the tympanic membrane. These effects might involve pain and a small hemorrhage within the tympanic membrane. Audiology demonstrates a cochlear type of sensorineural loss. Spontaneous nystagmus and positional vertigo may be present, especially with the involved ear down.

The patient should be put at bed rest with the head elevated 30 to 45 degrees, keeping the affected ear uppermost. When cases with a very clear history of abrupt pressure change show no improvement after a day or so of conservative management, arrangement for surgical exploration of the middle ear and repair of the leak is suggested.

VERTIGINOUS DISORDERS INVOLVING THE INNER EAR AND VESTIBULAR NERVE— NO HEARING LOSS

CUPULOLITHIASIS

Benign paroxysmal vertigo (cupulolithiasis) is a relatively uncommon, but very distinctive form of vertigo that should be known to all primary-care physicians (Fig. 4-3). It results when some otoconia from the utricular or saccular end-organs are loosened and tumble about in the endolymphatic space of one ear. When the affected ear is positioned towards the floor, the otoconia fall against the ampulla of the posterior canal, inciting the symptoms. This disorder occurs spontaneously, especially in the elderly—though it may affect any age group, particularly after head trauma.

ERECT POSITION

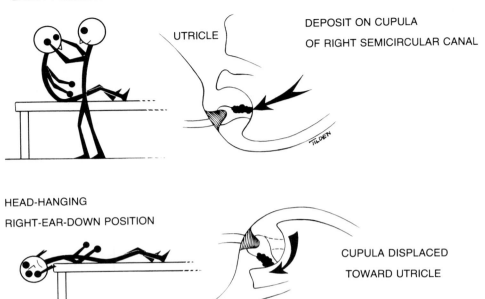

Fig. 4-3. Benign positional vertigo is the result of otoliths caught on the cupula of the ipsilateral posterior (cupulolithiasis). The canal is stimulated in the head-hanging position with the affected ear downward. When the test is positive, the patient will experience a frightening sensation of falling, associated with the onset of rotatory and horizontal nystagmus towards the undermost ear, that clears within a minute. On assuming the erect position, the rotatory nystagmus reverses direction for a few seconds.

The typical complaint is that of marked spinning a few seconds after lying down on one side. The spinning clears in a few moments or is improved by changing to another position. There is no associated hearing loss.

Examination will demonstrate normal ears. Hallpike positional tests should be done, preferably with Frenzel's glasses. The patient should be reassured that he will not be allowed to fall and reminded that he must keep his eyes open and look straight ahead. His head should be in the examiner's hands and should be placed briskly to the head-hanging position on the symptomatic side. In the characteristic response there is a several-second delay before the onset of the sensation of spinning vertigo and the fear of falling. At that time, the examiner will note the horizontal or rotatory nystagmus directed toward the undermost ear. The vertigo and nystagmus will crescendo in a few seconds and then gradually disappear within 30 seconds. Upon briskly resuming the upright position, the nystagmus reappears but is reversed, becoming horizontal rotatory in the opposite direction. Repeated attempts at provoking the vertigo will demonstrate fatiguing of the vestibular response.

Benign paroxysmal positional vertigo (BPPV) will usually resolve spontaneously in a matter of weeks or months. Because it can be controlled simply by avoiding the position that elicits it, no medication is required. In those patients who remain handicapped by unresolved BPPV, the branch of the vestibular nerve that runs to the posterior ampulla (singular nerve) can be sectioned by a middle-ear approach. The procedure, which has a high success rate, requires a few days hospitalization and the use of a general anesthetic for 1 to 2 hours. Complications might include some high-frequency hearing loss. Because this procedure is performed relatively infrequently, in most instances it would probably be done only by surgeons with a large volume of ear surgery.

VIRAL VESTIBULAR NEURITIS

Viral vestibular neuritis is a form of viral vestibular injury that involves the vestibular nerve exclusively. It is characterized by the abrupt onset of vertigo with nausea and vomiting that gradually diminishes over a several-day period, followed by a several-week period of improving imbalance. The ear appears normal, and the hearing remains unaffected. The ENG, however, will show a reduced caloric response in the involved ear, as well as spontaneous nystagmus that usually beats away from the involved ear. This disorder is self-limited and, like viral labyrinthitis, may occur as an outbreak in a community. It usually causes a single episode of vertigo. However, a chronic form exists that recurs over a period of years. Routine treatment for vertigo is employed.

VERTIGINOUS DISORDERS INVOLVING THE INNER EAR AND VESTIBULAR NERVE AS PART OF A LARGER SYNDROME

VESTIBULAR TOXICITY

Most ototoxic drugs affect primarily the cochlea. There are, however, substances and drugs that affect primarily the vestibular labyrinth. Among the common ones in daily use are caffeine, nicotine, alcohol, quinine, and certain tranquilizers and sleep preparations. Tranquilizers, barbiturates, and alcohol affect the vestibular system centrally as well. Their overuse may result in a sense of chronic imbalance or, if they have been used to an extreme, in vestibular ataxia.

Of the commonly used antibiotics, the aminoglycosides must be carefully monitored for ototoxicity. Streptomycin and gentamicin are primarily vestibulotoxic; tobramycin, kanamycin, and amikacin are more cochleotoxic. It is important to obtain an audiogram prior to beginning treatment with any of these antibiotics. Serum drug levels are useful guides to proper dosage. The earliest and best indication of ototoxicity for streptomycin and gentamicin is the onset of imbalance. At this point the dosage should be sharply reduced, or the medication should be discontinued. The vestibular effect is characterized by the onset of imbalance, not vertigo, because both end-organs are suppressed simultaneously. The other aminoglycosides are monitored by audiograms and serum drug levels.

Ototoxic effects are predisposed by renal failure, the combined use of ototoxic medications, advanced age, previous inner-ear disease, and high fever.

Certain diuretics, primarily ethacrynic acid and furosemide, are well-known ototoxic drugs that primarily affect the cochlea.

ACOUSTIC NEURINOMA

Acoustic neurinoma arises from the Schwann's sheath, most commonly of the superior vestibular nerve; it is often found in the internal auditory canal extending into the posterior fossa. The tumor will cause a progressive compression of the nerves and is therefore associated with the gradual onset of tinnitus and sensorineural hearing loss, as well as with intermittent unsteadiness or positional vertigo. Abrupt attacks of vertigo are only rarely seen. Any patient with unilateral progressive sensorineural hearing loss must be evaluated for acoustic neurinoma. The evaluation includes an electronystagmogram, x-ray films of the internal acoustic meatus, brain-stem evoked-response audiometry, and computed tomography (CT scan) with contrast. If the diagnosis still cannot be made with certainty, a posterior-fossa myelogram is done. Multiple acoustic neurinomas are sometimes seen in patients with von Recklinghausen's disease.

DYSEQUILIBRIUM AS A RESULT OF AGING

Dysequilibrium through aging results from a gradual deterioration of the vestibular system and is the vestibular equivalent of presbycusis.

Some patients in the seventh and eighth decades of life develop an instability when walking that causes them to walk with short shuffling steps and to be afraid of falling. These symptoms are very troublesome even to patients who are otherwise alert and vigorous. There is no treatment. Medications for vertigo are of no benefit and in fact may worsen the disorder by reducing mental alertness. Patients are benefited most by good light and a stabilizer, such as a cane or handrail.

MULTIPLE SCLEROSIS

Vertigo and nystagmus occur in over one third of the cases of multiple sclerosis. Hearing losses are not nearly so common; they are usually unilateral and may be of a sudden, profound nature. They may recover spontaneously. Vertigo is most probably due to areas of demyelinization located in the middle cerebellar peduncle of the flocculo-nodular lobe. The diagnosis is based on the finding of multiple, focal neurological deficits or injuries. The age of onset is generally in the third and fourth decades.

SYPHILIS: CONGENITAL AND TERTIARY

Ophthalmologic and auditory manifestations of congenital lues usually become evident in the third and fourth decades of adult life. Patients develop interstitial keratitis, and the otologic symptoms include a progressive sensorineural hearing loss that is usually bilateral but progresses at different rates in either ear. The hearing loss may be slowly progressive or may occur suddenly in one ear.

All patients with congenital syphilis develop symptoms of either spinning vertigo or imbalance at some point in the course of the disease and will develop a marked reduction in the function of the vestibular end-organs on caloric testing. The treatment consists of benzathine penicillin G, 1.2 million units IM weekly, for approximately 12 weeks. In addition, patients are placed on alternate-day prednisone therapy, approximately 40 mg, for 1 month. The rationale for this therapy is that after the *Treponema pallidum* has been sequestered in the ophthalmic or cochlear tissues for a long period of time, replication occurs only very slowly—approximately once every 90 days. Because penicillin is effective only at the time of bacterial cell division, it is necessary to keep adequate concentrations of the antibiotic available in the ophthalmic and cochlear tissues for that entire period of time. Cortisone is used to reduce the inevitable inflammatory response that accompanies the presence of *T. pallidum* in the cochlear tissues. The use of these medications will improve hearing significantly in approximately 15% of patients. In over half the patients it will have a beneficial effect upon the vestibular symptoms.

The otologic effects of tertiary syphilis are similar to those of congenital syphilis. The disorder is often confused with Meniere's disease because there may also be fluctuating hearing and episodes of sudden hearing loss associated with vertigo or marked imbalance. Patients being evaluated for hearing loss and imbalance should always have an FTA-ABS drawn in order to rule out either congenital or late tertiary syphilis.

RARE DISORDERS

WALDENSTRÖM'S MACROGLOBULINEMIA

Waldenström's macroglobulinemia is a rare cause of vertigo that is due to hyperviscosity of the serum secondary to an excess of monoclonal IgM. Treatment of hyperviscosity by plasmapheresis will correct the condition and control the vertigo and hearing loss.

RELAPSING POLYCHONDRITIS

Relapsing polychondritis is due to an inflammatory necrosis of the cartilaginous tissues of the body, most probably the result of anticartilage autoantibodies. Vertigo and hearing loss probably result from an inflammatory reaction involving the endochondral bone of the inner ear. They are sometimes improved by treatment with corticosteroids.

COGAN'S SYNDROME

Cogan's syndrome affects young adults—both sexes equally. Its clinical presentation mimics congenital syphilis. Progressive sensorineural hearing loss, vestibular upset, and interstitial keratitis are found, but serological tests for syphilis, including the FTA-ABS test, are negative. Despite treatment with high doses of steroids, hearing loss may become severe, and the vestibular function may progress to complete loss of response.

VERTIGO RESULTING FROM NECK INJURY

Patients who have suffered a severe neck injury, such as a whiplash, often complain of a sensation of vertigo when holding their head in certain positions. This is a verifiable complaint that can be documented by the presence of nystagmus on the ENG tracing when certain head positions are assumed by these patients. It is theorized that this dysfunction is due to an interruption of the proprioceptive nerve fibers to the injured muscles of the neck. These symptoms may require up to 6 months or more to resolve. Patients who have suffered a severe head injury frequently have a sense of imbalance for many months. This is due to small tears and areas of hemorrhage within the structure of the inner ear or to loose otoconia.

VERTIGO OF BRAIN-STEM ORIGIN

VASCULAR DISEASE

Vascular disease involving the blood supply to the inner ear usually arises in the anterior inferior cerebellar artery, which branches off from the inferiormost part of the basilar artery. The auditory artery branches off from the midportion of the anterior inferior cerebellar artery as it loops near the internal auditory meatus. This auditory artery supplies blood to the nerves to the internal auditory canal and then divides into the anterior vestibular artery and the common cochlear artery. The anterior vestibular artery supplies a major portion of the vestibular endorgan; the posterior vestibular artery supplies the remainder.

TRANSIENT BASILAR-ARTERY ISCHEMIA

Transient basilar-artery ischemia can result in a sudden loss of balance without loss of consciousness as a result of reduced blood supply to the vestibular nuclei in the brain stem.

WALLENBERG'S SYNDROME

Wallenberg's syndrome is characterized by a sudden onset of marked vertigo, usually accompanied by nausea and vomiting, hoarseness, aspiration and cough, and further voice changes secondary to hypernasal speech from palatal dysfunction. The patient may complain of double vision. On examination, there is ipsilateral analgesia of the face, ptosis and myosis of the ipsilateral eye, and ipsilateral paresis or paralysis of the palate, pharynx, and larynx. On the body trunk, there is a contralateral loss of pain and temperature sensation. These symptoms are related to either partial or complete occlusion of the vertebral artery or its largest branch: the posterior inferior cerebellar artery.

ANTERIOR INFERIOR CEREBELLAR-ARTERY SYNDROME

Anterior inferior cerebellar-artery syndrome presents with sudden onset of vertigo, hearing loss, facial paralysis, and cerebellar and sensory signs (see Chap. 2).

SUBCLAVIAN STEAL SYNDROME

Subclavian steal syndrome results in intermittent brain-stem ischemia, secondary to an occlusion of either the right or left subclavian artery proximal to the takeoff of the vertebral artery. Symptoms of vertigo are associated with exercise of the arm located on the side of the occlusion. The ischemia results from the shunting of the blood to the distal sub-clavian artery on the occluded side through the junction of the two vertebral arteries at the basilar artery. The treatment is surgical correction of the subclavian occlusion in markedly symptomatic patients.

NEOPLASTIC DISORDERS

Vertigo is a relatively common symptom associated with tumors of the brain stem. The most common types are astrocytoma, medulloblastoma, acoustic neurinoma, and occasionally meningioma and chordoma. Metastatic carcinomas involving the brain stem are most commonly those of the lung, the breast, or the bowel.

5

EAR EMERGENCIES

Joseph B. Nadol, Jr.

Auricle
  Hematoma
  Lacerations
  Perichondritis and chondritis
External auditory canal
  Foreign body
  Trauma
Tympanic membrane and middle
        ear
  Trauma
  Damage to the ossicular chain
        with or without peri-
        lymph leak

Barotrauma
Inner-ear trauma and temporal-
        bone fracture
Acoustic trauma
Rupture of the round window or
        oval window
Basilar skull fracture
Traumatic cerebrospinal fluid
        otorrhea
Sudden idiopathic hearing loss

The discussion of trauma and other emergencies is best approached from an anatomical orientation rather than from a symptom-oriented view. Because the inner ear is not easily examined, the challenge to the primary-care physician is to determine the extent of anatomical involvement in an injury. This is important, for example, in a case in which the danger from a traumatic rupture of the tympanic membrane may be greatly overshadowed by that from undetected ossicular fracture and perilymph leak. Primary infections of the external canal, middle ear, and mastoid are discussed in Chapter 3.

AURICLE

HEMATOMA

Hematomas of the auricle are usually the result of direct trauma. Once a hematoma has developed, the collection of blood elevates the perichondrium from the underlying auricular cartilage. This compromises the blood supply to the cartilage and if left undrained may result in a cauliflower ear owing to dissolution of part of the cartilaginous support of the auricle.

TREATMENT

The hematoma is evacuated using a large-bore needle and sterile precautions. A pressure dressing is required to prevent reaccumulation (Fig. 5-1). A conforming dressing is applied first, using cotton strips impregnated with benzoin, normal saline, or antibiotic ointment to fill in the interstices of the auricular cavities. A mastoid dressing is then applied using cotton, 4 × 4 surgical gauzes, and cling or preferably noneleastic rolled gauze. The ear should be reexamined and the dressing changed daily. If reaccumulation of the hematoma occurs, it may be reaspirated. If the hematoma has already organized so that needle aspiration is impossible, or if the hematoma accumulates repeatedly, incision of the overlying skin and evacuation of the hematoma cavity may be necessary. Although antibiotics are not strictly necessary, many practitioners prefer to use prophylaxis against *Staphylococcus aureus*. Some otologists believe that the use of a short, tapered course of corticosteroids will help prevent reaccumulation of a hematoma after aspiration.

LACERATIONS

In the case of a laceration of the auricle, standard surgical techniques for good wound repair are practiced. Macerated or clearly devitalized tissue is debrided. However, large segments of the auricle with little or no obvious vasculature may be reapproximated with hope for at least partial survival of the segment. Macerated cartilage and cartilage without good skin coverage should be debrided. The use of tetanus toxoid prophylaxis and antibiotics follows the usual surgical indications.

PERICHONDRITIS AND CHONDRITIS

ETIOLOGY

Infection of the perichondrium or auricular cartilage may occur secondary to infection of a hematoma and following surgical procedures and minor abrasions or burns of the auricular skin.

DIAGNOSIS

Local erythema and tenderness suggest the diagnosis. The edema often thickens and distorts the normal configuration of the auricle, giving it a doughy appearance. The usual organisms involved are *Pseudomonas aeruginosa* and *S. aureus*. Perichondritis and chondritis must be distinguished from relapsing polychondritis, a disease thought to be autoimmune in etiology and which results in recurrent episodes of pain, erythema, and inflammatory response in cartilaginous structures, including the nose and auricle. On the first occurrence of relapsing polychondritis, differentiating between it and suppurative perichondritis may be difficult, and the diagnosis may be based largely on the response to steroids—which usually produce a sudden and dramatic response in relapsing polychondritis. Biopsy of auricular cartilage may also be helpful in making this differentiation in difficult cases.

TREATMENT

The treatment of auricular perichondritis or chondritis requires the administration of parenteral antibiotics based on the results of a gram stain and culture. If no pus is available, antibiotic coverage for *Pseudomonas* and *Staphylococcus* is selected. Parenteral treatment is continued until all signs and symptoms have resolved, usually for 2 to 3 weeks. If little progress is made, or if obvious abscess formation occurs, drain-

(Text continues on p. 102)

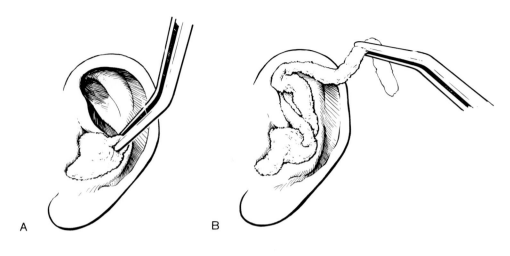

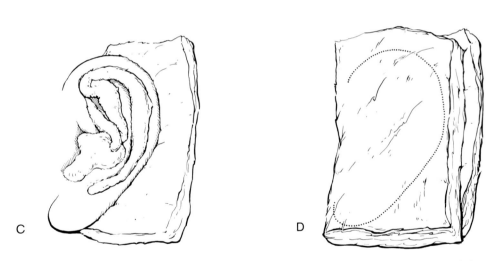

Fig. 5-1. (*A* and *B*) Cotton moistened in saline is placed in the concha and interstices of the auricular folds to prevent reaccumulation of the hematoma. This step is not necessary for the routine mastoid dressing, which begins with step *C*. (*C* and *D*) Sterile cotton cuts are placed behind the ear and over it to provide a comfortable bed of cotton. (*E*) Three or four 4 × 4 surgical gauzes are fluffed and placed over the cotton. A strip of 2-inch roller gauze is placed vertically over the temple, just lateral to the eye. (*F*) Roller gauze is wrapped around the head from the base of the occiput to the forehead. The dressing should not cover the opposite ear. (*G*) The dressing is tightened and moved away from the eye by tying the vertical strip.

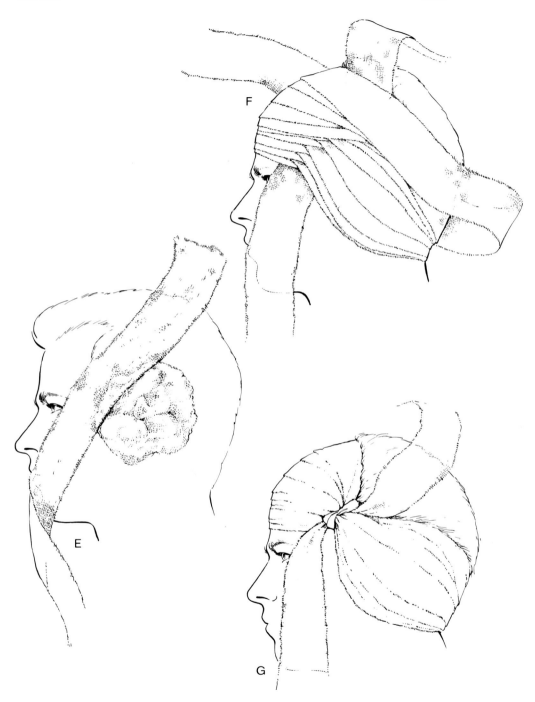

age, debridement of devitalized cartilage, and the insertion of drains may be necessary.

EXTERNAL AUDITORY CANAL

FOREIGN BODY

ETIOLOGY

The usual clinical situation for an ear emergency that results from the presence of a foreign body involves the accidental insertion of a small object or plaything into the external canal of a child. Foreign body emergencies also result from an insect gaining access to a patient's external auditory canal while the patient is asleep or unconscious.

DIAGNOSIS AND TREATMENT

The most important aspect of managing an emergency resulting from the presence of a foreign body is determining the extent of the injury. This is particularly true of injuries from penetrating objects such as pencils or paper clips. To determine the extent of injury, the following two questions must be addressed: Has there been damage to the tympanic membrane and the ossicular chain? Is there any evidence of inner-ear damage that might be caused by puncture of the round window, disruption of the stapediovestibular joint, or fracture of the promontory? Also, a sensorineural hearing loss, as determined by tuning-fork and whisper tests or by the presence of nystagmus, subjective unsteadiness, or vertigo, suggests inner-ear damage and may require emergency surgical intervention. During the initial evaluation the function of the facial nerve should also be assessed.

The second most important tenet of treatment is to avoid producing further damage in abortive attempts to remove a foreign body. Removal of a foreign body requires a cooperative patient. In an adult this may require the use of a local anesthetic; in a child a general anesthetic may be necessary. Proper otologic equipment and microscopic control are essential. Living insects may be drowned in otic drops or mineral oil before removal with alligator or Hartmann's forceps. Irrigation is generally avoided, especially with organic foreign bodies that may absorb water and expand. It is avoided, furthermore, because the extent of the damage to the tympanic membrane may not be easily assessed until the foreign body is removed; if a perforation is present, irrigation may produce otitis media or labyrinthitis. Round foreign bodies may be removed with a right-angle hook by passing it beyond the foreign body, or they may be removed with the Schuknecht foreign-body aspirator. Once the foreign body is removed, careful assessment is made of the tympanic membrane. Perforations are then treated as discussed in the section Tympanic Membrane and Middle Ear.

TRAUMA

Abrasions commonly occur in the external canal during attempts by either a patient or a physician to clean it because the skin of the bony external canal adheres tightly to the periosteum. Perfuse bleeding may occur, which prevents proper evaluation of the tympanic membrane.

TREATMENT

Good light, preferably under microscopic control, and suction with a No.-5 ear suction are used to determine the site of bleeding. The bleeding may be controlled by the application of silver nitrate to the external canal or by the use of an ear wick moistened with a few drops of epinephrine (1:1000). Once the bleeding is controlled, the prophylactic use of otic antibiotic drops is usually recommended for 5 to 7 days.

Lacerations of the external canal may result from longitudinal basilar skull fractures that pass through the squamous and tympanic portions of the temporal bone. These fractures also often cause the leak of cerebrospinal fluid (CSF). After an initial evaluation using a sterile suction tip, no immediate treatment is required other than occluding the ear with sterile cotton. Antibiotic drops or frequent manipulation are contraindicated to avoid contamination of the CSF. The use of prophylactic antibiotics to treat traumatic CSF leaks is controversial; if used, they should be administered in doses appropriate for meningitis.

TYMPANIC MEMBRANE AND MIDDLE EAR

TRAUMA

Direct trauma to the tympanic membrane may occur during attempts to clean the ear with a cotton-tipped applicator or bobby pin, or it may result from debris, such as slag from welding, falling into the external canal. Indirect trauma, such as a slap to the auricle, may also result in perforation of the drum.

DIAGNOSIS

Again, one of the most important aspects in evaluating a traumatic perforation of the eardrum is to determine the extent of injury and, in particular, whether there has been any injury to the ossicular chain or inner ear. Once the blood and debris have been removed by aspiration, the perforation is examined. Posterosuperior traumatic perforations are the most likely to result in damage to the ossicular chain. The presence of a sensorineural hearing loss, nystagmus, and significant vestibular symptoms suggests the possibility of a perilymph leak, and the case should be referred to an otologist for an emergent evaluation.

TREATMENT

Most uncomplicated perforations of the tympanic membrane will heal spontaneously. Some authors feel that large segments of infolded tympanic membrane should be returned to their normal anatomical position and should be held in place using cigarette paper impregnated in antibiotic ointment on the lateral surface of the drum. This may be done under a local anesthetic. If the perforation occurs in a contaminated situation, such as during swimming, or if it is caused by a grossly contaminated foreign body, scrupulous cleaning of the canal and middle ear is performed, and antibiotics are often prescribed. With a clean perforation of the tympanic membrane, neither topical nor oral antibiotics are necessary. However, the patient must allow no water to enter the ear canal. On a short-term basis this can be accomplished by occluding the external meatus with commercial ear plugs or with cotton impregnated with petroleum jelly during showering or bathing. The tympanic membrane should then be reexamined by an otologist within 10 days, or sooner if drainage occurs after the first 2 days. Unlike most acute traumatic perforations, those produced by hot slag during welding accidents seldom heal and may be complicated by superinfection with profuse otorrhea. Treatment consists of removing the foreign body if it can be located and allowing resolution of the intense inflammatory response and infection, followed by delayed tympanoplasty.

DAMAGE TO THE OSSICULAR CHAIN
WITH OR WITHOUT PERILYMPH LEAK

In the presence of significant injury to the ear, the initial examination should include assessment for possible ossicular damage, rupture of the round-window membrane, or dislocation of the stapes footplate resulting in perilymphatic leak. The ossicles may be visible if there is a perforation; if the drum is intact, a large, unexplained conductive hearing loss suggests discontinuity or fracture of a portion of the ossicular chain. Fracture or dislocation of components of the ossicular chain does not usually require emergency treatment. However, ossicular injuries may be associated with the rupture of either the stapediovestibular joint or the round window, either of which constitutes an otologic emergency. The presence of vestibular signs and symptoms, including nystagmus, subjective vertigo, and positional vertigo, and the presence of a high-tone sensorineural hearing loss with reduced discrimination suggest injury to the inner ear secondary to perilymphatic leak. If there is measurable hearing, many otologists prefer to hospitalize these patients, put them at bedrest, and follow the progression of their injury by daily audiograms, since many leaks will heal spontaneously. If there is no hearing at the initial evaluation, or if hearing deteriorates under such observation, urgent surgery is required to precisely ascertain the damage and to repair the leak with a fat graft. Ossicular fractures uncomplicated by perilymph leaks are usually better handled in a delayed fashion once the acute inflammatory response has resolved.

BAROTRAUMA

ETIOLOGY AND TREATMENT

Sudden, uncompensated pressure changes may occur during rapid descent in an aircraft or during scuba diving and may result in pain in the ear, bloody effusions in the middle-ear space, rupture of the tympanic membrane, or, less commonly, damage to delicate inner-ear membranes or rupture of the round or oval windows.

A hemotympanum resulting from barotrauma requires little treatment. Some practitioners use decongestants to improve eustachian-tube function and to achieve more rapid resolution of the effusion. Paracentesis or aspiration of the effusion is seldom necessary. Again, as with the treatment for other injuries to the ear, the examiner should include in his initial assessment the consideration of possible inner-ear injury by noting auditory and vestibular signs and symptoms. An acute hemotympanum is quite painful and may require narcotic analgesics for a few days. A hemotympanum may take several weeks to resolve, and all patients should be reexamined in 2 to 3 weeks both to check for resolution of the hemotympanum and to evaluate any residual hearing loss.

Rupture of the tympanic membrane by barotrauma is treated in the same way as other traumatic injuries to the eardrum.

INNER-EAR TRAUMA AND
TEMPORAL-BONE FRACTURE

ACOUSTIC TRAUMA

Acoustic trauma may result from exposure to a sudden loud noise, from the cumulative effects of protracted exposure to loud noise, or from a concussive injury to the skull. The usual rule of thumb is that a noise loud enough to be painful is loud enough to do temporary or permanent injury to the inner ear. A sharp blow to the skull may produce enough mechanical energy to produce hearing loss. This is usually more severe in the ear on the side of the injury, but a bilateral hearing loss may occur in such cases.

DIAGNOSIS

Immediately following acoustic trauma the patient will complain of a plugged or full feeling in the ear and tinnitus. Except in extreme cases, tuning-fork and whisper tests are normal or near normal because the hearing loss is almost always above 3000 Hz. Thus, adequate evaluation of acoustic trauma requires behavioral audiometry with particular attention to the high frequencies. Acoustic trauma usually has two components, a temporary threshold shift (TTS) and a permanent threshold shift (PTS). The temporary threshold shift is that part of the sensorineural hearing loss that resolves within 3 to 7 days. The permanent threshold shift connotes the permanent decrement of threshold for the high frequencies (Fig. 5-2). A hearing loss that is present 3 weeks after acoustic trauma occurs may be considered permanent. Audiometry may be performed acutely, but this is not essential since no treatment is required. All patients, however, should be examined after 3 weeks to evaluate permanent injury.

RUPTURE OF THE ROUND WINDOW
OR OVAL WINDOW

Rupture of the round window or oval window may occur in conjunction with barotrauma, direct trauma to the temporal bone, or a penetrating injury to the external canal and tympanic membrane. For diagnosis and treatment see the discussion of injuries to the tympanic membrane and ossicles.

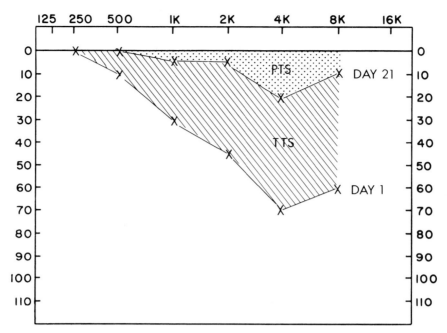

Fig. 5-2. Schematic illustration of temporary (*TTS*) and permanent (*PTS*) threshold shift following acoustic trauma of the left ear. An audiogram done immediately after exposure demonstrates a sensorineural loss of 70 db at 4 kHz. Part of this loss may be recovered over several days, leaving only a partial high-frequency sensorineural loss at day 21.

BASILAR SKULL FRACTURE

A blow to the head may produce a longitudinal, transverse, or mixed fracture of the temporal bone (Fig. 5-3). Primary longitudinal fractures occur most often, constituting approximately 75% of all fractures involving the temporal bone. Most of these fractures pass through the squamous portion into the tympanic portion of the temporal bone, resulting in fracture or fracture dislocation of the superior portion of the bony tympanic ring and perforation of the tympanic membrane. This will result in bleeding into the middle and external ear and perhaps CSF leak. Disruption of the ossicular chain may occur. Less commonly, the fracture may pass through the mastoid, bypassing the external canal and resulting only in bleeding into the mastoid and middle-ear space without rupture of the drum.

In transverse fractures, which constitute approximately 25% of fractures of the temporal bone, the fracture line passes transverse to the

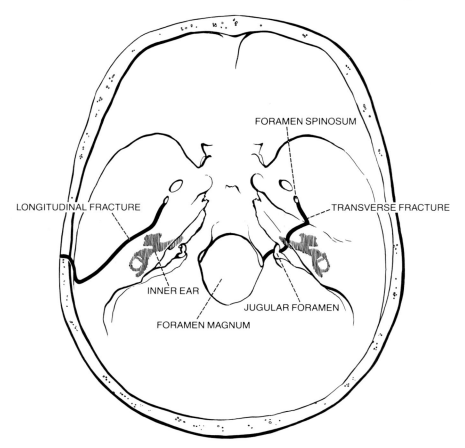

Fig. 5-3. Basilar skull fracture. On the left a longitudinal fracture passes along the axis of the petrous bone but does not enter the inner ear or internal auditory canal. On the right a transverse fracture, which usually begins at the foramen magnum, extends to the jugular foramen across the internal auditory canal or inner ear, passing anteriorly to the carotid canal and foramen spinosum area. Severe injury to the inner ear and facial nerve can be expected.

long axis of the petrous bone and hence across the internal auditory canal or inner ear. In this type of fracture, therefore, significant injury to auditory, vestibular, and facial nerves may occur. The tympanic membrane remains intact, and a hemotympanum is almost always present.

A mixed, or complex, fracture involves the presence of both transverse and longitudinal fractures. These often pass through the geniculate ganglion area and result in immediate or delayed facial paresis or paralysis.

DIAGNOSIS

A longitudinal fracture dislocation of the temporal bone is diagnosed when plain films of the skull and examination of the ear canal reveal a fracture step-off, laceration of the posterosuperior canal wall, rupture of the tympanic membrane, bloody otorrhea, or CSF otorrhea. However, in nondisplaced fractures or transverse fractures, radiographic assessment, including tomography, may fail to reveal a fracture line. Even if x-ray films do not reveal the fracture, the presence of a hemotympanum and a history of significant skull injury are sufficient to make a diagnosis of basilar skull fracture. The initial radiographic assessment may not reveal the fracture because of poor radiographic conditions, including time of day, cooperation of the patient, and other patient-care considerations. Such fractures may be more evident by tomographic evaluation at a later date, especially after some remineralization and early healing of a fracture site has occurred.

The evaluation of a patient with a suspected temporal-bone fracture should include consideration of (1) associated neurological status; (2) possible cervical-spine injuries; (3) the extent of injury to the tympanic membrane and ossicular chain; (4) evidence of inner ear injury, resulting either from perforation of the round-window membrane or dislocation of the stapes footplate, or from transection of the auditory nerve or fracture through the cochlea; (5) evidence of vestibular injury, such as subjective vertigo or nystagmus; and (6) status of the facial nerve. From an otologic perspective it is very important to know whether facial-nerve paralysis was immediate and complete or delayed and incomplete to accurately assess the need for further treatment, including exploration or decompression of the facial nerve. Many authors feel that immediate paralysis or even a delayed paralysis in which there is electrophysiologic evidence of rapid degeneration of the nerve requires surgical exploration. This is not a universally accepted opinion, and some otologists insist that there be clear-cut evidence that surgical exploration can be expected to help, such as a radiographic demonstration of a step-off in the fallopian canal or an injury from a bullet or other missile that can be expected to totally transect the facial nerve. Exploration of the facial-nerve canal, especially its intralabyrinthine portion, is a formidable surgical procedure and may require combined middle- or posterior-fossa and mastoid approaches.

An isolated injury to the round window or stapedial footplate may occur without fracture through the inner ear. Diagnosis of this injury is difficult or impossible to make without surgical exploration. The decision of whether to proceed with surgical exploration is based on the individual clinical situation. Delayed treatment of trauma to the temporal bone may include repair of perforations of the drum and fracture dislocations of the bony tympanic ring and reconstruction of the ossic-ular chain.

TRAUMATIC CEREBROSPINAL FLUID OTORRHEA

Fracture through the temporal bone involving the floor of the middle cranial fossa often results in profuse CSF otorrhea. The role of antibiotics in treating such cases is controversial. There is some evidence that antibiotics should be withheld until there is clear-cut evidence of infection, and the best evidence suggests that if antibiotics are used they should be given in doses appropriate for meningitis. In most cases, profuse CSF otorrhea due to a fracture will cease spontaneously within the first 10 days, but repair of a CSF leak is required if it is persistent. The surgical approach to repairing a persistent leak depends on the site of injury. Some leaks are best repaired by a neurosurgical approach; others are best repaired by an otologic approach.

SUDDEN IDIOPATHIC HEARING LOSS

The usual presenting clinical situation in sudden idiopathic hearing loss involves a patient who suddenly hears a pop in his ear or who states that his hearing has been turned off. A subjective sense of plugging and fullness also occurs. Less commonly, the hearing may be lost over several hours or days. The patient may or may not have vestibular symptoms.

DIAGNOSIS

The diagnosis of sudden idiopathic sensorineural hearing loss is arrived at by excluding other possible causes. Most other treatable causes of sudden hearing loss can be eliminated from consideration simply by history and physical examination. These include the obvious examples of acoustic trauma to the temporal bone, the presence of obvious middle-ear or mastoid infection, surgical trauma, or the administration of ototoxic drugs. Other less common causes of sudden sensorineural hearing loss may require laboratory assessment. These include, for example, primary or secondary syphilis, which may cause sudden loss of auditory and vestibular function, and tumors of the cerebellopontine angle, which may rarely cause sudden deterioration of hearing, perhaps by hemorrhage into the tumor and compromise of the vascular supply to the inner ear.

Initial evaluation of sudden hearing loss should include a thorough history to eliminate traumatic and toxic causes and medical disorders, including blood dyscrasias and malignancies. A serology should be done. Temporal-bone x-ray films may be useful to detect the presence of a vestibular schwannoma (acoustic neuroma) and to rule out a lytic lesion in the temporal bone. Some authors believe that certain metabolic conditions, such as arteriosclerotic cardiovascular disease, diabetes mellitus, thyroid disease, renal disease, or hyperlipidemia, may produce deterioration of hearing. However, because conclusive proof is wanting at this time, screening tests for these entities are of questionable importance in management. A history consistent with injury, including strain that may result from heavy lifting or from straining at stool, may suggest the possibility of a rupture of the round-window membrane. In such a case, an otologist should be consulted concerning the advisability of exploring the middle ear. Once other possible causes of sudden hearing loss have been excluded by history, examination, and a limited number of laboratory tests, a diagnosis of sudden idiopathic sensorineural hearing loss is made. The etiology of this disorder is unknown. A primary viral infection of the inner ear or a complex virus–host immune interaction may be the cause.

TREATMENT

The treatment of sudden idiopathic hearing loss is controversial. The literature abounds with various treatment protocols, including the use of anticoagulants, antihistamines, vasodilators, steroids, Hypaque, CO_2 rebreathing, and plasma expanders. There is little or no convincing evidence that any of these treatments are effective, with the exception of steroids. In a double-blinded study, Wilson has recently demonstrated that certain subcategories of sudden idiopathic sensorineural hearing loss need no treatment, that others will not benefit from any treatment, and that a third subgroup may be alleviated significantly by the administration of corticosteroids. Mild midfrequency or flat sensorineural hearing losses up to 30 db almost always recover spontaneously. Immediate profound losses rarely recover spontaneously and are not influenced by steroid therapy. The chance of recovery in idiopathic sudden hearing loss of moderate degree, 30 db to 90 db, is enhanced by corticosteroid therapy. For an adult the usual dosage is 80 mg of prednisone per day for 5 days, followed by a tapered course over the next 7 days.

SELECTED READING

WILSON WR, BYL FM, LAIRD N: The efficacy of steroids in the treatment of idiopathic sudden hearing loss. Arch Otolaryngol 106:772–776, 1980

6

A BRIEF REVIEW OF NASAL ANATOMY AND PHYSIOLOGY

William R. Wilson

Anatomy of the external nose
Anatomy of the internal nose and
paranasal sinuses
Anatomy of the upper respiratory
tract
The neural supply of the nose
The vasculature of the nose
The nasal examination
Differential diagnosis
Nasopharyngeal examination
Sinus examination
Radiographic examination of the
nose, nasopharynx, and
paranasal sinuses

The nasopharynx
Anatomy
Chronic nasal obstruction and
adenoidal hypertrophy
Carcinoma
Cysts
Chronic nasopharyngitis exclu-
sive of adenoiditis
Diagnosis of palatal dysfunction

The nose is a relatively complex organ that functions as a portal for air into the respiratory system and that serves to warm, humidify, and cleanse the air as it passes through. It also aids in the control of infection in the airway. It is the center of olfaction (the sense of smell and fine taste) and is vital in lower animal forms for the procurement of food and a mate.

ANATOMY OF THE EXTERNAL NOSE

In discussing the anatomy of the external nose (Fig. 6-1), the following terms are useful for the description of injuries and tumor sites: the *root* is where the nasal and frontal bones articulate, it is divided into the nasion and glabella; the *dorsum* is the ridge line from root to apex; the *apex* is the tip of the nose; the *base* is the triangular portion between the apex and the lip; the *anterior nares* are divided by the columella and bounded by the alae; the *columella* is the membranous portion of the nasal septum; the *bridge* is the bony structure of the nose, the frontal portion of the maxilla plus the nasal bones; the *alae* are the lateral rounded eminences at the base of the nose, formed by the lower lateral cartilages; the *nasal septum* is made up of the septal cartilage plus the vomer and the perpendicular plate of ethmoid.

ANATOMY OF THE INTERNAL NOSE
AND PARANASAL SINUSES

The lateral wall of the nose has three *turbinates,* or conchae; however, the third turbinate is very small, located high and posterior, and cannot be seen on examination. Turbinates have a thin, bony framework but are covered with highly vascular subcutaneous tissue that is composed of a dense arterial network and venous plexuses (lakes) similar to erectile tissue. This covering is particularly evident on the inferior turbinate. The turbinates can swell by means of vascular engorgement to occlude the nose.

Beneath each turbinate lies a meatus. The *inferior meatus* receives drainage from the nasolacrimal duct only, at a point about one third of the way back from the anterior margin. The *middle meatus* receives drainage from the nasofrontal duct and anterior ethmoid cells anteriorly, from the middle ethmoid cells and maxillary sinus ostium medially, and from

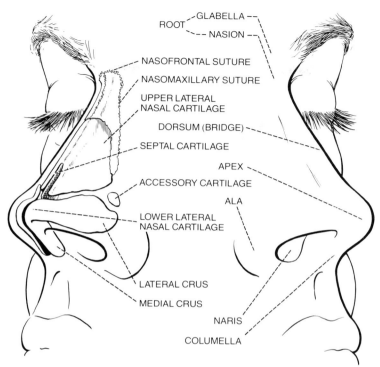

GLABELLA
ROOT
NASION
NASOFRONTAL SUTURE
NASOMAXILLARY SUTURE
UPPER LATERAL
NASAL CARTILAGE
DORSUM (BRIDGE)
SEPTAL CARTILAGE
APEX
ACCESSORY CARTILAGE
ALA
LOWER LATERAL
NASAL CARTILAGE
LATERAL CRUS
MEDIAL CRUS
NARIS
COLUMELLA

Fig. 6-1. The structures of the external nose.

the posterior ethmoid cells posteriorly. Mucopurulent material can often be seen draining from these regions during acute sinus infections, thereby identifying the site of the infection.

The *sphenoethmoidal recess* is a long, narrow space located between the upper portion of the middle turbinate and the nasal septum. The cribriform plate forms the roof of this area, and the posterior limit is the anterior face of the sphenoid sinus. The sphenoid ostium empties into this region. More importantly, the olfactory epithelium is located here.

The *nasal septum* is formed by cartilage anteriorly and by bone posteriorly. It may grow irregularly or may be traumatized so that it obstructs breathing on one or both sides of the nose. If the deviation is severe enough, it will inhibit proper drainage or will obstruct sinus ostia by putting pressure on the turbinates.

The function of the paranasal sinuses is unknown. The *ethmoid sinuses* are a complex of 10 to 25 small sinuses that form a roughly rectangular shape front to back. The posterior length is 4 cm to 5 cm, the height is 2.5 cm to 3 cm, and the width bilaterally between the eyes is 1 cm to 1.5 cm. Some of these sinuses are present at birth, and they are often involved in nasal infections and allergic diseases in children. As the head enlarges, the ethmoid sinuses increase in size and complexity.

The *maxillary sinuses,* sometimes present at birth, remain small until the development of permanent teeth. At that time the maxillary sinuses gradually enlarge to their full size. The small ostium (2 mm to 3 mm in diameter) is located high on the medial wall of the sinus under the middle turbinate, and for these anatomical reasons, this sinus drains very poorly once it is infected. The bony canal encasing the infraorbital nerve travels through the roof and the roots of the second premolar, and first and second molars often project into the sinus floor. Localized pain and pain in the distribution of the infraorbital nerve are common symptoms of maxillary-sinus infections due to neural irritation.

The *sphenoid sinuses* begin to develop by the sixth year. They are highly variable in size and ramifications. The ostium is located high on the anterior wall, and, therefore, as with the maxillary sinuses, there is no dependent drainage from this sinus.

The *frontal sinuses* are the last to develop and continue to enlarge during the teen years. Not uncommonly, the frontal sinuses may be absent or, in the other extreme, may be very large with multiple ramifications. No particular size or configuration of the frontal sinuses portends frontal-sinus disease.

The nasal and sinus mucous membrane is pseudostratified columnar epithelium. Like the skin, the mucosa has nociceptors: free, naked nerve endings that respond to chemicals and to changes in temperature, humidity, and pressure. These receptors serve to alert and protect the lower airway following exposure to extremes of temperature or to pollutants. They stimulate nasal vasodilation, mucous production, and bronchial constriction.

ANATOMY OF THE UPPER RESPIRATORY TRACT

The *upper respiratory tract* is an irregular, double-tubed structure, but even in normal circumstances it is not static. Eighty percent of individuals have a cycle of congestion and decongestion involving first one side of the nose, then the other, known as the nasal cycle. In the normal nose, one nasal passage opens up, accompanied by secretion by the serous and mucous glands, while the opposite side closes down with increasing obstruction and decreasing secretion. There is a shift of autonomic balance, occurring every $\frac{1}{2}$ to 4 hours. However, the combined or total airway resistance is unchanged. This cycle becomes evident to most people when they try to sleep. Inspiratory air currents fan out superiorly, while expiratory currents swirl in the nose. The nasal cycle ensures that air "sheets" are formed in the nose and that at some point these sheets are no more than 1 mm in thickness; it therefore becomes more likely that inspired foreign particles can be trapped by the nasal mucous coat. Patients with cause for a reduced airway secondary to a deviated septum, or with a chronically engorged mucous membrane from perennial allergy, will complain that their nose is never completely open and that the airway shifts from side to side. In other words, they become aware of the nasal cycle because of their abnormally limited nasal space, while patients with normal nasal patency do not.

The blocked nose creates *hyponasal* (denasal) speech, recognizable by the substitution of other sounds for the normal nasal consonants of m, n, and ng. Smaller changes in resonance are noted with minor nasal swelling, as with a mild cold. Experienced rhinoplasty surgeons know the resonance is changed most by narrowing of the alar region, not the dorsum.

The nose will efficiently warm cold air, no matter what the temperature of the air. Warming the air permits humidification up to 95% before the air reaches the trachea. Experience with laryngectomized patients, however, indicates that this process is not vital. The nasal mucosa and the sinus linings are comprised of respiratory epithelium that is covered by a sticky, mucoid layer. This mucous blanket is produced at a rate of approximately one liter per day by the goblet cells and the submucosal serous–mucinous glands. The mucus serves to waterproof the nose, preventing loss of water outward and drying of the mucosa. It is a thin, sticky, clear sheet with a *pH* of 7 or slightly lower (more acidic), and is composed of mucin, a long molecule of mucopolysaccharide that forms a spongelike meshwork (2.5% to 3%); salts (1% to 2%); water (95%); and proteins, among which are included lysozymes and immunoglobulins. The mucus is propelled posteriorly in the nose by the nasal cilia, 10 to 20 cilia per cell. Mucus and particulate matter advance slowly in the anterior of the nose, but more rapidly in the posterior, taking 20 to 30 minutes in all to reach the nasopharynx.

The mucus serves to protect the nose from infection. The lysozymes present in the mucus cause weakening of bacterial cell walls. Of the immunoglobulins, IgA is the most prominent; there are lesser amounts of IgG. IgA is produced locally by mucosal plasma cells and is secreted as a dimer into the nasal mucus. It can inhibit viral growth and is probably a significant factor in immunity to viral infections. In the case of bacterial infection, the usefulness of IgA is unknown because it does not fix complement and therefore will not lyse bacteria. There is some evidence that it may work in concert with lysozymes. IgG and IgM are routinely observed in the connective-tissue spaces beneath the mucous membrane. Increasing amounts of IgG occur in the mucus in association with inflammatory reactions. The outpouring of this antibody represents the principal host defense once an infection has been established. IgE is present in the nasal mucus of individuals with allergies, generally in proportion to the serum value. It is manufactured locally by submucosal plasma cells.

THE NEURAL SUPPLY OF THE NOSE

The first and second divisions of the fifth nerve are responsible for sensation, and, hence, these are the nerves responsible for the referred pain patterns of the nose and sinuses.

The preganglionic fibers of the sympathetic nervous system arise from the cervical spinal cord and synapse in the middle or superior cervical ganglia with 30 or more postganglionic fibers. Fibers travel by way of the carotid plexus—the deep petrosal nerve that forms the vidian nerve—and pass through the sphenopalatine ganglion to the arterioles of the nasal mucosa. Stimulation of the sympathetic plexus produces vasoconstriction and mucinous secretion. Following sympathetic-nerve injury, as occasionally occurs following a sympathectomy for Raynaud's phenomenon, there is unopposed activity of the parasympathetic nerve supply and subsequent vasodilation, mucosal swelling, nasal obstruction, and hypersecretion. The result is a nasal disorder characterized by nasal obstruction and rhinorrhea that resembles nasal allergy and is known as vasomotor rhinitis (VMR).

The path of the parasympathetic nerves is as follows: they arise in the superior salivary nucleus, form the nervus intermedius, join the facial nerve, pass to the greater superficial petrosal nerve, go through the vidian nerve, and synapse in the sphenopalatine ganglion. The postsynaptic fibers are distributed to the nose. Sectioning of the vidian nerve (vidian neurectomy) results in a pale, dry, shrunken mucosa and is used as a treatment for severe cases of vasomotor rhinitis.

THE VASCULATURE OF THE NOSE

The principal arterial supply to the internal nose is through the sphenopalatine arteries, which enter through the sphenopalatine foramen at the back of the middle meatus. Here posterior lateral branches spread in dense, parallel rows over the turbinates at two levels. The deeper vessels supply venous sinuses or lakes. The superficial arterioles supply a submucosal capillary network and are responsive to changes in temperature. The ethmoid, labial, and palatine arteries also contribute to the nasal blood supply.

THE NASAL EXAMINATION

The tools for an office examination are shown in the Appendix (Fig. A-1). In a child, an examiner can view the anterior of the nares by pushing the nasal tip up with his thumb. The anterior septum and tip of the inferior turbinate are then in view. However, with a cooperative child or an adult, a nasal speculum is preferable. The proper technique is to place the speculum blades under the ala to the desired depth; then the blades are opened down to the nasal floor, and the nares is gently spread. With a headmirror or headlight, the inferior turbinate and septum will be in immediate view. If the mucosa is swollen, a vasoconstricting nasal spray, such as oxymetazoline (Afrin), is administered. The examiner reexamines the nose after a few minutes, looking for inflammation or discharge, deviations, masses, and so forth.

DIFFERENTIAL DIAGNOSIS

The nasal mucosa should be pink to dull red in color. Thickened, bright red mucosa suggests an inflammatory reaction, often owing to a viral or bacterial infection. Discharge from a viral infection is mucoid, copious, and gray. Bacterial infections result in yellow-tinged secretions. Old mucus, as is found in nasal stasis, develops a greenish discoloration; but this change does not necessarily mean that an infection is present. Allergic rhinitis may present as bright red, inflamed mucosa, or with a reddish blue or bluish white mucous membrane. Allergic patients and those with vasomotor rhinitis have copious, watery, yet ropy, crystal-clear secretions.

Any odor to the drainage, whether noted by the patient or perceived by the examiner, suggests a bacterial infection, such as a dental root abscess, chronic nasal infections, or atrophic rhinitis. In general, there is no odor to the drainage from acute viral rhinitis or sinusitis.

NASOPHARYNGEAL EXAMINATION

The nasopharyngeal examination is facilitated, if necessary, by the administration of tetracaine HCl spray (Cetacaine) to the soft palate and oropharyngeal wall. The patient should attempt to breathe through his nose while his tongue is depressed sufficiently to permit a small mirror to slide behind the soft palate. If available, a nasopharyngoscope or fiberoptic laryngoscope are helpful.

SINUS EXAMINATION

The sinuses are best tested clinically by gentle tapping with the examiner's third finger. Beginning laterally on the forehead, the examiner taps across the patient's brow. An infected frontal sinus will be tender locally. There will also be rather marked tenderness with pressure placed on the sinus floor by the examiner's index finger. The maxillary sinuses are gently tapped over the malar eminences. In addition, the first and second molars may be sensitive to gentle tapping or pressure from a wooden tongue depressor. The ethmoids can be only very superficially visualized on nasal examination. The sphenoid is best examined radiographically. Drainage from the nasofrontal duct can be seen streaming from under the anterior end of the middle turbinate and over the inferior turbinate. Drainage from the maxillary sinus would be found more posteriorly (Fig. 6-2).

RADIOGRAPHIC EXAMINATION OF THE NOSE, NASOPHARYNX, AND PARANASAL SINUSES

When the source of nasal obstruction and discharge is not apparent, and sinusitis, tumor, polyps, foreign body, or choanal atresia are suspected, a sinus x-ray series should be obtained. In most radiology departments this series consists of the following four basic views (see Fig. 14-1), which, within the limits of practicality, should be obtained in the upright position so that secretions within the sinuses will form fluid levels. The *upright Water's view* is the best all purpose film, giving a particularly good view of the maxillary and sphenoid sinuses, and less satisfactory visualization of the ethmoid and frontal sinuses. The *Caldwell view* gives the best visualization of frontal and ethmoid sinuses. The *lateral* and *submental vertex views* round out the series.

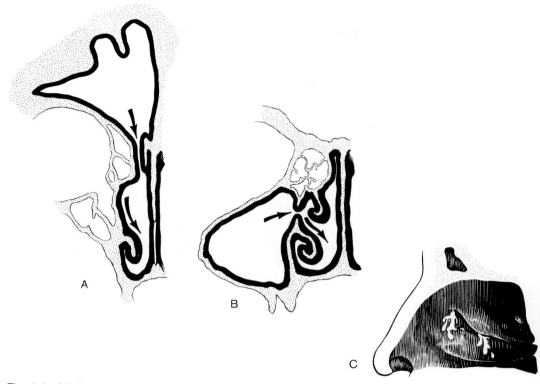

Fig. 6-2. (*A*) Frontal-sinus drainage by way of the nasofrontal duct. (*B*) Maxillary-sinus drainage from the maxillary-sinus ostium. (*C*) Relative location of drainage from the frontal and maxillary sinuses.

THE NASOPHARYNX

ANATOMY

The *nasopharynx* (Fig. 6-3) is formed superiorly by the inferior surface of the sphenoid sinus, posteriorly by the cervical vertebrae, and anteriorly by the posterior portion of the nasal septum and posterior choanae, with the tips of the inferior and middle turbinates immediately adjacent to it. The lateral wall of the nasopharynx is the most complex portion. The eustachian-tube orifices are located immediately posterosuperior to the soft palate, and immediately posterior to the inferior turbinate. The surrounding eustachian-tube cartilages form a moundlike structure around the orifice itself. Immediately above the eustachian-tube cartilages is a depression known as the fossa of Rosenmüller. For some reason, as yet

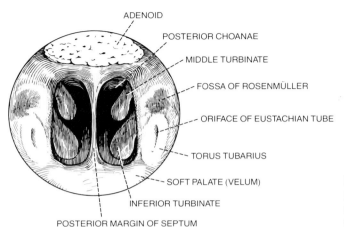

ADENOID

POSTERIOR CHOANAE

MIDDLE TURBINATE

FOSSA OF ROSENMÜLLER

ORIFACE OF EUSTACHIAN TUBE

TORUS TUBARIUS

SOFT PALATE (VELUM)

INFERIOR TURBINATE

POSTERIOR MARGIN OF SEPTUM

Fig. 6-3. Mirror view of the nasopharynx, looking from the posterior end toward the anterior end.

unknown, it is in this area that carcinoma of the nasopharynx usually arises.

The nasopharynx is a relatively dirty region, and positive cultures can be obtained in this area more often than not. Therefore, the vestibule of the nose and the nasopharynx are similar in that they often harbor pathogens, while the nasal cavities are relatively free of disease-producing organisms. Therefore, when culturing the nose, take care that the culture is obtained from well within the nasal cavities.

In children and young adults, the pharyngeal tonsil, or adenoid, may be present. It is a mass of lymphoid tissue adherent to the roof of the nasopharynx. In some children, the adenoid becomes markedly enlarged and may obstruct the posterior choanae of the nose. Also, a chronically enlarged and inflamed adenoid will result in irritation and edema of the surrounding eustachian-tube orifice. The primary disorders involving the nasopharynx include adenoid hypertrophy and chronic adenoiditis.

CHRONIC NASAL OBSTRUCTION AND ADENOIDAL HYPERTROPHY

When children are affected by *chronic nasal obstruction* and *adenoidal hypertrophy*, it is not possible in most cases to determine which problem is leading the other. Allergic children with chronic nasal obstruction and mucous retention and infection will develop adenoidal hypertrophy in response to the chronic nasal inflammation. The treatment for this problem is, first, medical. Therapy should include a combination of antihistamines and vasoconstrictors, such as Dimetapp, Actifed, or Triaminic syrup, and a short course of antibiotics based on cultures taken from within the nasal cavity at the outset. If this course of treatment fails to resolve the problem, a surgical approach should be considered. This would include, first, an adenoidectomy to remove the obstructing lymphoidal tissue in the posterior of the nose and nasopharynx and, second, deep electrocautery of the inferior turbinate to produce scarring of its submucosal vascular tissue and thereby achieve mucosal retraction and improvement of the airway and mucous flow. A combination of these procedures will result in a resolution of the problem of nasal obstruction.

Children with serous otitis media secondary to eustachian-tube obstruction who also have a large adenoid may require an adenoidectomy. Serous otitis, discussed earlier, is a fickle disorder that comes and goes, and that is often related to the onset of a respiratory infection or allergy problems. Patients who do not respond to conservative therapy—namely, the combinations of antihistamines and vasoconstrictors listed above—should undergo myringotomy with aspiration of fluid from the middle ear. If the fluid is thin and serous, most surgeons defer placement of pressure-equalization tubes in the tympanic membrane. However, if the fluid is thick and mucinous (*e.g.*, gluelike) a pressure-equalization tube is placed in the tympanic membrane in order to prevent the reaccumulation of mucus. If myringotomy and the placement of pressure-equalization tubes are followed by a recurrence of middle-ear fluids, an adenoidectomy is combined with the reinsertion of pressure-equalization tubes. In most instances, this combination of procedures will result in resolution of the problem.

CARCINOMA

Carcinoma of the nasopharynx is not an uncommon disorder. It affects men and women equally and is found in patients of approximately 20 years of age and upward, with a peak incidence between 40 and 60 years of age. For some reason, as yet poorly understood, the tumor is most common among the Chinese. There is a relationship between carcinoma of the nasopharynx and the Epstein-Barr virus; patients with nasopharyngeal carcinoma have been found on serodiagnostic studies to have high titers against the EB virus.

Carcinoma of the nasopharynx in general is a silent tumor, causing few symptoms. In approximately half the cases, the presenting symptom is a lymph-node metastasis in the neck. Nasopharyngeal carcinoma has the propensity to metastasize to the lymph nodes of the posterior cervical chain, which is palpated just anterior to the margin of the trapezius muscle. A second, common presenting symptom is the presence of unilateral serous otitis media or bacterial otitis media, and for this reason any adult with either of these should have a careful examination of the nasopharynx.

The most common nasopharyngeal tumor is lymphoepithelioma, although lymphoma makes up approximately 10% of the cases. Treatment involves administering radiation therapy to the nasopharynx and also to the regions of lymphatic drainage. Tumors in the nasopharynx cannot be locally resected, and if they fail to respond to radiation therapy, they will slowly extend through the foramen lacerum into the cavernous sinus and middle fossa, eventually involving the third, fourth, and sixth nerves. Less commonly, the tumor spreads into the lateral pharyngeal space and involves the tissues and nodes surrounding the carotid and jugular foramen, and here may involve the ninth, tenth, and eleventh nerves. Persistent metastatic tumors in the neck can be removed by block dissection of the neck.

CYSTS

Cysts of the nasopharynx can arise either from a bursa that lies on the undersurface of the sphenoid, or from Rathke's pouch, the site of invagination of embryonic tissues into the region of the pituitary. These cysts present with foul nasopharyngeal discharge and, at times, occipital headache. They are treated by surgical marsupialization of these areas and removal of as much of the cystic tissue as possible. Once opened, the cysts cause little or no further trouble.

CHRONIC NASOPHARYNGITIS EXCLUSIVE OF ADENOIDITIS

Chronic nasopharyngitis exclusive of adenoiditis may result from a chronic bacterial or allergic condition, causing an irritated sensation above the palate, a chronic postnasal drip, and recurrent sore throats. It is a common sequela of nasopharyngeal radiotherapy. Control of associated disorders, such as sinusitis, and judicious use of antibiotics is helpful in treating this disorder.

DIAGNOSIS OF PALATAL DYSFUNCTION

The palate forms a dynamic valve between the pharynx and oropharynx, preventing saliva and food from entering the nasopharynx when swallowing. In addition, the palate is vital to the production of intelligible speech because of its role in maintaining the patency of the nasopharynx and nose. Obstruction of the nose and nasopharynx and failure of the normal amounts of air to pass through them results in hyponasal speech. The nasal sounds that require patency of the nose and nasopharynx are those represented by the letters m, n, and ng. These are impossible to pronounce with an obstructed nose, and the inability to make these sounds characteristically accompanies a cold.

There are five pairs of muscles that are responsible for the structure and function of the soft palate. Included in these pairs are the tensor veli palatini, the levator veli palatini, the palatoglossis, the palatopharyngeus, and the constrictor pharyngis superior, which insert into an aponeurosis in the palatal midline and are innervated from the nucleus ambiguus by way of the glossopharyngeal and vagus nerves. Improper functioning of the palate, producing hypernasal speech, can result either from an anatomical defect, such as a congenital cleft palate or a congenitally short palate, or from the shortening of the palate by tumor surgery. It may also occur secondary to neuromuscular disorders, such as myasthenia gravis or amyotrophic lateral sclerosis. Excessive amounts of air escape through the nose, and the patient is unable to articulate those sounds requiring sealing of the nasopharynx. Marked hypernasal speech is unintelligible; however, slight to moderate hypernasal speech can be difficult to distinguish from other disorders of articulation. The distinction is made most easily by placing a small wisp of cotton just anterior to the patient's nares, and asking him to say "school." If the cotton is blown, a diagnosis of palatal dysfunction is made.

Repairs of the cleft palate are done by means of a palatal pushback procedure and the use of a posterior pharyngeal flap. A palate shortened by tumor surgery may require a flap reconstruction or an obturator to occlude the defect in order to allow intelligible speech.

7

NASAL AND SINUS CONGESTION AND INFECTION

William R. Wilson

Nasal infections
  Nasal furunculosis
  Recurrent nasal vestibulitis
  Viral rhinitis
Unilateral nasal obstruction
  Choanal atresia
  Meningoencephalocele
  Foreign bodies
  Trauma
Bilateral nasal obstruction
  Allergic rhinitis
  Vasomotor rhinitis
  Rhinitis medicamentosa
  Polypoid rhinosinusitis
Sinus headache, pain, and drainage
  Acute sinusitis
    Acute frontal sinusitis
    Acute sphenoid sinusitis
    Acute maxillary sinusitis
    Acute ethmoiditis
  Chronic sinusitis

Chronic frontal sinusitis
Chronic sphenoid sinusitis
Chronic maxillary sinusitis
Chronic ethmoiditis
Sinus surgery
  Caldwell-Luc procedure
  Ethmoidectomy
  Osteoplastic frontal-sinus
    obliteration
Unusual causes of nasal obstruction and drainage
  Tuberculosis
  Sarcoidosis
  Syphilis
  Wegener's granulomatosis
  Midline granuloma
  Mucormycosis
Olfaction
  Disorders of the sense of smell
  Evaluation of olfactory disorders

NASAL INFECTIONS

NASAL FURUNCULOSIS

Nasal furunculosis is a minor *Staphylococcus aureus* infection involving the follicles of the vibrissae of the nares. Redness, swelling, and pain are usually limited to the inner surface of the vestibule, and any drainage occurs spontaneously into the vestibule. However, prompt antibiotic treatment plus incision and drainage are required if the infection becomes more than superficial. The reason for special concern is that infections involving this portion of the nose may seed the cavernous sinus by way of the facial veins, occasionally leading to a cavernous-sinus thrombosis. In general, patients with severe nasal furunculosis are hospitalized for several days for intravenous antibiotic therapy.

RECURRENT NASAL VESTIBULITIS

A chronically irritated nasal vestibule may be the result of recurrent staphylococcal infections. Patients should be evaluated for rhinologic or sinus infections, although often these are not present. A patient can control vestibulitis by keeping his hands away from his nose and face, by washing his hands and face twice daily with hexachlorophene soap, and by applying bacitracin ointment to the nasal vestibule twice daily with a sterile cotton applicator. Patients with a mustache may have to remove it to control vestibulitis.

VIRAL RHINITIS

Viruses are spread by droplet dissemination or by fomite transfer from a patient's hands to his nose. There are a host of viruses responsible for occurrences of the common cold: rhinovirus will cause about one third, parainfluenza types 1-4 and influenza A and B are responsible for 15% to 20%, and respiratory syncytial virus, adenovirus, enterovirus, and all others combined are each responsible for 5% or less.

During the first 24 hours of a viral cold, there is a significant increase in the IgA level of nasal mucus due to the release of stored specific and nonspecific IgA into nasal secretions. During the secretory phase of viral rhinitis (days 2 to 5), there is necrosis and shedding of epithelial cells, accompanied by marked transudation of serum albumin and IgG. At this point, the nose is most inflamed and obstructed, and bacterial rhinitis and sinusitis may occur secondary to stasis of mucus.

The normal flora of the anterior of the nose and nasopharynx include many pathogens that live symbiotically but that under altered conditions of anatomy and physiology can become pathogenic to the host. These include *Staphylococcus aureus, Hemophilus influenzae, Streptococcus pneumoniae,* and beta streptococcus. In general, although the nasal vestibule and the nasopharynx will often culture positively for potential pathogens regardless of the state of the patient's health, the intervening mucosal surfaces should be pathogen free. For this reason, when culturing the nose it is best to place the tip of the cotton applicator along the lower surface of the middle turbinate because this is an area bathed by drainage from the sinuses as well as the nose. Care should be taken to avoid touching the vestibular surfaces during this procedure.

Cultures are taken when the mucus becomes thickened and creamy or tinged with yellow. In small children this is an indication of bacterial rhinoethmoiditis and should be treated with appropriate antibiotics, although some physicians would choose not to use antibiotics for these symptoms. In an adult, these symptoms will be accompanied by complaints of nasal discomfort, namely obstruction, copious rhinorrhea, and headache or facial pain, and the indications for antibiotics are more apparent. Five to seven days of antibiotic treatment is sufficient to resolve rhinitis. However, sinusitis requires a longer course of treatment.

The treatment for viral rhinitis often includes a mild analgesic for the accompanying achy malaise as well as an antihistamine–vasoconstrictor combination for the nasal symptoms. Most antihistamines have an atropinelike drying effect; the vasoconstrictor reduces congestion by reducing vascular engorgement. Further relief of congestion is obtained from the temporary use of vasoconstricting nasal sprays.

Our preference of medication for viral rhinitis includes acetaminophen 325 mg to 650 mg q. 4 hr p.r.n. and chlorpheniramine (Chlor-Trimeton) 4 mg to 8 mg q. 4 hr for 3 days, in addition to steam inhalations through a hot towel. There are many similar medications that will accomplish the same therapeutic goals. When bacterial infections are present, an antibiotic is added to the regimen.

UNILATERAL NASAL OBSTRUCTION

Unilateral nasal obstruction may present as a continuous discharge or as an irritation about one nares of the nose. This symptom requires a thorough evaluation. The diagnostic possibilities include the following *congenital anomalies.*

CHOANAL ATRESIA

Undetected *unilateral choanal atresia* is an unusual anomaly that can result from bony or membranous obstruction of the posterior nose. The diagnosis can be made readily in the office by attempting to pass a soft catheter through the nose or by instilling a small amount of methylene blue in the nostril being examined. Failure of the dye to appear in the pharynx strongly suggests the presence of choanal atresia. X-ray films must be obtained to confirm the diagnosis. A small amount of radiopaque dye in the nose will help outline the structures during that procedure. Treatment is surgical correction.

MENINGOENCEPHALOCELE

Meningoencephalocele may present extranasally or intranasally, and, when intranasal, it will at times present as a mass involving the septum or as a pedunculated structure resembling a polyp. Careful x-ray evaluation will demonstrate a bony defect in the floor of the anterior or middle cranial fossa. Biopsy should *not* be considered. Patients should be referred for neurosurgical and otolaryngological evaluation.

FOREIGN BODIES

A *foreign body* in the nose may be one of an endless variety of inanimate objects. By far the most common objects are bits of toys, such as wheels, beads, and buttons. Pebbles, bits of cotton, beans, peas, and nuts may also be found. Persistent unilateral fetid mucopurulent discharge should arouse clinical suspicion. To prevent aspiration of the dislodged object, a cooperative child should be placed in a supine position with his head down. The nose should be carefully anesthetized topically before forceps or a wire loop are introduced. Other methods, such as passing a Foley or Fogerty catheter beyond the object, inflating the catheter slightly, and withdrawing it, are occasionally useful. The use of a general anesthetic may be required in uncooperative children. It is prudent when removing one foreign body to make a quick check for other sites.

TRAUMA

Nasal obstruction may result from a traumatic dislocation of the caudal cartilage of the nasal septum or from a septal hematoma (Fig. 7-1).

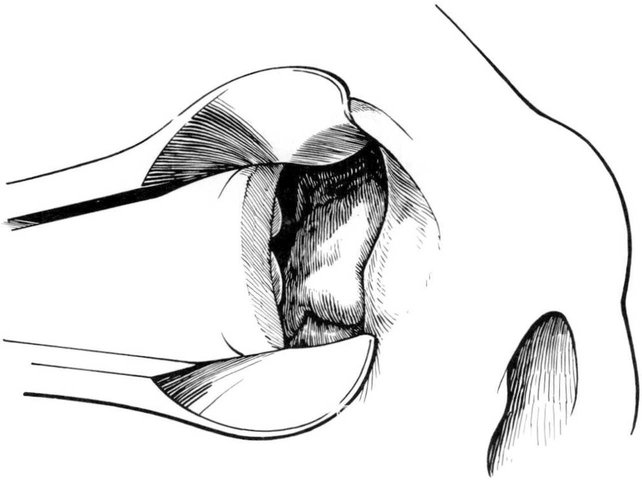

Fig. 7-1. Nasal speculum exam. One of the most common findings is a deviated nasal septum, which may obstruct breathing. It may also become a source of bleeding due to trauma or excessive drying from the air stream.

BILATERAL NASAL OBSTRUCTION

ALLERGIC RHINITIS

Allergic rhinitis is very common and affects at least 10% of the population to some degree. It takes two forms: seasonal and perennial. *Seasonal allergy* may be recognized as hay fever and is associated with inflamed conjunctival membranes as well as nasal and, in some patients, bronchial symptoms. In the Northeast, patients who are sensitive to tree pollen will begin to notice symptoms beginning in late March or early April. Grass-sensitive patients will be symptomatic from mid-May to the end of June. July and the first 2 weeks of August is a good, relatively allergy-free period for most of these patients. Ragweed and other summer weeds pollinate from the end of August until the first frost, usually early in October.

The first treatment program for seasonal allergy involves the antihistamines. These medications can be used alone or in combination in a standard-release or sustained-release form. The patient should be made aware that these medicines prevent the effects of histamine release by competing with histamine for binding sites, and that, therefore, they should be taken in a regular prophylactic manner. The side-effect of drowsiness often abates after several days of use. The standard dosage form may be too strong for women or for persons with low body weight; therefore, the dose should be titrated by breaking the pills or by using the liquid form. Vasoconstrictors can be used in combination or separately. Because of the relatively long symptom period of seasonal allergy, vasoconstricting nasal sprays should be avoided. The rebound phenomenon may develop or be made worse in these patients, owing to rhinitis medicamentosa, by the use of these sprays. On the other hand, topical steroid nasal sprays such as dexamethasone and beclomethasone are often helpful.

Patients who are so uncomfortable that they are unable to function normally despite these measures can be given corticosteroids for the duration of their allergy season if the allergy season is short—a few weeks to a month—and if there are no medical contraindications. For nasal allergy, 20 mg of prednisone on *alternate* mornings is usually very effective and has minimum supressive effects on the adrenal-pituitary axis. Prednisone should be withdrawn gradually as the end of the season approaches.

Skin testing or antigen-specific serum IgE levels (PRIST test) should be undertaken in order to determine sensitivities. By combining the results of these tests with an allergic history, the physician and patient can better understand the etiologic basis of the patient's symptoms and develop an appropriate plan of allergen avoidance and therapy. When allergic rhinitis becomes sufficiently troublesome, many physicians attempt allergic hyposensitization. This form of therapy is successful in providing partial or complete relief to approximately 80% of allergic patients. There are a variety of materials and techniques employed. In general, injections should be begun soon after the allergic season and should be gradually increased to the highest tolerable dose prior to the next allergic season.

The largest amounts of antigen, as measured by protein nitrogen units, can be administered with alum-precipitated extracts of pollens because they are absorbed more slowly by the patient. The host responds by producing antigen-specific IgG that serves as a blocking antibody by combining with the antigen in the respiratory tissues, thus preventing the combination of the antigen with IgE fixed to the surface of mast cells.

Perennial nasal allergy is also very common, and patients suffering from it complain of year-round nasal stuffiness, particularly at night when they try to sleep, although there may be exacerbations during pollen seasons. Sleep is often fitful, and patients awaken early in the morning with a blocked nose and begin to sneeze immediately upon arising. There is some gradual, but not complete, improvement during the day. Thick postnasal drip accompanies this disorder. Other common symptoms are intermittent loss of smell and taste, frontal headaches, and a dry throat and cough. Common allergens include house dust, house-dust mites, molds, feathers, and animal danders. The role of food allergy in allergic rhinosinusitis is controversial and poorly understood. When these patients are questioned closely, many describe an increased incidence of symptoms following the social use of alcohol and exposure to cigarette smoke, perfumes, exhaust, and paint fumes. In general, it is this group of patients that develops polypoid degeneration of the mucous membrane of the nose and paranasal sinuses (nasal polyps).

An evaluation of these patients should include full skin testing, testing for serum IgE level, and sinus x-ray films. The films should include several polytomographs through the sinuses in order to better assess the amount of mucosal thickening.

Skin testing in these patients usually demonstrates a diffuse sensitivity to many antigens, but principally to those from house dust and pets. Based on this information, the patient should be instructed on how to eliminate sources of irritation from his environment. If there is little or no polypoid degeneration of the mucosa of the nose and paranasal sinuses, hyposensitization may be tried. Allergy injections will not reverse polypoid degeneration. Most patients with perennial nasal allergy have suffered for many years and have tried almost every form of antihistamine and vasoconstrictor. Although these medications are beneficial to some patients, many patients are not helped because thickened secretions become thicker and the mucosa becomes refractory. Topical medications, such as cromolyn sodium (Aarane and Intal), dexamethasone (Decadron Turbinaire), and beclomethasone (Beconase and Vancernase) are of some value. Patients with perennial allergy are difficult to help medically.

VASOMOTOR RHINITIS

Symptomatically, *vasomotor rhinitis* (VMR) seems identical to nasal allergy. Although it is approximately ten times less common than allergy, it is not mutually exclusive and at times is seen in conjunction with allergy. In pure VMR, skin tests are negative and there is no elevation of IgE level. Unlike allergy, this condition is not improved by a short clinical course of cortisone, such as prednisone 20 mg p.o., every morning for 5 days. A course of treatment such as this is useful when doubt exists as to how much nasal symptomatology is due to allergy, and how much is due to vasomotor rhinitis or structural dysfunction, such as a deviated septum. The allergic symptoms will clear, leaving residual symptoms secondary to other nasal disorders.

In general, VMR is poorly controlled by medications, although an antihistamine–vasoconstrictor combination should be tried. In our experience, Ornade is the most effective of these preparations for treating this disorder because, since an anticholinergic is added, it has the most drying effect. If obstruction persists despite therapy, one of a number of surgical treatments becomes necessary. In patients bothered primarily by obstruction, cryosurgical treatments of the inferior and middle turbinates (cryoturbinectomy) or electrocautery plus surgical trimming of the inferior turbinate are useful. For profuse rhinorrhea, sectioning of the parasympathetic nervous supply to the nose may be necessary (vidian neurectomy).

RHINITIS MEDICAMENTOSA

Rhinitis medicamentosa is a common disorder associated with the chronic use of vasoconstricting nasal sprays. The mucosa becomes red and swollen, and the nose becomes completely obstructed with engorged turbinates because of irritation from the continual use of nasal spray and the recurring rebound phenomenon. Initially, the use of nose spray gives the patient relief, but in time the periods of improvement become shorter and shorter. Treatment consists of complete abstinence from nose spray for 2 weeks or more.

Corticosteroids, such as prednisone 20 mg every other morning for 2 weeks, are helpful in reducing some of the inflammation associated with this disorder, and they will help the patient do without the spray. If the obstruction fails to clear, and there is no underlying nasal disorder, a procedure such as electrocautery and trimming of the turbinates or cryoturbinectomy is required to establish a satisfactory airway.

POLYPOID RHINOSINUSITIS

Both allergic and nonallergic patients may develop hyperplastic, boggy, thickened mucosa of the ethmoid, maxillary, and, less frequently, the other sinuses. The causative factor is unknown. The majority of allergic patients never develop polyps, but there may be increased polyp formation in the presence of viral or bacterial infections. Also, there is a relationship between aspirin sensitivity, nasal polyps, and bronchial asthma (aspirin triad syndrome). Patients with this condition should be advised to avoid tartrazene (US FD & C yellow #5) and indomethacin as well. Polyps should be removed as often as is necessary to maintain a satisfactory airway and to prevent obstruction and interruption of mucous flow and infection from stasis. Repeated or chronic infection compounds the problem by leading to increased inflammation and polyp formation. In most instances, polypectomy is a short office procedure, and in most patients it is best to remove polyps as soon as they become obstructive. If nasal polyps become too numerous, they require removal in the operating room with the patient under a general anesthetic. When polypoid sinus disease becomes complicated by constant sinus headache pain or chronic infection, sinus surgery may be often required.

The surgery for polypoid rhinosinusitis should be as limited in extent as possible, but it must also achieve the goals of providing an airway, reducing infection, preventing recurrence of polyps, and relieving sinus headaches and discomfort. In general, this surgery always includes an ethmoidectomy, because the polyps commonly arise from the ethmoidal sinuses. The sphenoid sinus may be opened for polyp removal and drainage. The maxilla should be opened if there is a choanal polyp because choanal polyps arise from that structure. Sinuses need not be disturbed unless they are symptomatic.

SINUS HEADACHE, PAIN, AND DRAINAGE

ACUTE SINUSITIS

All forms of paranasal sinusitis are usually precipitated by nasal congestion from a viral, upper-respiratory-tract infection or nasal allergy, or both. Although occasionally acute sinusitis is a pure viral infection, much more commonly it is the result of a bacterial acute superinfection. Whether it occurs in the frontal, maxillary, or ethmoid sinuses, the most frequent causative pathogens are: *Streptococcus pneumoniae, H. influenzae, Staphylococcus aureus,* and beta streptococcus. (Anaerobes are frequently found in chronic sinusitis.)

For patients with the clinical symptoms of sinusitis, a sinus x-ray study should be done to establish the diagnosis. As a minimum, the views should include an upright, open-mouth Water's view (so that air–fluid levels will be seen), a Caldwell view, a submental vertex view, and a lateral view. Transillumination is too inexact a technique to use for diagnosis, but it is helpful in assessing the progress of therapy. Cultures are also helpful, but only if pus is cultured as it streams from the sinus ostium; otherwise, contamination from nasal flora makes the results open to question. Therapy should not await the culture report. Antibiotic selection is based upon the known frequency of occurrence of the pathogens and regional bacterial sensitivities, but it may be adjusted on the basis of clinical progress and the culture report. Ampicillin is effective in most instances against all common sinus pathogens. A suggested regimen is ampicillin 500 mg p.o., q. 4 hr for 48 hr, then 250 mg q. 6 hr for 10 days, and then 250 mg q. 12 hr for 10 days. Cephalexin is also effective. Along with the antibiotic, a long-acting, vasoconstrict-

ing nasal spray, such as xylometasoline hydrochloride (Otrivin) or oxymetazoline hydrochloride (Afrin), should be prescribed. The most
effective way to use these sprays is to spray the nose once, wait 5
minutes for the nose to clear, then spray again so that the second spray
can reach the swollen sinus ostia. Following this, the patient should
breathe through a very hot, wet towel for several minutes. The warm,
moist air helps to liquify the secretions. A patient with maxillary sinusitis should be instructed to lie across his bed and hang his head over
the other side, with the affected sinus uppermost to promote drainage.
This routine should be followed for 5 minutes three times a day for 3
to 4 days after the initiation of therapy. Oral antihistamines are not
recommended in the treatment of acute sinusitis because they tend to
thicken, rather than to liquify, the purulent material trapped within the
sinus. Analgesics are used on a p.r.n. basis.

Acute sinusitis may resolve slowly because of a narrowed nasofrontal duct or because of the lack of dependent drainage from the
maxillary sinuses. A follow-up x-ray study consisting of one film, the
upright Water's view, should be obtained after 2 to 3 weeks of antibiotic
therapy to ensure complete resolution of the infection. This is an important film for the following reasons. First, acute sinusitis often resolves slowly, and the film may show only partial resolution of the
infection. At this point the decision to continue antibiotic therapy for
another 2 weeks should be made. Failure to adequately treat an acute
sinus infection may result in troublesome chronic sinusitis. Second, this
x-ray film occasionally reveals an underlying mechanism for the infection that is obscured by the inflammation and the secretions on the
original films. Acute sinusitis that fails to clear after 3 to 4 weeks of
treatment should be reevaluated for further medical and surgical treatment. There are special diagnostic and therapeutic considerations that
pertain to each sinus.

ACUTE FRONTAL SINUSITIS

Acute frontal sinusitis causes pain in the forehead immediately over the
sinus. This pain is intensified by bending forward or by tapping with a
finger over the sinus. In general, the diagnosis of acute frontal sinusitis
is simple to make; the difficulty lies in determining how much of a risk
the infection represents to the patient. An infection of a frontal sinus
that is not draining through the nasofrontal duct may potentially induce
bacterial phlebitis of the diploic veins of the posterior wall of the sinus;
therefore, it may spread centrally and result in an epidural, subdural,
or brain abscess. In other words, because the frontal sinuses, and sphenoid sinuses as well, are contiguous with the cranial vault and can
become completely obstructed, when infected they represent a greater

hazard to patients than infected maxillary and ethmoid sinuses. Also, improperly treated acute frontal sinusitis may become chronic sinusitis, a more difficult problem to treat.

If a patient with frontal sinusitis is febrile or has intense pain associated with edema of the overlying skin and tissues of the upper lid, he should be hospitalized, intravenous antibiotics and topical vasoconstrictors should be administered, and an otolaryngology consultation should be obtained. When rapid improvement fails to occur within 24 hours, surgical drainage by means of a trephine procedure is recommended. This procedure, done with the patient under a local or general anesthetic, requires a 2-cm incision along the inferior medial edge of the eyebrow. The floor of the sinus is exposed (in the roof of the orbit), and a 5-mm to 7-mm opening is made in the bone. The contents are cultured for aerobes and anaerobes and aspirated, and a small catheter to be used for irrigation with an antibiotic solution is sutured in place for several days. The wound heals without significant scarring.

A common cause of acute frontal sinusitis is from water being forced into the sinus during diving into fresh water. These patients are often hospitalized because of the difficulty encountered with antibiotic therapy for an enteric bacterial infection from swimming water.

ACUTE SPHENOID SINUSITIS

Acute sphenoid sinusitis occurs in otherwise healthy adults in conjunction with pansinusitis. In general, because the sphenoid sinuses will clear as the other sinuses clear, there is no cause for particular concern. However, acute sphenoid sinusitis can present as an isolated and potentially lethal infection in immunosuppressed, diabetic, or elderly debilitated patients. The early signs are few, and, therefore, the physician must have a high index of suspicion. Symptoms include fever, headache referred to the vertex of the skull, and some purulent nasopharyngeal secretions. If the symptoms do not resolve rapidly upon institution of antibiotic therapy, the sphenoid sinus should be opened, cultured, and drained through an external ethmoidectomy–sphenoidotomy approach. If acute sphenoid sinusitis is not quickly recognized and treated, there is risk of central spread of infection either by direct extension through phlebotic veins or by the development of osteomyelitis of the sphenoid bone, particularly if the sphenoid sinus is well pneumatized. Because the lateral sinus wall is contiguous with the superior orbital fissure and the cavernous sinus the infection may spread to these areas. The superior orbital fissure syndrome consists of panophthalmoplegia involving the third, fourth, and sixth cranial nerves. In addition, the first division of the fifth and sympathetic nerves may also be involved. Cavernous sinus thrombosis is associated with spiking fever, exophthalmos and edema of the orbit and lids, decreased vision, papilledema, and panophthalmoplegia.

ACUTE MAXILLARY SINUSITIS

Acute maxillary sinusitis causes tenderness over the sinus that is also felt in the teeth that are contiguous with the sinus. These include the ipsilateral second premolar and the three molars. (In some patients the tooth roots protrude into the antrum and are covered by only a thin layer of bone.) The teeth may be sensitive to hot and cold liquids. Also, achy pain is referred to the orbital, zygomatic, and temporal regions. Unilateral, isolated maxillary sinusitis requires increased diagnostic attention because it can arise secondary to carcinoma of the maxillary sinus or to a dental-root abscess. X-ray films of the sinus should be carefully examined for any bone destruction indicative of a tumor. A survey x-ray film of the teeth that includes the roots should be obtained as well.

Patients in whom acute maxillary sinusitis does not resolve may require antral irrigation. This procedure is performed in the doctor's office. The lining of the nose is anesthetized, and a trocar needle is placed in the inferior meatus and pushed into the antrum. Warm sterile saline is then used to irrigate the sinus. Persistent infections will require surgical exploration, such as creating a nasal-antral window or performing a Caldwell-Luc procedure (see Chronic Maxillary Sinusitis).

ACUTE ETHMOIDITIS

Viral ethmoiditis accompanies many severe upper respiratory infections. It can produce frontal or orbital headache and a reduced sense of smell and taste. There are no additional symptoms associated with a bacterial infection, other than an observable change in the nasal secretions from a mucoid consistency to a yellow gray purulence. Acute ethmoiditis is the only form of sinusitis that occurs in young children because the other sinuses are yet to develop.

The ethmoid sinuses are separated from the orbital contents by a very thin plate of bone, the lamina papyracea. As a result, ethmoid sinusitis is occasionally complicated by orbital cellulitis. Patients with this complication are immediately hospitalized for intravenous antibiotic therapy. If the infection fails to resolve rapidly (in 24 to 48 hours), the ethmoid sinus and orbit are explored and drained as a combined ophthalmology–otolaryngology procedure. Orbital cellulitis must be differentiated from cavernous sinus thrombosis.

CHRONIC SINUSITIS

CHRONIC FRONTAL SINUSITIS

Chronic frontal sinusitis takes several forms. It may result from improperly treated acute frontal sinusitis, allergic polypoid sinus disease, or obstruction of the nasofrontal duct secondary to scarring or fracture of the sinus wall. The sinus membrane is thickened and infected secretions are retained. Patients may complain of a steady headache associated with dull, localized tenderness and intermittent, purulent nasal and postnasal drainage. The sinus x-ray films of these patients demonstrate opacification of the sinus and sclerosis of the bony sinus margins.

Chronic frontal sinusitis may take the form of a mucocele, an expanding mucosal cyst filled with mucinous secretion. When infected, this cyst becomes pyocele. Mucoceles slowly erode the walls of the sinus, and can reach the dura or expand into the orbit. Physical symptoms include headache and, at times, a soft mass protruding below the medial aspect of the brow or into the upper lid. Because the expanding cysts cause rarefaction of the bony walls of the sinus, radiological determination of chronic sinusitis is often difficult to make.

The treatment for chronic sinusitis or mucopyocele is surgical extirpation of the disease from the sinus, and obliteration of the sinus cavity with fat (osteoplastic frontal sinus obliteration).

CHRONIC SPHENOID SINUSITIS

Chronic sphenoid sinusitis occurs as an isolated infection in the chronically ill and the elderly. Physical findings are scant, except for a headache deep to the eyes and to the vertex of the skull, in conjunction with complaints of intermittent purulent nasopharyngeal drainage. X-ray films will demonstrate thickened mucosa, sometimes an air–fluid level, and sometimes complete opacification plus sclerosis of the surrounding bone. Cases that are refractory to medical care require surgical drainage.

CHRONIC MAXILLARY SINUSITIS

Chronic maxillary sinusitis presents with a generalized facial ache in the region of the sinus, in addition to intermittent ipsilateral mucopurulent discharge. In the absence of a dental-root abscess, carcinoma, or very thick allergic or hyperplastic sinus mucosa, the condition may respond to a series of antral-wash procedures along with a 3- to 4-week course of treatment with a properly selected antibiotic based upon the antral cultures. Otherwise, a Caldwell-Luc procedure to remove the diseased sinus membrane and to establish improved drainage through a large window between the sinus and the nose is often curative.

CHRONIC ETHMOIDITIS

Chronic ethmoiditis is seen most commonly as a complication of polypoid allergic sinusitis or polypoid hyperplastic sinusitis in which mucus and bacteria become entrapped. Patients suffer recurrent or continuous mucopurulent nasal discharge and headache. Blockage of the upper portions of the nose produces headache and a diminished or absent sense of smell or taste. X-ray films demonstrate a dissolution of the bony ethmoid septa and replacement by soft tissue. Infections are often difficult to satisfactorily treat medically; therefore, consideration must be given to ethmoid-sinus surgery.

SINUS SURGERY

Surgery for chronic sinusitis is indicated for chronic pain, chronic purulent drainage, and osteomyelitis, and for biopsy if there is a possibility of a tumor. Asymptomatic sinuses, opacified on x-ray film by polypoid mucosal linings, do not require surgery.

CALDWELL-LUC PROCEDURE

The *Caldwell-Luc procedure* is the most common surgical procedure used in the treatment of chronic maxillary sinusitis. In this operation, a 4-cm incision is made at the buccogingival junction above the canine and premolar teeth. The tissues of the cheek are then elevated, and an opening of 1 cm to 2 cm in diameter is made in the anterior bony wall. After culturing the contents of the sinus, the diseased membrane lining is removed, and a permanent opening is made between the inferior meatus and sinus (a nasal antral window) to provide dependent drainage. Several days of hospitalization are required for this procedure. The incision heals rapidly, but an occasional oral antral fistula may require secondary closure. Patients can be left with temporary or permanent numbness of the cheek in the area of distribution of the inferior orbital nerve. More commonly, there may be some numbness of the one or two teeth that are adjacent to the area of bone removal.

ETHMOIDECTOMY

The *ethmoidectomy* can be done through the nose (intranasal ethmoidectomy) or by way of a $1\frac{1}{2}$-cm to 2-cm vertical incision placed halfway between the medial canthus of the eye and the dorsum of the nose (external ethmoidectomy). The external ethmoidectomy provides better exposure than the intranasal procedure, and as a rule a more thorough exenteration of the sinus cells can be achieved by this method. It is the method of choice when a mucocele or tumor is present. Wounds from ethmoidectomy heal well with little scarring. Ethmoidectomy can be bloody, because the only method of controlling bleeding is by tamponade and electric cautery; therefore, transfusions are not unusual. Gauze packing is usually left in the sinuses for several days postoperatively. Complications, though rare, may be of a serious nature, and may include cerebrospinal-fluid leak, epiphora, ophthalmoplegia, and blindness. The usual hospital stay is 3 to 4 days following surgery, followed by a 1 to 2 week convalescent period at home.

The external ethmoidectomy provides an approach to the sphenoid sinus for sphenoidotomy and hypophysectomy. A sphenoidotomy includes removal of the anterior wall of the sphenoid and exenteration of the contents of the sinus. The complications and hospital stay are the same as for ethmoidectomy. Intranasal and external ethmoidectomy can be combined with the Caldwell-Luc procedure and others when necessary.

OSTEOPLASTIC FRONTAL-SINUS OBLITERATION

Osteoplastic frontal-sinus obliteration is the procedure of choice for chronic frontal sinusitis. The incision can be hidden in the scalp or hair, or, less satisfactorily, it can be placed above the eyebrows. The anterior bony wall of the sinus is elevated as a flap based on the periosteum inferiorly. The infected lining of the sinus is completely removed, and the sinus is obliterated with subcutaneous abdominal fat. This is an effective and relatively complication-free procedure with a high success rate. The patient is hospitalized for approximately 4 to 5 days, followed by several weeks of convalescence.

UNUSUAL CAUSES OF NASAL OBSTRUCTION AND DRAINAGE

TUBERCULOSIS

Tuberculosis is very rare and presents as beefy red edema, an ulceration, or a granulomatous growth or polyp. It probably does not occur in the absence of pulmonary tuberculosis. Diagnosis is made by skin test, smears, cultures, and biopsy.

SARCOIDOSIS

Sarcoidosis occasionally presents as, or includes, nasal congestion and rhinitis. The diagnosis should not be seriously considered in the absence of generalized sarcoidosis or evidence of 1-mm to 3-mm nodular lesions of the turbinal or septal mucosa. Diagnosis is made based on biopsy information that fits the general clinical picture of the disorder.

SYPHILIS

Primary syphilis may rarely present as a chancre on the nasal epithelium–mucosa junction. Diagnosis requires a darkfield examination because serological, reagin, and specific treponemal tests are negative for the first 8 to 12 weeks. Syphilis can be an occupational hazard to medical personnel.

Secondary syphilis can present as gray, mucinous patches on the nasal mucous membrane as well as on the oral mucosa. The lesions are highly infectious. Rhinitis, nicknamed "the snuffles" in infants, is classically seen in early congenital syphilis and is characterized by mucosal inflammation and bloody, mucopurulent discharge.

Congenital syphilis is analogous to secondary syphilis in the adult, and, if unrecognized, it can lead to nasal saddle deformities from luetic chondritis and osteitis.

Late syphilis presents as a gummatous reaction of the bony septum and foul-smelling drainage.

WEGENER'S GRANULOMATOSIS

Wegener's granulomatosis is an uncommon disease characterized by focal necrotizing vasculitis that most commonly affects the upper respiratory tract initially, followed by the lower respiratory tract, skin, joints, and kidneys. Patients may present with a secondarily infected and painful ulceration of the nose or a granular draining otitis media—both of which are unresponsive to therapy. Nasal or otic, as well as pulmonary and renal, biopsies are often necessary to confirm the diagnosis. Cytotoxic drugs, primarily cyclophosphamide, have produced remissions and revolutionized the treatment of this previously lethal disorder.

MIDLINE GRANULOMA

Midline granuloma is very rare. It presents in a manner similar to Wegener's granulomatosis but tends to remain localized. The underlying disorder is an atypical lymphoid and reticulum-cell proliferation in granulation tissue, identified by deep biopsy. Treatment is high-dose (4000 to 6000 rad) radiation therapy.

MUCORMYCOSIS

Mucormycosis is an opportunistic fungal infection caused by *Rhizopus* in patients with diabetic ketoacidosis or blood dyscrasias, immunosuppressed patients, or patients requiring long-term treatment with high doses of steroids and antibiotics. Patients complain of nasal pain and have a serosanguineous nasal discharge. Examination of the nose reveals a black, necrotic turbinate. Biopsy and smear for *Mucor* are diagnostic. The treatment of mucormycosis is prompt debridement and immediate initiation of amphotericin B. The prognosis is grave. *Aspergillosis* can present in a similar manner but is generally unresponsive to amphotericin B.

OLFACTION

In lower animals, including fish, the olfactory organs are used for the recognition of food and for procreation. In man, however, reliance on smell has been superseded by reliance on sight.

The olfactory region is a small, yellow brown area made up of the superior turbinate and the nasal septum opposite from it. The epithelium is made up of 10 to 20 million bipolar olfactory cells, each an olfactory rod extending into the mucous blanket. From each rod extend hundreds of fine cilia known as olfactory hairs. These are the sensors. The central process of each olfactory cell joins with the neighboring processes to form bundles, which, as they become larger, are sheathed in myelin and pass through the cribriform plate to the olfactory bulb. Following synapse there, connections are complex and run to the hypothalamus and brain stem.

At present, there is no adequate explanation of the transducing mechanism that determines the quality or quantity of an odor. In order to be smelled, a substance must not only be volatile, but also soluble in water and lipids. The fine discrimination tasks of taste, such as distinguishing veal from lamb, are mediated by a combination of taste and smell.

DISORDERS OF THE SENSE OF SMELL

Complaint: Reduction or absence of the sense of smell (hyposmia, anosmia) and taste (ageusia, hypogeusia). This may be caused by

Congenital anosmia: resulting from birth trauma or, rarely, agensis of the olfactory bulb, and at times can be associated with hypogonadism

Injury: such as cribriform fracture, frontal-lobe laceration or hemorrhage, or complication of intranasal or intracranial surgery

Nasal obstruction: caused by mucosal swelling from upper respiratory infection (URI) (viral or bacterial); allergy (the most common cause); nasal polyps; chronic ethmoiditis; or neoplasia in the region of the cribriform plate

Mucosal injury: from atrophic rhinitis, or such as a chemical injury or viral injury after influenza

Intracranial lesions: caused by a meningeal neoplasm in the frontal lobe, or resulting from intracranial surgery

Hysteria

Complaint: Enhancement (hyperosmia) or perversion of the sense of smell or taste (parosmia, dysgeusia). Normal smells become putrid, and food smells rotten. The patient finds it difficult to eat or cook. This disorder may result from idiopathic, viral, or drug-related causes, or from a vitamin deficiency or trauma. It may also occur because of olfactory hallucination (in schizophrenic and obsessional patients) or from an injury to the uncus of the temporal lobe.

EVALUATION OF OLFACTORY DISORDERS

1. History: fracture, infection, allergies
2. Careful examination of the nose
3. Cranial-nerve exam, including funduscopy
4. Testing of olfactory sense with vials of coffee grounds, lemon extract, and ammonia (each side of the nose is tested separately)
5. Sinus x-ray films with polytomographic sections through the cribriform plate
6. Allergy testing
7. Therapeutic trials
   a. Prednisone
   b. Vitamin A

8

NASAL AND FACIAL EMERGENCIES

William R. Wilson

Epistaxis
  Anterior septal bleeding
  Rare disorders
  Arterial epistaxis
Treatment for persistent nasal
      bleeding
  Nasal tampons
  Nasal balloons
  Anterior and posterior nasal
      packs
  Surgical options
  Treatment of rare disorders as-
      sociated with epistaxis
Nasal fractures: Office or emer-
      gency-room repair
  Examination
  Treatment
Septal drainage procedures
  Septal hematoma
  Septal abscess
Repair of soft-tissue lacerations of
      the head and neck
  Evaluation
  Preparation of the wound for
      closure
  Repair of facial lacerations
  Repair of mucosal lacerations
  Repair of through-and-through
      lacerations of the lip
Differential diagnosis of disorders
      of the facial nerve
  Inflammatory disorders
    Bell's palsy
    Melkersson-Rosenthal syn-
      drome

Infectious disorders
  Viral disorders
  Bacterial disorders
Central causes
  Cerebellopontine-angle neo-
      plasms
  Intratemporal neoplasia: Rare
      causes of facial palsy
  Trauma
The facial nerve: Stages of degen-
      eration and diagnostic
      tests and treatment
  Stages of facial-nerve degenera-
      tion
    Neurapraxia
    Axonotmesis
    Neurotmesis
  Electrodiagnostic testing
    Nerve excitability testing
    Conduction-latency tests and
      strength-duration tests
    Electromyography
  Therapy for Bell's palsy
  Therapy for persistent facial pa-
      ralysis: Surgical options
    Facial-nerve decompression
    Hypoglossal transplant
    Autogenous nerve grafts
    Muscle transposition tech-
      nique
    Cross-facial nerve grafting
    Nerve–muscle pedicle transfer

EPISTAXIS

ANTERIOR SEPTAL BLEEDING

Anterior septal bleeding from Kiesselbach's plexus (Fig. 8-1), primarily venous, is by far the most common variety of nosebleed. Almost without exception, it is the type of nosebleed seen in children, and it is the most common site of bleeding in adults.

Often there is a history of trauma or hay fever, and most commonly there are repeated episodes of bleeding. The possibility of clotting disorders should be ruled out, and familial histories of epistaxis should be sought.

Examination demonstrates venous bleeding from one side of the nasal septum. A check should be made for septal spurs and deviations, ulcerations, septal perforations, granulomas, foreign bodies, and tumors.

There is a great deal of folklore regarding the *treatment* of epistaxis. Patients, and in the case of children their parents, should be questioned about treatment methods because many old tricks or misconceptions, such as lying down, merely serve to prolong bleeding.

Taking the time to teach patients the principles of treatment for minor epistaxis will help them have fewer bleeding episodes.

The patient should sit up and lean forward to reduce venous pressure in the head and to prevent the swallowing of blood. A small piece of cotton soaked with a vasoconstricting nose drop such as phenylephrine hydrochloride (Neo-synephrine) or oxymetazoline hydrochloride (Afrin) is placed in the vestibule of the nose and pressed against the bleeding site for 5 to 10 minutes. This will stop almost all venous bleeding of this type. The patient should be given precautions to prevent retraumatizing the area: children's nails should be trimmed; humidity is helpful in dry weather or homes; and a lubricant, such as bacitracin ointment or petroleum jelly, helps promote healing.

If these remedies fail, the mucous membrane can be anesthetized using cotton soaked with 4% cocaine or 4% lidocaine (Xylocaine) for 5 minutes. A silver nitrate stick can be applied to the membrane over the bleeding site and to any vessels that appear prominent.

Occasionally, a small artery in the septal mucous membrane either will fail to stop bleeding or will rebleed a short time later. These episodes can usually be controlled by anesthetizing and recauterizing the area, and by placing a small amount of oxidized regenerated cellulose (Surgicel) against the bleeder, or a small packing of petrolatum gauze strip in the nasal vestibule for 24 hours.

Problems that may require an otolaryngologic consultation include chronic nasal ulcerations due to bony septal spurs, or septal deviations

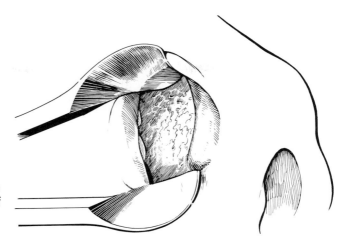

Fig. 8-1. Speculum exam. Venous plexus located on the anterior nasal septum is the most frequent source of epistaxis, particularly in children.

that become dried and easily traumatized by the flow of air through the nose. Correction may require a *submucous resection* or septoplasty in order to remove the spurs and correct the deflection.

Patients with clotting disorders or liver or renal disease require especially careful treatment so that the mucous membrane does not suffer further abrasions. These cases are best handled with soft cotton tamponades wetted with long-acting nasal vasoconstricting drops, such as oxymetazoline hydrochloride 0.1% (Afrin nasal solution), humidity, and copious lubricants. Packing should be avoided at all costs, but, if necessary, it can be accomplished with a piece of Surgicel or Oxycel, which does not require removal.

RARE DISORDERS

Bleeding secondary to granulomas is uncommon, but if it is seen, the patient should be referred for biopsy and further management. *Osler-Weber-Randu disease,* or *familial hereditary telangiectasia,* presents with frequent epistaxis, up to several times daily in extremely severe cases. If local measures do not control the bleeding, a surgical procedure involving skin grafting of the nasal septum (septal dermoplasty) can be used. *Long-standing nasal foreign bodies* can cause epistaxis. They are usually impacted and often require removal by a nasal surgeon with the patient under a general anesthetic.

ARTERIAL EPISTAXIS

Arterial epistaxis is a less common variety of epistaxis involving primarily middle-aged or elderly adults. The patient's history may include hypertension, nasal trauma, or surgery. When arterial epistaxis presents in young males, examination for a vascular tumor is required in order to rule out juvenile nasopharyngeal angiofibroma.

Examination for arterial epistaxis requires a headmirror or surgical headlight and a large nasal suction. The most common finding is unilateral brisk arterial epistaxis from a branch of the sphenopalatine artery on the posterolateral wall of the nose, either below or above the inferior turbinate. Less commonly, the bleeding is from an ethmoid artery; if this is the case, bleeding is commonly seen from the superior aspect of the nose, above the level of the middle turbinate.

Treatment of arterial epistaxis involves the following steps: (1) The patient must be seated and leaning forward slightly so that the blood runs from his nose. This permits an assessment of the bleeding and helps prevent nausea in the patient from ingested blood. (2) A vasoconstrictor such as phenylephrine hydrochloride (Neo-synephrine) or oxymetazoline hydrochloride (Afrin) must be sprayed into the nose. (3) Using bayonet forceps, the nose is packed gently with long cotton pledgets soaked in 4% cocaine or 4% lidocaine (Xylocaine solution) in order to induce anesthesia and to temporarily tamponade the bleeding for 10 to 30 minutes. A hematocrit is obtained. (4) Upon removing the pledgets, the bleeding site is electrocauterized, and a small piece of Surgicel is placed over the area. Recent reports indicate that a specially designed nitrous oxide cryosurgical probe* that is capable of −90°C will control the bleeding in some cases if placed on the site for 30 to 60 seconds. If the equipment is available, this method constitutes a relatively simple measure with low morbidity.

Once the bleeding is controlled, the patient is given the following instructions to help prevent recurrence. Do not blow your nose forcibly. If you must sneeze, expel the sneeze through your open mouth. Avoid strenuous exercise and stooping. Sleep with two or three pillows to elevate your head at night. Avoid hot drinks, alcohol (a nasal vasodilator), and smoking. Do not take aspirin or medications that contain aspirin. Use a laxative if constipated. It is advisable to use a long-lasting vasoconstricting nasal spray, such as xylomethazoline hydrochloride 0.1% (Otrivin nasal solution) or oxymetazoline (Afrin) for several days.

TREATMENT FOR PERSISTENT NASAL BLEEDING

If bleeding persists or recurs, the nose must be packed or tamponaded. There are several varieties of tampons and balloons available commercially.

*Frigitronics Corporation

NASAL TAMPONS

Nasal tampons, made of compressed Merocel sponges,* are sometimes useful in the treatment of epistaxis. The sponge swells with hydration and acts as a tamponade. They come with or without a silicone-cannula airway through the packing. Tampons are most effective when the bleeding is in a relatively confined space, such as under the inferior turbinate, where they can be wedged into position. These sponges must be anchored anteriorly to prevent slippage into the pharynx. If the tampon is placed in the posterior portion of the nose, the patient should be hospitalized for observation. Tampons should be removed after 5 days. They may be regularly soaked with vasoconstricting nasal sprays, antibiotic solutions (1 ml of bacitracin 1:1000), and thrombin. All patients treated with tampons should receive antibiotic coverage.

NASAL BALLOONS

In general, a nasal balloon is placed more easily, and without as much discomfort for the patient, than nasal packing. Unfortunately, balloons are not always as successful as packing in controlling bleeding, because they cannot conform as well to the nasal interstices. Balloons often cause mucosal ulcerations from pressure necrosis, and they have a tendency to leak and, occasionally, burst. Balloons, and to a lesser degree packing, can result in intranasal scarring and partial nasal obstruction. This becomes apparent several weeks after their removal.

Before a balloon or pack is put in place, the patient's nose must be well anesthetized with a topical anesthetic. Premedication with morphine sulfate, IM, or diazepam (Valium) is recommended. In general, the balloons leak less when inflated with normal saline than when inflated with air. The balloons must be carefully secured anteriorly in order to prevent their displacement into the lower airway.

It is our practice to hospitalize patients with balloons or posterior nasal packing. Arterial hypoxemia and hypercapnia are frequent sequelae of posterior nasal packs, and arterial blood gases should be monitored in some patients. Obstructed airways can occur secondary to a slipped packing or balloon, swelling of the palate, or relaxation of the tongue secondary to exhaustion and pain medication. Nurses must be aware of these potential airway problems. A rubber nasopharyngeal airway placed in the opposite side of the nose can be of benefit. Patients must be placed on antibiotics, such as penicillin, erythromycin, or cephalexin, in order to prevent sinusitis. In addition, good mouth care should

*Americal Corporation

be maintained with lemon and glycerine drops and oral irrigations with half-strength hydrogen peroxide q.i.d.

The packing or balloon is removed after 5 days. Ferrous sulfate, 300 mg p.o. every day, helps to replenish lost hemoglobin. In general, our patients are transfused only if they are symptomatic from blood loss, or if the stabilized hematocrit is below 25% to 30%.

ANTERIOR AND POSTERIOR NASAL PACKS

A method of cinching an anterior packing tightly into the nose has recently been described, which accomplishes a tight packing that does not slip into the nasopharynx* (Fig. 8-2). This *modified anterior pack* eliminates the need to place a packing into the posterior choana through the mouth and is more comfortable, and probably as effective, as standard anteroposterior (AP) packing for the patient. Other advantages include less eustachian-tube blockage and less nasopharyngeal obstruction, permitting less respiratory obstruction through the opposite nares.

When a nasal balloon or tampon is not available or has not been effective, an *anterior* or *posterior nasal pack* should be put in place. The patient must be well-medicated beforehand, and the nose and palate must be anesthetized (Fig. 8-3).

The packing is prepared by folding a 4 × 4 gauze to a size estimated to be slightly larger than the posterior choanae. It is secured with two heavy silk sutures. The four ends of the sutures are left about 1 foot in length. Bacitracin ointment is worked into the pack to act as a lubricant and to inhibit infection.

A soft rubber catheter is inserted through the side of the nose that is bleeding until the end is seen in the oropharynx; it is then grasped with a Kelly clamp and brought out through the mouth. Two ends of the sutures are secured to the catheter, which is now withdrawn from the nose as the pack is placed into the mouth and around the soft palate, and is cinched into the posterior choana. The physician can use his fingers or a Kelly clamp to facilitate placement of the pack in the choana.

With the posterior pack held tightly in place by the silk sutures, petrolatum gauze packing ½ inch wide and approximately 6 feet in length is packed in the nose. This packing should be placed tightly and should completely surround the silk sutures to keep them from coming in contact with, and cutting, the mucous membrane. More than one of the petrolatum gauze packings may be required. Once the nose is packed, the posterior pack is secured into position by tying the ends of the suture over a rolled 1-inch × 1-inch gauze placed at the anterior nares. The other suture is brought out through the mouth and taped to the

*M. Joseph, M. Strome: Personal communication

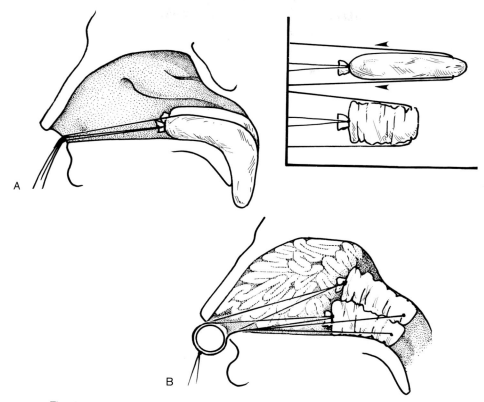

Fig. 8-2. An alternate method of placing an anterior nasal pack. (*A*) Two finger cots are prepared by placing a second heavy silk suture, which is cut approximately 12 inches long, through the distal end (tip). After the patient has been premedicated and the nose has been anesthetized with topical anesthetics, such as 4% cocaine solution on wrung-out cotton sponges, the finger cots are placed partway through the posterior choana. (*B*) The anterior nose is then packed with ½-inch petrolatum (Vaseline) gauze in a layered fashion so that the silk sutures do not come in contact with mucosa or skin. When completed, the sutures through the tip of the finger cot are pulled tight, and all sutures are tied over a gauze in the nares. This maneuver creates a pressure packing at the posterior end of the turbinates, the region where the sphenopalatine artery enters the nose.

cheek. Its purpose is to facilitate removal of the pack. The patient is hospitalized with the same medications and precautions as those patients treated with nasal balloons.

SURGICAL OPTIONS

If the bleeding persists, the patient should be advised about further treatment. Referral to an otolaryngologist should be made at this point.

(Text continues on p. 154)

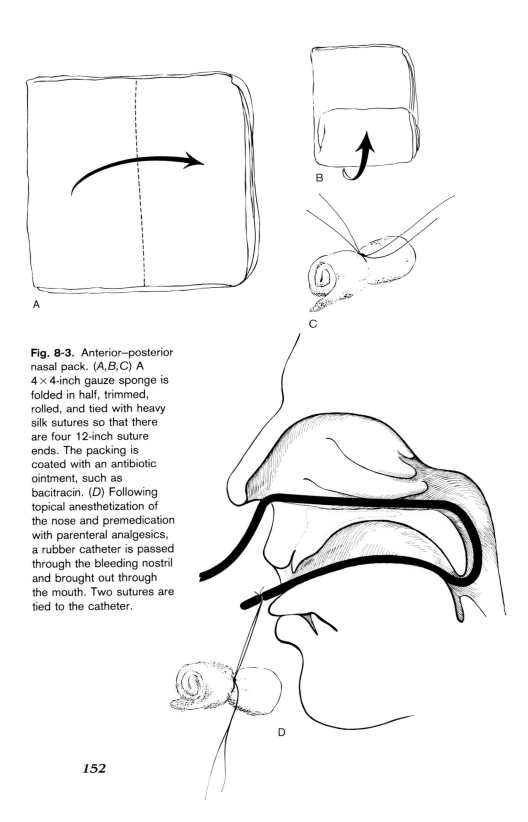

Fig. 8-3. Anterior–posterior nasal pack. (*A,B,C*) A 4 × 4-inch gauze sponge is folded in half, trimmed, rolled, and tied with heavy silk sutures so that there are four 12-inch suture ends. The packing is coated with an antibiotic ointment, such as bacitracin. (*D*) Following topical anesthetization of the nose and premedication with parenteral analgesics, a rubber catheter is passed through the bleeding nostril and brought out through the mouth. Two sutures are tied to the catheter.

A

B

C

D

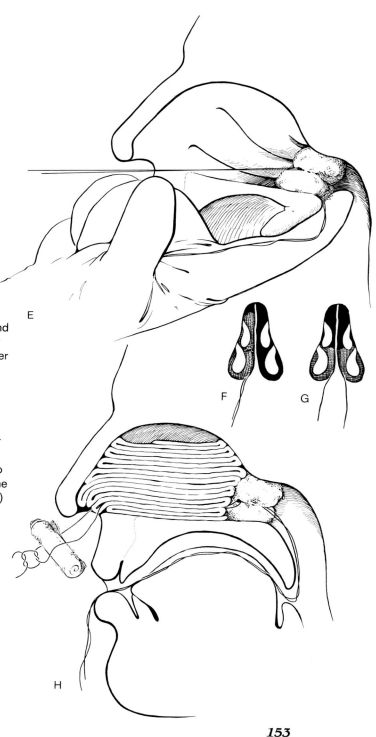

Fig. 8-3 *Continued.* (*E*) The catheter is carefully withdrawn from the nose, and the pack is guided and pressed into the posterior choana with an index finger or Kelly clamp. (*F*) The proper position of the posterior nasal pack. (*G*) A frequent error, demonstrated here, is to place one suture on either side of the septum. This does not allow the pack to be drawn tightly against the posterior bleeding site. (*H*) One-half-inch petrolatum gauze is packed by layers into the nose, inferiorly to superiorly, against the posterior pack. Care is taken to completely surround the sutures with the layering gauze so that neither the nasal mucosa nor the nasal ala can be cut by them. The sutures are pulled tight and tied over a soft, rolled gauze at the nares.

The surgical options are listed below in relative order of popularity, and depend in part on the facilities available.

1. *Transantral ligation of the internal maxillary artery and ligation of the anterior and posterior ethmoidal arteries* is almost uniformly successful and leaves only a small scar adjacent to the medial canthus of the eye and in the buccogingival sulcus. The risks are slight when this procedure is performed by an experienced surgeon, but they include possible eye injury and occasional numbness in the area of the infraorbital nerve, in the ipsilateral hard palate, or in adjacent teeth. Because of the relative safety of this procedure, coupled with the elimination of the need for packing and the associated complications and hazards, many surgeons recommend this surgery as the initial treatment. The success rate is approximately 80% to 90%.

2. *Ligation of the ipsilateral external carotid artery* is a simple procedure, but it has a lower success rate because of the large, collateral blood supply in the head and neck.

3. *Selective internal maxillary arteriography and embolization* is an elegant method available in large medical centers. A skilled head-and-neck arteriographer is required. The success rate is approximately the same as that of arterial ligation.

TREATMENT OF RARE DISORDERS ASSOCIATED WITH EPISTAXIS

Juvenile nasopharyngeal angiofibroma (JNA) is a benign vascular tumor unique to postpubescent adolescent males (13 to 21 years of age) that most often presents with a very brisk epistaxis. Once the bleeding is controlled, the diagnosis is made by x-ray studies of the paranasal sinuses. Biopsies are not to be done because of the risk of excessive hemorrhage. Removal should be attempted following arteriography and embolization of the feeding vessels.

Intracranial aneurysms secondary to trauma or infection occur spontaneously. They have been known to rupture into the sphenoid sinus or, from a pulsating mass, into the nasopharynx. The hemorrhage is massive and usually fatal.

NASAL FRACTURES: OFFICE OR EMERGENCY-ROOM REPAIR

Patients with a history of nasal injury, some epistaxis, and a question of nasal fracture are frequently seen in emergency areas. Palpation of the nasal bridge, an intranasal examination, and an x-ray evaluation constitute a complete examination. Severely injured noses involving comminuted bone fractures and cartilage breaks or tears will require referral to an ENT surgeon.

EXAMINATION

1. If there is little or no swelling, it is particularly useful to palpate the nasal bones and orbital rims in order to identify small fractures. Ascertain whether the paired upper and lower lateral cartilages are torn.

2. Inspect the nasal septum both externally and with a nasal speculum for evidence of fracture, dislocation, or hematoma formation. The correction of internal deformities must accompany the correction of external deformities. Failure to drain a septal hematoma will result in gradual resorption of the septal cartilage and a saddle deformity of the nose. In addition, a septal hematoma may lead to a septal abscess and subsequent meningitis. Septal hematomas can occur gradually, and, therefore, patients should be told to return in 24 hours if nasal breathing becomes obstructed.

3. Ask the patient to lean forward in order to identify any cerebrospinal fluid (CSF) leakage. A brief check should be made for the presence or absence of the sense of smell.

4. X-ray views for nasal fractures should include lateral projection, Water's view, hyperextended Water's view, and superinferior tangential view. For the superinferior tangential view, a bite-wing film is placed between the tongue and palate, providing an excellent view of the nasal bones (Figs. 14-22 and 14-23). Care must be taken not to overinterpret the x-ray films because the nasal suture lines as well as the impression made by the angular vessels in the nasal bones can be misinterpreted as fractures.

5. Injuries in the region of the nasal bones and the nasal process of the frontal bone may lead to a fracture through the cribriform or ethmoid bones. Patients with such injuries should be asked whether they have noted a small amount of clear drainage after their injury. The drainage is most commonly unilateral and may be intermittent, coming in short, rapid gushes, or may present as a steady flow. CSF is perfectly clear, has a slightly salty taste, and, unlike nasal mucus, contains protein (15 mg/dl to 40 mg/dl) and glucose (50 mg/dl to 80 mg/dl). A clue to CSF leak is the formation of a characteristic "bulls eye" when CSF is mixed

with blood and dried on a white sheet. Clear fluid can be differentiated from watery nasal secretions by means of a positive glucose test using a commercial dipstick designed for testing urinary sugar. Situations in which CSF leakage is possible, for example, when there is a fracture through the cribriform area, should be evaluated with AP and lateral tomography and, if indicated, through a computed tomography (CT) scan with metrizamide. Further evaluation might require injection of markers, such as fluorescein or I-131 albumin, by way of a lumbar puncture.

In general, CSF leakage should be treated by keeping the patient at bed rest with his head elevated at all times, and by maintaining prophylactic antibiotic coverage until the leak seals spontaneously. Leaks that do not stop in 6 weeks require repair. In general, intranasal repair techniques, by way of the external ethmoidectomy approach, work well for small defects. Large tears may require an intracranial approach.

TREATMENT

1. Nondisplaced nasal fractures require no treatment. However, patients should be warned to return for treatment promptly if they experience increasing nasal obstruction, unusual pain or swelling, or clear drainage through the nose.
2. Simple nasal fractures involving depressed fractures of the nasal bones or septal fractures and dislocations can be reduced in a properly equipped emergency area. And nasal fractures in adults can be reduced at any time up to 10 days. It is not uncommon to defer reduction in adults if nasal swelling at the time of the initial visit is severe enough to obscure the adequacy of reduction. In children, reduction should not be delayed more than a few days, if at all.
3. For reduction of a nasal fracture, the patient is premedicated with Demerol or morphine. Intranasal anesthesia is achieved by packing the nose with cotton strips soaked with 4% cocaine or an appropriate substitute. An external field block is obtained by injecting 2% lidocaine with epinephrine 1:100,000 subcutaneously with a No.-27 needle introduced at the root of the nose. Additional injections can be made at the lateral margins of the nose and at the base of the columella if necessary.

Upon removal of the anesthetic packing, a blunt nasal elevator wrapped with moistened cotton to decrease intranasal trauma is introduced into the nose under the nasal fracture and lifted until the deformity can no longer be felt. Most reduced fractures require stabilization with an intranasal Iodoform gauze-strip packing for several days.

Fractures involving the septum or a fracture of both nasal bones may require the use of Asch forceps or Walsham forceps to achieve proper reduction. If after a week, when the swelling is decreased, it is apparent that the reduction is less than satisfactory, the fracture can be corrected further by a nasal surgeon. The technique of treatment varies with the surgical problem and the surgeon's preferences; resetting, packing, internal or external splints, and reduction by means of septorhinoplasty are among the options.

Immediate referral should be made for torn cartilages and for a comminuted fracture involving either intranasal or external laceration or the nearby bony structures, such as the ethmoid, the ascending processes of the maxilla, or the nasal process of the frontal bone (nasal-frontal-ethmoid complex). These patients usually require an open reduction and external nasal splinting to prevent a root-depression deformity. Every effort should be made to achieve the best possible functional and aesthetic results initially because, in general, it is more difficult to achieve excellent results with chronically twisted or distorted noses.

SEPTAL DRAINAGE PROCEDURES

SEPTAL HEMATOMA

A *septal hematoma* should be treated as soon as it is identified. The septal mucosa is cocainized and 1-cm incisions are made on the right and left sides. In order to avoid the risk of septal perforation, the incisions are placed so they are not apposed to one another (Fig. 8-4). Following culture of the accumulated blood, the remaining blood is aspirated from both sides of the nose using a Frazier suction. The status of the septal cartilage can be assessed at this time. A small Penrose drain or piece of ½-inch wide Iodoform gauze is placed in each drainage site to prevent reaccumulation of the hematoma. Finger-cot packings are placed bilaterally to reapproximate the mucosal flaps. We make a practice of hospitalizing patients with a septal hematoma and place them on antibiotics for several days until the danger of infection is past. Patients must be warned of the possibility of saddle deformity, even if the hematoma has been treated expeditiously.

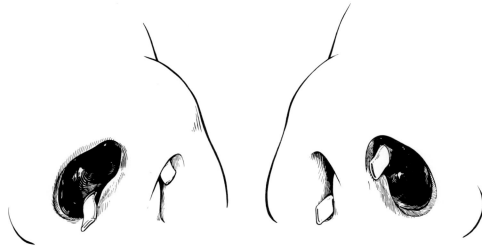

Fig. 8-4. Placement of submucosal Penrose drains for septal hematoma or septal abscess.

SEPTAL ABSCESS

A *septal abscess* almost always evolves from an unrecognized septal hematoma 2 to 14 days following nasal trauma. Patients present with nasal pain and swelling, elevated temperature, headache, and, occasionally, meningitis. Bacterial cultures most often grow a variety of nasal pathogens, including *Hemophilus influenzae, Staphylococcus aureus,* and *Streptococcus pneumoniae.* Therefore, following culture, the antibiotics of choice for treatment are synthetic penicillins, such as nafcillin. The drainage procedure is identical to that described for a septal hematoma. Parenteral antibiotics are maintained for approximately 10 days. Invariably, the caudal cartilage is destroyed, and a marked saddle deformity occurs. These are best repaired by augmentation rhinoplasty, using autogenous cartilaginous or bony implants 6 months or more after the infection.

REPAIR OF SOFT-TISSUE LACERATIONS OF THE HEAD AND NECK*

Although they have had little formal training in surgery, many primary-care physicians, such as family-care practitioners, pediatricians, and in-

*This section was written with suggestions from Howard M. Ecker, M.D., Clinical Instructor in Otolaryngology (Plastic Surgery), Massachusetts Eye and Ear Infirmary, Boston.

ternists, master and understand the techniques of laceration suturing and wound repair and are capable of superior closures of minor wounds in the head and heck. The difference between fair and superior results is often a matter of attention to detail prior to and during the surgery, as well as of appropriate follow-up care.

A minor-surgery room or emergency room must have good lighting, cooperative help, appropriate supplies, and instruments suitable for the work that is to be done. If a physician is frequently called upon to do suturing, a small investment in a few plastic surgery instruments for his own set will ensure the availability of the proper tools. His skill will be enhanced and his confidence will grow as his case volume increases, and familiarity with his own instruments will further increase his surgical skill. (For instance, it is very difficult to close a facial laceration while trying to hold a 6-0 suture in a long, serrated jaw needle-holder designed for abdominal surgery.)

This list of instruments is included only as a guide for selection. Two fine skin hooks are useful (a single and a double). These are the simplest of instruments and most atraumatic to skin. It is also important to have a fine-toothed forceps, such as a Lester forceps, or Bishop Harmon forceps (both with tying platforms). These are used *primarily* to grasp *subcutaneous* tissue to avoid crushing margins of the epidermis. Four very fine, curved mosquito hemostats should be enough. For trimming tissues, a No.-15 or No.-11 Bard Parker surgical blade is the most useful. A few pair of scissors are most helpful. The set should include a good-quality, blunt, curved scissors (very delicate Metzenbaum type), a curved, sharp iris scissors, and a straight, sharp iris scissors. A good marking pen with a fine point is a frequently omitted instrument that can be used for planning alignment, margin refinement, or even a simple flap. A comfortable fine-tipped needle holder, such as the Gilles right or left handed or the Olsen-Hegar needle holder, both with built-in scissors that can readily grasp 5-0 and 6-0 suture material during tying, is a vital and useful instrument.

Finally, binocular loops (1.8 to 2 power is sufficient) are recommended. These also have to be given a short trial but prove their worth with brief use. Delicate margins and sutures become much easier to handle with this simple optical aid.

EVALUATION

When evaluating a head-and-neck laceration, the physician must consider the possibility of injury to underlying neural, vascular, ductal, cartilaginous, bony, or mucosally lined structures. The wound must be examined thoroughly to its depths and must be cleansed by gentle irrigation with sterile saline. A local anesthetic, 1% Xylocaine with epinephrine as medically appropriate, can be used to achieve anesthesia with relatively little discomfort for the patient if it is administered to the subcutaneous tissues through the skin dehiscence. Then the wound can be thoroughly cleansed with a dilute soapy solution, such as Septisol or Hibiclens, dried, draped, and reexamined for severed neural and ductal structures and foreign bodies. Impacted debris must be meticulously removed to prevent traumatic tattoo. Photographs should be taken to document the injury, and tetanus immunization (booster of immune globulin as medically indicated) should be administered.

PREPARATION OF THE WOUND FOR CLOSURE

Ragged lacerations require debridement of obviously nonviable subcutaneous tissue. Cutaneous margins must be judiciously trimmed with a scalpel so they appose well. Wounds should be closed along skin-tension lines whenever possible, a technique that is more easily achieved with older patients, who have lax, mobile skin and readily apparent skin creases. The degree of tension on the closure determines the amount of undermining required; wounds running across lines of skin tension may require greater undermining and increased attention to the subcutaneous and dermal closure. Ideally, the wound should close with little or no tension. Loss of skin may require the use of a local flap or flaps or grafting for coverage.

REPAIR OF FACIAL LACERATIONS

The choice of suture material and suture techniques for repairing facial lacerations varies depending on the wound and the preference of the surgeon. The following is a description of one method that we use with success for facial wounds (Figs. 8-5 and 8-6).

After the wound is prepared for closure, the subcutaneous tissues are judiciously approximated with a few absorbable sutures (mild chromic or Vicryl), on a curved needle (the use of a noncutting one is possible) in order to eliminate any dead space. Next, the dermis is approximated with 5-0 mild-chromic sutures or 5-0 Vicryl sutures, which are placed to slightly evert the edges. This row of sutures usually provides the strength to the closure. Physicians should practice placing all the stitches at precisely the same depth (or at compensating levels) in order to learn to appose the skin with the edges everted perfectly. In most cases, after the subcutaneous closure is completed, the wound should appear closed.

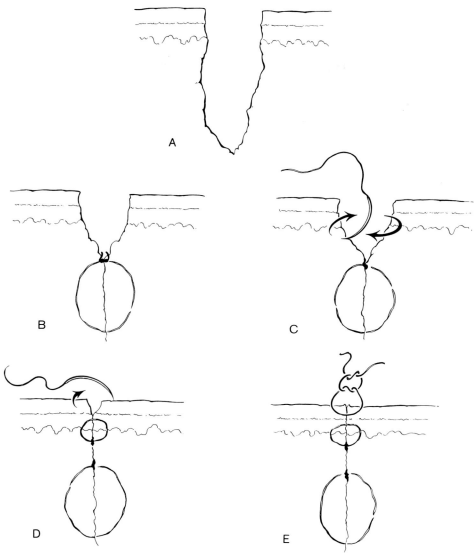

Fig. 8-5. (*A*) Laceration through the skin and subcutaneous layer. (*B*) Closure of the subcutaneous fat layer with a few large, simple stitches of chromic gut tied just tightly enough to approximate but not strangulate. (*C*) A subcuticular stitch with the knot buried closes the dermal layer and places the knot at the deepest portion of the suture tract. (*D*) A small cutting needle with a 6-0 suture may be used for the skin surface layer. The needle must enter the skin 2 mm to 3 mm from the wound margin at an obtuse angle in order to slightly evert the edges. (*E*) The skin stitches are shallow and should be placed 2 mm to 3 mm apart. Sutures should just approximate the edges with as little tension as possible to allow for swelling. Square knots are preferred.

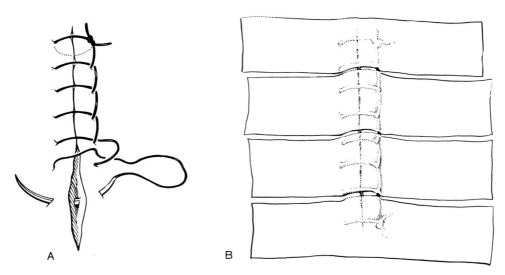

Fig. 8-6. (A) Each stitch or every second or third stitch must be locked. Locked stitches should *not* be used when drainage is expected (*e.g.*, if there are contused surfaces or if there is a diffuse surface and wound-edge bleeding). (B) The wound is then covered, and tension released, with a Steristrip, and the wound is kept dry. A return appointment is given after 4 to 5 days. Antibiotics appropriate to the medical circumstance are used.

The skin sutures ensure that the wound margins remain in perfect alignment despite the swelling and movement that will occur over the next few days. A fine 5-0 or 6-0 monofilament suture, such as nylon on a cutting needle, may be used with a simple stitch, a running subcuticular stitch, or a running locking stitch. We also sometimes use a 6-0 mild-chromic suture, Davis and Geck No. 351-13.

The advantages of this 6-0 mild-chromic closure, used only in areas of little mobility, low concentration of sebaceous glands, and little tension, are that the sutures usually weaken in 4 to 5 days, thus reducing the chance that noticeable stitch marks will form. In addition, the necessity for stitch removal is eliminated, which saves office time, and is of great benefit when dealing with children. Most importantly, the results from using this technique are excellent. The physician must remain aware that occasionally patients have a sensitivity to gut suture.

A tension-releasing, moderate-pressure, antibiotic dressing that is appropriate to the area is the last (but a crucial) part of the closure, because it protects and supports the wound and absorbs drainage. Components of the dressing from inward out are antibiotic ointment, Xeroform gauze, an absorbent gauze layer, and supportive adhesive materials such as Steri-strip.

REPAIR OF MUCOSAL LACERATIONS

Mucosal wounds are often closed with gut suture. Silk sutures are also used; they provide longer lasting alignment strength, but require removal. A tapered needle should be used rather than a cutting one because the latter will cause mucosal teats. The mucosal margins should be joined loosely. Knots must be square, and at least three to four throws of the knot are used in the mouth because the movement of the surfaces and moisture tend to untie the sutures. Any laceration that passes through the vermilion border must be perfectly joined at that border (mucocutaneous junction) by the initial stitches of the repair. Mucosal surfaces heal rapidly, usually without complication and with little or no scarring.

REPAIR OF THROUGH-AND-THROUGH LACERATIONS OF THE LIP

In the repair of a through-and-through laceration of the lip, the principles of repair for the skin and subcutaneous tissue are identical to those described earlier (see Fig. 8-5); however, the mucosal layer of the lip should be approximated by means of a deep-layer closure and a loosely closed surface layer. This technique provides for intraoral drainage and prevents abscess formation from contamination by oral flora that might disrupt the skin closure.

DIFFERENTIAL DIAGNOSIS OF DISORDERS OF THE FACIAL NERVE

The facial nerve (Fig. 8-7) is a mixed nerve with a large motor root that arises from a nucleus located in the caudal portion of the pons. The root loops around the nucleus of the sixth nerve before leaving the brain stem. The fibers of this root innervate the muscles of facial expression as well as the stapedius muscle and the auricular muscles, and the posterior belly of the digastric, stylohyoid, and platysma muscles.

The motor root is joined in the brain stem by a smaller portion of the nerve that arises from the superior salivary nucleus, the *nervus intermedius* of Wrisberg, consisting of preganglionic parasympathetic secretomotor fibers for the submaxillary, sublingual, lacrimal, and nasal glands. The nervus intermedius also includes special sensory (taste)

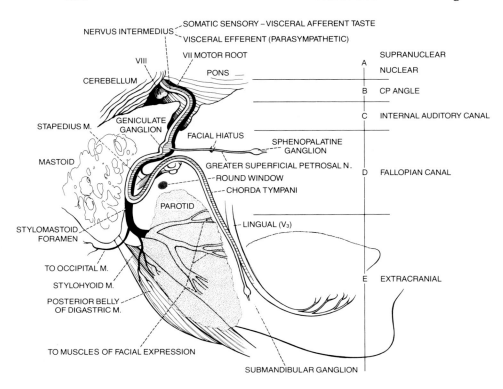

Fig. 8-7. Differential Diagnosis of Disorders of the Facial Nerve.

	Structures	Symptoms	Disorders
A.	Supranuclear	Incomplete facial weakness	Stroke, multiple sclerosis, Guillain-Barré syndrome, amyotrophic lateral sclerosis, tumor
		Emotional facial response more active than voluntary	
		More paralysis in lower face than upper face	
		Associated neurological involvement	
	Nuclear	Complete upper and lower facial palsy	Meningitis, tumors including neuroma, meningioma, cholesteatoma, metastatic tumor
		Associated 6th-nerve palsy (failure of lateral gaze)	
B.	Cerebellopontine (CP) Angle	Lesions may involve auditory and vestibular nerves as well. Large lesions can involve 5th, 9th, 10th, or 11th nerves. The 7th nerve is able to withstand a large amount of stretching without loss of clinical function.	Acoustic neurinoma, meningioma, congenital cholesteatoma, metastatic cancer to CP angle.

Fig. 8-7. Differential Diagnosis of Disorders of the Facial Nerve (*Continued*).

	Structures	*Symptoms*	*Disorders*
C.	Internal auditory canal	The nervus intermedius is involved before there are *clinical* signs of 7th-nerve palsy. Symptoms include decreased tearing, decreased salivary flow, or taste changes. Subtle changes in motor neuron conduction rates can be measured. Associated 8th-nerve signs.	
D.	Fallopian canal	Facial weakness at this level may be associated with decreased taste on the ipsilateral anterior tongue or diminished stapedius muscle reflex testing depending on the location of injury.	Bell's palsy, herpes zoster oticus, Melkersson-Rosenthal syndrome, temporal bone fracture, acute or chronic otitis media, or tumor; 7th-nerve neuroma, glomus jugulare, squamous cell carcinoma
E.	Extracranial	The nerve involves only the branches affected by that tumor or traumatic event.	Trauma, malignant parotid tumor

fibers for the ipsilateral anterior two thirds of the tongue, arising from unipolar cells in the nucleus of the tractus solitarius.

After passing through the cerebellopontine angle of the posterior fossa, the two roots of the facial nerve enter the internal auditory canal, travel in the anterior superior quadrant, and, upon reaching the terminus, enter a 3½-cm-long narrow channel in the temporal bone called the *fallopian canal*. Thus, the seventh nerve is the most encased of the cranial nerves. Paradoxically, it is in the fallopian canal, as it passes through the middle ear and mastoid, that the nerve is most susceptible to injury. During this bony route, prior to emerging from the stylohyoid foramen, the branches comprising the nervus intermedius leave the motor portion of the nerve. The site of lesion in the fallopian canal can at times be localized by careful testing of lacrimation, submaxillary salivation, and taste because the complex anatomy of the nerve aids in the localization of injury and in the differential diagnosis (see Chap. 1).

INFLAMMATORY DISORDERS

BELL'S PALSY

Bell's palsy is an acute facial paralysis of undetermined etiology that each year affects approximately 20 out of every 100,000 persons. Possible causes include viral neuropathy with inflammatory swelling and secondary ischemia due to compression within the fallopian canal. Other possibilities include diabetic and neural ischemia caused by microvascular disease. There is an 80% good-to-excellent spontaneous recovery rate, but it is difficult to identify those patients who will recover and those who will not, and to decide upon a subsequent choice of therapy. Opinions regarding methods of testing, interpretation of tests, and choice of treatment vary widely and are the source of some controversy in the medical literature.

Presenting symptoms include progressive facial weakness that involves all divisions of the peripheral motor nerve relatively equally. There is sometimes accompanying facial pain and often an antecedent history of viral infection or exposure to drafts.

MELKERSSON-ROSENTHAL SYNDROME

Melkersson-Rosenthal syndrome is a recurrent facial paralysis characterized by simultaneous facial palsy and facial edema. Rosenthal noted a fissured tongue in some patients.

INFECTIOUS DISORDERS

VIRAL DISORDERS

Herpes zoster oticus is an occasional cause of facial paralysis. It is identified by the associated painful vesicular eruption of the external auditory canal and auricle, as well as by associated sensorineural hearing loss and vestibular injury of some degree. This is a true viral infection, with neural and intraneural round-cell infiltration. Treatment includes the administration of oral steroids, unless precluded by corneal ulceration.

Rubella and *infectious mononucleosis* are other viral infections reported to have occurred in association with facial paralysis; presumably the pathophysiology and therapy would be identical to that for herpes zoster oticus.

BACTERIAL DISORDERS

Acute suppurative otitis media is occasionally associated with facial-nerve palsy in children and adults. The facial palsy always resolves. In addition to the usual antibiotic regimen, a myringotomy should be performed in order to rapidly remove purulent material and keep it away from the inflamed neural sheath. It is presumed that these patients have an area of dehiscence of the covering of the nerve in the middle ear;

retrograde infection by way of the chorda tympani is a less likely possibility.

Facial paralysis in conjunction with *chronic suppurative otitis media,* indicated by a chronically infected ear with purulent, foul-smelling drainage, represents a surgical emergency. Unlike facial paralysis associated with acute otitis media, it will not resolve. The infected tissue must be removed by a mastoid tympanoplasty, and the facial nerve is uncovered (decompressed) in the middle ear and mastoid from the geniculate ganglion to the stylomastoid foramen. The success rate for resolution of paralysis is high when surgery is performed within a day of onset.

Malignant otitis externa is a virulent form of chondritis and osteitis caused by *Pseudomonas* in diabetics, resulting from an initial superficial otitis externa. Facial palsy is a sign of advanced bone involvement.

CENTRAL CAUSES

Central causes of seventh-nerve paralysis include stroke, multiple sclerosis, Guillain-Barré syndrome, and amyotrophic lateral sclerosis. These are rare forms of facial-nerve paralysis involving incomplete as well as complete facial paralysis associated with other neurological complications.

CEREBELLOPONTINE-ANGLE NEOPLASMS

1. *Acoustic neurinoma:* Sensorineural hearing loss and unilateral vestibular dysfunction occur prior to any loss of facial function. In fact, facial-nerve paralysis is an unusual finding with acoustic neurinoma.
2. *Meningioma:* Other than the fact that acoustic neuromas occur far more frequently, there is no other way to differentiate acoustic neurinoma from meningioma in the posterior fossa. The treatment, surgical extirpation, is the same.
3. *Congenital cholesteatoma:* Congenital cholesteatoma is a rare congenital lesion that may involve the facial nerve medial to the middle ear. It arises from an epithelial rest of the petrous portion of the temporal bone.
4. *Metastatic cancer of the cerebellopontine (CP) angle or temporal bone:* Metastatic cancer of the CP angle or temporal bone is a rare

cause of seventh-nerve paralysis, usually apparent on temporal bone x-ray films.

INTRATEMPORAL NEOPLASIA: RARE CAUSES OF FACIAL PALSY

1. *Glomus jugulare* is an unusual tumor arising from the non-chromaffin-staining cell masses found along Jacobson's or Arnold's nerves in the jugular fossa or middle-ear space. Because facial paralysis is a late complication, the diagnosis is suggested by the presence of a red mass behind the tympanic membrane or in the ear canal, plus a conductive hearing loss. Treatment requires referral to a qualified ear surgeon for extirpation of the tumor and, in most cases, subsequent radiation therapy.
2. A *facial-nerve neuroma* is sometimes recognizable by a bony defect in the auditory canal or fallopian canal. It rarely occurs.
3. *Squamous cell carcinoma* presents as a painful, foul-smelling, draining ear, and at times as seventh-nerve paralysis.
4. *Sarcoma (rhabdomyosarcoma)* often presents with ear symptoms and as a lytic lesion on x-ray film.
5. *Histiocytosis X and leukemic infiltrates* result in osteolytic lesions of the temporal bone that require biopsy by an otologic surgeon.
6. *Malignant parotid-gland tumors* are also associated with facial paralysis.

TRAUMA

1. *Temporal-bone fractures:* Temporal-bone fractures associated with immediate facial-nerve paralysis require surgical exploration as soon as possible. A fracture that passes through the fallopian canal may crush or sever the nerve. The nerve must be uncovered (decompressed) and, if severed, reapproximated with microsutures. Nerve-grafting techniques are used when a portion of the nerve is missing.
2. *Facial injury or laceration:* Laceration of the face with injury to a branch or branches of the facial nerve requires immediate referral to a surgeon familiar with the techniques for repair of the nerve. The distal nerve endings respond to stimulation for 24 to 72 hours after injury.
3. *Surgical trauma:* Occasionally the nerve is injured during surgery involving the parotid gland or temporomandibular joint.

THE FACIAL NERVE: STAGES OF DEGENERATION AND DIAGNOSTIC TESTS AND TREATMENT

STAGES OF FACIAL-NERVE DEGENERATION

The following are stages of degeneration of the facial nerve based upon the neurophysiology and micropathologic changes taking place in the nerve.

NEURAPRAXIA

Neurapraxia is a partial nerve paralysis (paresis) or a complete nerve paralysis during which no change in the results of nerve excitability testing occurs. It is the most minor of the clinically apparent facial-nerve injuries. Neurapraxia is due to a partial obstruction of the flow of axoplasm distally. If the neural injury does not advance beyond this stage, recovery is complete within a few weeks to a month.

AXONOTMESIS

Complete blockage of axoplasm will result in degeneration of the axon distal from the injury. Unfortunately, a change in the results of nerve excitability testing occurs gradually, usually a day or so after this process has begun. In the presence of axonotmesis, the time for recovery of facial movement will be lengthened to 4 to 8 weeks.

NEUROTMESIS

Neurotmesis is a severe lesion that results in injury to the Schwann's cells and in the breakdown of the myelin sheath. This injury often results in a recovery with incomplete reinnervation of the facial musculature and a high incidence of synkinesis, or mass movements of the face. These phenomena are due to the inability of the regenerating axons to find their way entirely to the terminus of the nerve. In other cases they become misdirected, such as when a few nerve fibers from the orbicularis oris reinnervate the orbicularis oculi. For these patients, a smile becomes a wink. Similarly, "crocodile tears" occur when the parasympathetic fibers to the submaxillary gland find their way to the lacrimal gland.

ELECTRODIAGNOSTIC TESTING

There is no simple, reliable test for facial-nerve function. The nerve excitability test is the most universally used because it is easily administered and requires only a few moments, and because the equipment, a nerve stimulator (Hilger nerve stimulator), is compact and relatively inexpensive.

NERVE EXCITABILITY TESTING

Nerve excitability testing measures the difference in the nerve stimulation threshold between the normal and the affected side of the face. A stimulating probe is first placed over the trunk or over one of the branches of the affected nerve. The intensity of 1-millisecond electrical pulses is gradually increased until the facial nerve has become sufficiently stimulated to respond with perceivable twitches. The position of the probe is adjusted slightly until the probe elicits the maximal response at this setting. The setting is then adjusted downward to the slightest perceptible muscular movement and then recorded. This process is repeated on the opposite, paralyzed side. Experience has taught us that a difference of 4 milliamperes (ma) or less is consistent with neurapraxia or a physiological block, and the incidence of recovery is very high. A difference of greater than 4 ma indicates the presence of axonotmesis or neurotmesis, and recovery is less certain and less complete. Complete denervation is often defined as a loss of up to 10 ma in nerve excitability. The major failing of excitability testing is that nerve excitability of the distal segment can be normal for up to 3 days after nerve transection. The test is useful primarily as an aid in advising the patient of the prognosis for recovery and in determining the timing for possible facial-nerve decompression.

Electroneuronography is a new nerve excitability test being employed in some medical centers. It involves computer-assisted comparison of the summating potentials from the involved and noninvolved facial nerves following a super maximal nerve stimulus. This technique provides an evaluation of the percentage of functioning nerve fibers that remain. It improves prognostic reliability.

CONDUCTION-LATENCY TESTS AND STRENGTH-DURATION TESTS

Conduction-latency tests and *strength-duration tests* are also of limited value in predicting which nerves are destined to fully degenerate in time to institute preventative measures, such as surgical decompression.

ELECTROMYOGRAPHY

Electromyography provides early indications of facial-nerve recovery. When inserted into facial muscles, the needle electrode will measure resting electrical activity and activity during facial movement. The fibrillation of denervation begins 14 days after the nerve injury. Motor-unit potentials occur during attempts to move the face and indicate functioning nerve fibers. Polyphasic, or recovery, potentials occur during reinnervation and are a good prognostic sign.

THERAPY FOR BELL'S PALSY

Because inflammation undoubtedly plays an early role in the pathophysiology of Bell's palsy, treatment with corticosteroids instituted within a few days of partial or complete paralysis is probably beneficial, although the medical literature is not absolutely clear on this point. Sudden idiopathic hearing loss and hearing loss from herpes zoster do respond to cortisone therapy, and it is likely that Bell's palsy often represents a viral neuritis as well, although this has not been proven.

We do not use decompression of the facial nerve for the treatment of Bell's palsy except in a patient with neurapraxia, as diagnosed by nerve excitability testing, who fails to improve after a several-month wait. Routine decompression does not improve the recovery rate for patients with axonotmesis or neurotmesis, in our experience.

Eye care is very important and involves the use of methylcellulose drops (artificial tears) during the day and patching of the eye at night to prevent corneal injury.

THERAPY FOR PERSISTENT FACIAL PARALYSIS: SURGICAL OPTIONS

FACIAL-NERVE DECOMPRESSION

Facial-nerve decompression is used to treat facial-nerve palsy following trauma and temporal-bone fracture with immediate loss of facial-nerve function. In these instances the nerve has been transected or crushed in the fallopian canal and must be freed-up for recovery to occur. Also, some surgeons will employ facial-nerve decompression for cases of Bell's palsy with loss of nerve excitability.

Tarsorrhaphy can be done simultaneously with facial-nerve decompression and can be temporary or permanent. This procedure is required only occasionally in Bell's palsy and, because it is quite disfiguring, is employed only when daytime protection of the cornea is necessary.

Atrophy of the facial muscles followed by fibrosis occurs after a period of months. It is likely that physical therapy helps inhibit this process and, therefore, should be instituted. When electromyographic fibrillation potentials indicate that viable muscle fibers remain, it is appropriate to initiate procedures to rehabilitate neural function. Timing, therefore, is important, but no procedure or combination of procedures can totally restore normal facial function.

HYPOGLOSSAL TRANSPLANT

Hypoglossal transplant is probably the most commonly employed method of restoring facial function. It is technically the simplest procedure and usually provides good facial movement. Unfortunately, it results in an initial loss of function of the small strap muscles of the neck, as well as of the ipsilateral muscles of the tongue. Therefore, the patient's condition is worsened before recovery begins. The procedure involves the transection of the ipsilateral hypoglossal nerve, which is then anastomosed to the facial nerve just before it divides at the pes anserinus. A similar procedure has been performed using the spinal accessory nerve, but this leaves the patient with a noticeable and uncomfortable shoulder deformity and has not been a popular technique.

AUTOGENOUS NERVE GRAFTS

Autogenous nerve grafts are used when portions of the nerve are missing. If long grafts are required, the sural nerve is used; for short grafts, the greater auricular nerve is used. Grafting may begin near the brain stem or in the temporal bone, or it may consist of short repairs for soft-tissue defects of the face. Repair of the facial nerve involves microsurgical techniques and has a moderately good success rate. Repairs made within 30 days or less after onset produce the most satisfactory results. However, up to 6 months are required for noticeable improvement to begin.

MUSCLE TRANSPOSITION TECHNIQUE

A method of facial rehabilitation that is employed for longstanding facial paralysis is transposition of the temporalis and masseter muscles. These muscles are divided into functional strips, in which the neuromusculature is maintained, and they are sutured to the appropriate facial muscle groups. The temporalis can rehabilitate the eye and corner of the mouth. The masseter is generally sutured to the orbicularis oris. There may be some renervation of the denervated facial musculature, particularly if muscle atrophy and fibrosis are not advanced. This technique is frequently combined with fascia lata slings and rhytidectomy (face lift).

CROSS-FACIAL NERVE GRAFTING

Cross-facial nerve grafting is a bold procedure. Following dissection and selective sectioning of small branches of the intact facial nerve, a sural-nerve graft is tunneled subcutaneously and anastomosed to branches of the nonfunctional facial nerve. To date, experience with this procedure is limited. The drawback is that recovery is slow and both sides of the face are weakened.

NERVE–MUSCLE PEDICLE TRANSFER

Nerve–muscle pedicle transfer is a newer technique that involves taking very small muscle pedicles based on the ansa hypoglossi from the sternohyoid, sternothyroid, and omohyoid muscles in the neck and tunneling them to and implanting them in the levator anguli oris, depressor anguli oris, and orbicularis oris. This procedure is still in the developmental stage.

9

PAIN SYNDROMES IN THE HEAD AND NECK

Joseph B. Nadol, Jr.

Sources of referred ear pain
  Dental pain and the temporo-
        mandibular-joint syn-
        drome
  Salivary glands
  Nose and paranasal sinuses
  Nasopharynx
  Oropharynx
  Laryngopharynx and esophagus
  Neck
  Neuralgia-causing otalgia
    Ramsay Hunt syndrome
        (herpes zoster oticus)
    Glossopharyngeal neuralgia
        (tympanic neuralgia)

Trigeminal neuralgia
Sphenopalatine neuralgia
Geniculate neuralgia
Eagle's syndrome
Carotidynia
Sources of referred head and fa-
        cial pain
Ear
Nose and paranasal sinuses
Teeth
Neck
Orbit
Other sources of referred pain

Recurrent or chronic pain is one of the most challenging diagnostic problems in the head-and-neck area. Proper diagnosis requires a familiarity with anatomy and the common sources of referred pain. It also requires that the physician have self-confidence in his diagnostic abilities in the head-and-neck area to exclude significant occult causes of pain.

SOURCES OF REFERRED EAR PAIN

Several cranial nerves and part of the cervical plexus contribute to the sensory innervation of the auricle, external canal, and middle ear. Hence, it is not surprising that disease processes in quite distant sites may refer pain to the ear. In order to determine the cause of ear pain the physician must develop a search strategy, such as is suggested below.

1. *A careful history* should be done to determine whether the pain is primary in the ear or is referred. The history of physiological disturbances in the head and neck, including such disorders as malocclusion, salivary-gland disturbances, significant sinus disease, recurrent bleeding from the nose, pain in the oropharynx and hypopharynx, dysphagia, hoarseness, or masses in the head-and-neck area, will give the first indication of a probable origin of referred pain.
2. *A careful ear examination* will rule out a primary disorder of the ear. This should include otoscopy, manipulation of the external canal and auricle to rule out tenderness in this area, and tests of auditory function. If no local dysfunction or source of referred pain is found, x-ray films of the mastoid and temporal bones will help rule out the presence of a neoplasm in the petrous bone or along the petrous ridge.
3. If primary otologic disease is not found, the examiner must then rule out significant diseases in the head-and-neck area that may refer pain to the ear.

I prefer to investigate referred pain in a systematic way, proceeding from the auricle to the most common sites of referred pain.

Sensory Innervation of the Ear

Cranial nerve V (auriculotemporal portion of V_3) innervates the skin of the tragus, the anterior wall of the external auditory canal, a portion of the helix, the tympanic membrane, a portion of the middle ear, and the tympanic plexus.

Cranial nerve VII supplies cutaneous sensory innervation to the concha, a portion of the posterior canal wall, and the posterior aspect of the auricle. There may be interconnections with nerves VII and IX.

Cranial nerve IX (tympanic nerve, or Jacobson's nerve) innervates the medial aspect of the tympanic membrane and forms a major component of the tympanic plexus on the medial wall of the middle ear.

Cranial nerve X, by way of its auricular branch (Arnold's nerve), mediates cutaneous sensation in a portion of the concha, the posterior aspect of the auricle, and part of the posterior wall of the external auditory canal. Some anatomists believe that there are interconnections between the sensory branches of nerves VII, IX, and X. A portion of the postauricular skin over the mastoid is also supplied by the auricular branch of the tenth nerve. And it is probable that the cough reflex commonly seen when manipulating the external auditory canal is mediated by the auricular branch of cranial nerve X as well.

Cranial nerves C2 and C3, by way of the posterior branch of the greater auricular nerve (C3), supply most of the posterior aspect of the auricle and its lateral surface. The lesser occipital nerve (C2) innervates the posterior aspect of the auricle and the adjacent skin overlying the mastoid cortex.

DENTAL PAIN AND THE TEMPOROMANDIBULAR-JOINT SYNDROME

By far the most common causes of nonotogenic otalgia are disorders of the teeth and temporomandibular joint. Malocclusion, ill-fitting dentures, caries, periapical abscesses, fractures and dislocations of the mandible, unerupted molars, bruxism, and ulcerative lesions of the oropharynx may cause pain in the ipsilateral ear by way of the auriculotemporal branch of V_3.

In temporomandibular-joint syndrome, palpation over the joint while opening and closing the patient's mouth may reveal clicking, subluxation, lateral displacement of the mandible during opening, and tenderness. X-ray results are negative except in the most advanced cases, in which there is also trismus related to advanced degenerative changes in the temporomandibular joint. Examination of the dental arches may reveal abnormalities predisposing to the temporomandibular-joint syndrome or other sources of dental origin for referred otalgia.

SALIVARY GLANDS

Disorders of the salivary glands, including infection, and other inflammatory and neoplastic disorders in the parotid, submandibular, sublingual, and minor salivary glands may be the source of referred pain in the ipsilateral ear.

A careful history and an examination for masses and tenderness are sufficient to exclude this possibility. Sialography is unnecessary unless there is some positive finding in the salivary tissues.

NOSE AND PARANASAL SINUSES

Structural abnormalities, inflammatory disorders, and neoplasms in the nose and paranasal sinuses may cause otalgia. Tumors of the nose and paranasal sinuses and acute, and occasionally chronic, sinusitis, particularly of the maxillary and sphenoid sinuses, may be the source of such pain. Most commonly, sphenoid-sinus pain radiates to the vertex or occiput, but the pain may radiate by way of the vidian nerve to the ear. Some authors believe that spurs of the nasal septum impinging on the middle turbinate may also cause ear pain.

A careful inquiry for suggestive symptoms, such as chronic drainage, tenderness, intermittent swelling, and recurrent epistaxis, is followed by a thorough, careful anterior and posterior examination of the nose. X-ray films of the sinuses are usually deferred unless there are other suggestive symptoms or findings.

NASOPHARYNX

Inflammatory disorders and, especially, neoplasms of the nasopharynx are common causes of pain referred to the ear.

The history may include suggestive symptoms such as bleeding from the nose into the pharynx or chronic discharge. However, the most common presenting signs are ipsilateral serous otitis media and the presence of a node in the anterior or posterior cervical triangles. Cranial-nerve paresis, especially of the sixth nerve, is not uncommon. There is a much higher than average incidence of nasopharyngeal carcinoma among young adult males from mainland China.

Tumors of the nasopharynx are most commonly diagnosed by way of a mirror or transnasal nasopharyngoscopy. Some tumors of the nasopharynx spread out in a submucosal plane, and the physical findings by endoscopy may be extremely subtle or nonexistent. Therefore, if there is a high suspicion of nasopharyngeal tumor, radiography, including a lateral view of the nasopharynx, tomography of the skull base to look for bony erosion, and direct nasopharyngoscopy and biopsy, may be indicated.

OROPHARYNX

Inflammatory or neoplastic disease of the oropharynx may refer pain to the ear by way of the ninth and tenth cranial nerves that form the pharyngeal plexus. In children, tonsillitis is a common cause of otalgia, even, paradoxically, when the child does not complain of throat pain. Parapharyngeal and retropharyngeal tumors or inflammation are other common sources of ear pain. Neoplasms of the lateral pharyngeal wall and the base of the tongue very commonly refer pain to the ear.

Careful examination of the oropharynx with proper light to check for asymmetry, masses, and inflammatory disorders of the posterior oropharyngeal area and mirror examination of the hypopharynx and the base of the tongue are essential. Because neoplasms of the tongue base may spread submucosally and show little or no visual evidence of tumor, palpation of the tongue base and the floor of the mouth is also essential.

LARYNGOPHARYNX AND ESOPHAGUS

Disorders in the area of the laryngopharynx and esophagus may cause referred ipsilateral otalgia by way of cranial nerves IX and X. The most common causes are neoplasms of the epiglottis, pyriform sinus, and postcricoid area. In advanced neoplastic disease, otalgia is considered a negative prognostic sign because it suggests deep invasion.

A careful history should be taken of functional disorders of this area. A careful mirror examination is performed, particularly of the laryngeal surface of the epiglottis, pyriform sinus, and postcricoid area. Appropriate x-ray studies, including fluoroscopy, barium swallow, and tomography of the larynx, are usually not performed unless there is positive symptomatology, or unless the physician has a high index of suspicion of disorders in this area or is unable to accomplish a thorough examination. If a good mirror examination can be accomplished and there is not significant suspicion of a disorder, x-ray films are not usually necessary in the evaluation of otalgia. Even when they are performed, x-ray studies, including barium swallow, are not sufficient to rule out neoplasms of the laryngopharynx and esophagus. Relatively large tumors can be missed even by sophisticated radiographic techniques. Mirror examination is still essential in the diagnosis of neoplasms of the hypopharynx and larynx.

NECK

Disorders of the muscles, spine, and organs of the neck may refer pain to the ear by way of nerves C2 and C3. Such disorders include arthritis of the spine and tumors of the thyroid gland.

A careful history of dysfunction in the area and palpation of the neck, including assessment of mobility of the spine, are usually sufficient to rule out disorders in this area.

NEURALGIA-CAUSING OTALGIA

RAMSAY HUNT SYNDROME (HERPES ZOSTER OTICUS)

Ramsay Hunt syndrome is easily recognized once the herpetic lesions have developed. However, severe pain may precede the vesicular eruption by several days.

GLOSSOPHARYNGEAL NEURALGIA (TYMPANIC NEURALGIA)

Glossopharyngeal neuralgia consists of attacks of intense, deep, boring pain at one or more sites along the course of the distribution of the ninth cranial nerve. Typical locations of pain include the base of the tongue, the soft palate, the tonsillar area, and deep within the ear. The pain may be triggered by certain acts, such as swallowing. The character of the pain is usually described as severe, intense, and boring and lasts only seconds. A few cases of glossopharyngeal neuralgia associated with syncope have also been described. *Tympanic neuralgia* is considered a subcategory of glossopharyngeal neuralgia in which pain is limited to the ear. The pain is usually felt deep within the ear and may be triggered by the stimulation of other areas innervated by the glossopharyngeal nerve, particularly in the throat. If there is a trigger point within the throat, local anesthesia of the area may prevent pain. If there is no trigger point within the throat, glossopharyngeal neuralgia is diagnosed by excluding other possible causes of pain.

If pain is limited to the ear, transection of Jacobson's nerve by way of a transcanal tympanotomy may be curative. The glossopharyngeal nerve may also be approached through an external cervical route or an oral route through the tonsillar fossa.

TRIGEMINAL NEURALGIA

A classical presentation of trigeminal neuralgia includes paroxysmal, severe, lancinating pain in the face. However, in a typical case the pain may be limited to an area near the ear.

SPHENOPALATINE NEURALGIA

Pain characteristic of sphenopalatine neuralgia is located in the lower aspect of the external ear, mastoid, occipital area, neck, or shoulder. The pain is described by the patient as deep and boring and may last minutes to hours. Associated symptoms may include unilateral or bilateral lacrimation, nasal congestion, and pain and tenderness in the upper teeth.

Local anesthesia of the sphenopalatine ganglion may abort the pain during an attack. This may be accomplished through the use of 10% cocaine on a nasal pledget or the injection of 1% Xylocaine by way of the greater palatine foramen. If pain is frequent or severe enough to warrant a surgical procedure, the sphenopalatine ganglion may be removed by a transantral approach.

GENICULATE NEURALGIA

There have been a few reports of pain caused by neuralgia originating in the geniculate-ganglion area. The pain is characterized as deep within the ear, but it may radiate to other parts of the face. If analgesics are not successful in controlling the paroxysms of pain, relief may be achieved by sectioning the nervus intermedius portion of the facial nerve intracranially. Certainly, the diagnosis of geniculate neuralgia is one of exclusion, and some authors consider this another manifestation of tympanic neuralgia.

EAGLE'S SYNDROME

An elongated styloid process or a calcified stylohyoid ligament may cause referred otalgia, in addition to difficulty with swallowing, owing to pain in the lateral aspect of the posterior oropharynx. The diagnosis of Eagle's syndrome is confirmed by the presence of tenderness over an elongated styloid process and calcification verified by radiography.

Often the pain will regress spontaneously, but if it persists, the styloid process may be removed either by an external cervical or a transoral approach.

CAROTIDYNIA

Pain associated with carotidynia is usually localized to the neck and may radiate to the ear. It may be aggravated by head movement or swallowing. After other possible causes of pain have been excluded, the diagnosis of carotidynia is confirmed by reproducing or aggravating the pain by putting pressure on the carotid in the area of its bifurcation. The artery will feel otherwise normal. The injection of a local anesthetic should relieve the pain temporarily.

Most cases of carotidynia are self-limited and regress spontaneously within a year. To treat severe cases, the use of a short course of corticosteroids has been recommended.

If, as will occur in a great number of cases, a thorough head-and-neck examination and evaluation of all possibly significant symptoms has failed to lead to a reasonable, working diagnosis or a cause of otalgia, the test of time may be invaluable. That is, it is not unreasonable to inform a patient that no significant disease has been found but that the symptoms should not be ignored. The patient should be reexamined in 2 to 3 months or sooner if the pain worsens or new symptoms develop.

SOURCES OF REFERRED HEAD AND FACIAL PAIN

It is not the purpose of this section to review all the various causes of headache and facial pain. It is assumed that the reader is familiar with the fact that headache may be caused by inflammatory or vascular disturbances of the scalp, blood vessels of the head, muscles, and meningeal structures, and that common syndromes include migraine, cluster headaches, lower-half headaches, tension headaches, an increase in intracranial pressure, irritation of the meninges, and cranial neuralgias.

In the evaluation of headache, it must be understood that referral of pain to the head may occur in disorders of the ear, nose, paranasal sinuses, dental structures, neck, orbit, and even the heart.

EAR

Inflammatory or neoplastic diseases of the ear may refer pain to the postauricular, or mastoid, area and the temporal area of the head. Severe pain in the presence of infection of the ear may be a sign of impending serious complications. With acute or chronic active otitis media, headache may be an early sign that the disease has spread to the petrous apex, meninges, or lateral venous sinus. Chronic active otitis media is almost never painful, and severe pain almost always suggests a serious complication. The differential diagnosis is based on the spread of infection to surrounding cranial structures or the presence of squamous cell carcinoma within the middle ear or mastoid, which occurs most frequently in the setting of chronic drainage.

NOSE AND PARANASAL SINUSES

Pain from inflammatory and neoplastic disorders of the nose and paranasal sinuses is usually well-localized to the area of disease, but some referred pain is not unusual. For example, a patient with a disorder of the maxillary sinus will often complain of pain in his upper teeth. With ethmoid-sinus disease, the pain may be localized behind the patient's eyes or deep between the eyes. With sphenoid-sinus disease, the pain may be referred to the vertex or occiput.

TEETH

Disorders of the teeth and temporomandibular joint may refer pain to other areas in the trigeminal distribution or to adjacent structures, such as temporalis musculature.

NECK

Disorders of the cervical spine may refer pain to the distribution of the upper cranial nerves, particularly of C2 and C3.

ORBIT

Disorders within the orbit are a frequent source of headache. The most common of these is an increase in intraocular pressure. The most common problem in differential diagnosis is determining whether the pain is of frontal-sinus origin or ocular origin. Other suggestive symptoms in the history, x-ray films of the sinuses, and an ophthalmologic exam will almost always differentiate between the two.

OTHER SOURCES OF REFERRED PAIN

Occasionally, structures distant from the head and neck may refer pain to the head area. An example of this is *atypical angina pectoris*, in which intense pain is felt in the throat, jaw, or lower teeth.

10
SALIVARY-GLAND DISORDERS

Joseph B. Nadol, Jr.

Anatomical considerations
  Major salivary glands
    Parotid gland
    Submandibular gland
    Sublingual gland
  Minor salivary glands
Diagnostic strategy for disorders of the salivary glands
  Clinical history
  Physicial examination
  Categories of salivary-gland disorders
    Acute inflammatory disorders
    Mumps
    Acute bacterial sialadenitis

Obstructive salivary-gland disease (strictures and stones)
Chronic progressive inflammatory disorders
Benign lymphoepithelial infiltration of the salivary glands
Granulomatous infiltration of the salivary glands
Metabolic disorders
Discrete mass within a salivary gland (salivary neoplasm)

ANATOMICAL CONSIDERATIONS

The daily salivary output of approximately 1500 ml is formed in both major and minor salivary glands. The paired parotid, submandibular, and sublingual glands are termed *major* salivary glands. *Minor* salivary glands are found in the oral cavity, including the tongue and soft palate, and in the nasopharynx. Saliva consists of a variable amount of water, mucin, and digestive enzymes. Columnar cells are responsible for the production of mucin, and cuboidal cells are responsible for the production of serous fluid, which contains enzymes. These two principal cell types are found within all salivary glands. The parotid gland produces a predominantly serous saliva, while the sublingual glands produce a predominantly mucinous saliva. The submandibular gland produces a mixed secretion. Minor or accessory salivary glands produce a primarily mucinous saliva.

MAJOR SALIVARY GLANDS

PAROTID GLAND

The normal parotid gland is barely palpable. It is located in the lateral aspect of the face and extends superiorly to the zygomatic arch, inferiorly to the level of the mandible, posteriorly to the cartilage of the external auditory canal, and anteriorly to approximately the anterior margin of the ascending ramus of the mandible. The tail of the parotid gland lies between the mastoid tip and the posterior aspect of the ascending ramus of the mandible in the infratemporal fossa (Fig. 10-1). Clinically, the gland is divided into superficial and deep lobes by the branches of the facial nerve and its major divisions to the muscles of facial expression. The two lobes are actually interconnected between the branches of the facial nerve, and anatomically there is not a true lobular structure. The salivary duct (Stensen's duct) extends from the anterior aspect of the gland, lateral to the masseter muscle, and pierces the buccinator muscle, opening into the buccal mucosa at approximately the level of the second mandibular molar.

Salivary secretion is controlled by an autonomic nerve supply. The preganglionic parasympathetic fibers originate in the inferior salivatory nucleus and reach the gland by way of the ninth cranial nerve. The ninth cranial nerve crosses the middle-ear space as Jacobson's nerve and synapses at the otic ganglion. Postganglionic fibers follow the third

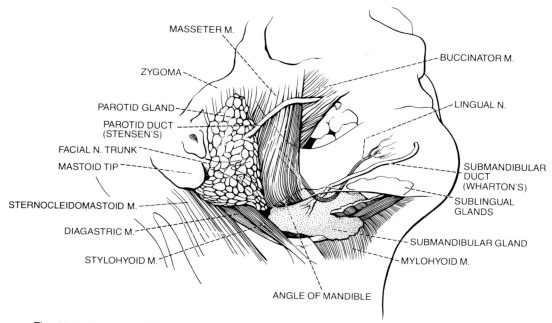

Fig. 10-1. Anatomy of the parotid and submandibular glands.

division of the fifth cranial nerve to innervate the gland. The sympathetic innervation is derived from the carotid plexus.

SUBMANDIBULAR GLAND

The submandibular gland lies in the submandibular triangle and is normally palpable. In the aged, it may become ptotic, which suggests the presence of a mass in the neck. Superiorly, the gland extends under the mandible; inferiorly, it overlays the diagastric muscle; and anteriorly, it extends medial to the mylohyoid muscle (Fig. 10-1). The salivary duct (Wharton's duct) originates on the medial surface of the gland between the mylohyoid and hyoglossus muscles, crosses the lingual nerve, and opens at a papilla in the anterior floor of the mouth lateral to the frenulum of the tongue.

The salivary secretion of the submandibular gland is under autonomic control. Preganglionic parasympathetic fibers originate in the superior salivatory nucleus and reach the submandibular ganglion by way of the nervus intermedius and chorda tympani divisions of the facial nerve and the lingual branch of the fifth cranial nerve. The sympathetic innervation is derived from the carotid plexus.

SUBLINGUAL GLAND

The sublingual gland is located in a submucosal plane in the floor of the mouth and extends anteriorly along the medial aspect of the mandible to the midline. There are usually multiple-duct orifices in the floor of the mouth. The autonomic nerve supply is shared with the submandibular gland.

MINOR SALIVARY GLANDS

It has been estimated that there are between 500 and 1000 minor salivary glands in the oropharynx, tongue, soft palate, and nasopharynx. These are not under obvious autonomic control.

DIAGNOSTIC STRATEGY FOR DISORDERS OF THE SALIVARY GLANDS

A wide variety of inflammatory, infiltrative, obstructive, and neoplastic disorders may be found in the salivary-gland tissue. The practitioner must develop a diagnostic strategy that helps him separate these lesions into smaller categories so that he may intelligently select further diagnostic procedures. For example, although radiopaque sialography may be diagnostic in cases of suspected strictures or stones, it is contraindicated in acute suppurative sialadenitis.

A working diagnosis, whether specific or for a broad category of disorders, is made on the basis of a clinical history and an initial examination.

CLINICAL HISTORY

The clinical history is an essential element in assessing salivary-gland disorders. The patient's complaint is almost always of a fullness or mass within the salivary-gland tissue that may or may not be painful. The following elements of the history should be determined:

1. How long has the mass or fullness been present? Development over a course of hours suggests an infectious disorder, whereas a mass that enlarges slowly over months or years may suggest some infiltrative or neoplastic disorder.

2. Does the fullness or mass fluctuate in size? Intermittent obstruction will often cause great variations in the size of a mass, whereas neoplastic disorders progressively enlarge in size. Postprandial swelling suggests duct obstruction with a stone or stricture.
3. Is there pain? Infectious and other inflammatory disorders often cause pain, whereas benign neoplastic disorders are generally painless unless they cause secondary obstruction of the duct. Malignancies of the salivary glands may cause pain.
4. What is the general health of the patient? Are there acute or chronic illnesses that may relate to the salivary-gland disorder? For example, suppurative parotitis is most commonly seen in a debilitated, poorly hydrated patient with poor dental hygiene. Or the medical history may suggest that a rapidly enlarging mass within the parotid gland may be a local manifestation of lymphoma or leukemia. Enlargement of the gland may also occur in metabolic disorders, including alcoholism, cirrhosis, endocrinopathy, diabetes mellitus, and malnutrition. Systemic granulomatous diseases, such as tuberculosis and sarcoidosis, may also affect salivary-gland tissue.

PHYSICIAL EXAMINATION

The following questions help the physician determine the physical characteristics of a salivary lesion and assign it to a specific category of disease process:

1. Is the swelling or enlargement localized to one gland, or are several glands involved? Multiple-gland involvement even to varying degrees suggests systemic illness, such as an endocrinopathy or an inflammatory disorder (*e.g.,* Sjögren's syndrome).
2. Does the mass or swelling constitute a diffuse increase in the size of the gland, or does the swelling represent a nodule or mass within the anatomical confines of the gland? A diffuse increase suggests an inflammatory disorder, such as an infectious or obstructive disease, Sjögren's syndrome, endocrinopathies, or infiltration of the gland, such as is occasionally seen in leukemia. On the other hand, a mass within but not filling the anatomical confines of the gland suggests a neoplasm or, in rare cases, granulomatous infiltration. A well-encapsulated mass that is easily mobile and possesses a smooth contour suggests a benign lesion; a more infiltrative, poorly mobile, irregular mass suggests a malignant lesion. Facial-nerve paresis or

paralysis in the presence of an irregular or poorly mobile infiltration lesion of the parotid is further evidence of malignant disease.

3. Is there a stone? If so, it may be revealed by palpation of the duct, which is often best accomplished by bimanual examination.

Once a specific working diagnosis has been reached, or at least a category of disease process has been identified, a decision is made as to the need for additional radiographic, chemical, cytological, or serological studies, skin tests, or culture of expressed salivary secretions.

CATEGORIES OF SALIVARY-GLAND DISORDERS

On the basis of history and examination, a salivary-gland disorder can be placed into one of three diagnostic categories, thus reducing the differential diagnostic possibilities.

ACUTE INFLAMMATORY DISORDERS

In acute inflammatory disorders, the clinical history consists of an abrupt onset, pain, tenderness, and erythema over the gland. Fever may be present.

Mumps

Mumps is recognized as a systemic illness with an obvious predilection for children. One or more of the major salivary glands may be involved, and the involved gland is diffusely and acutely swollen and tender to palpation. Trismus and fever are common. In contrast to bacterial sialadenitis, in which purulent material is expressed, salivary secretions expressed from the duct will be clear. Serum amylase is elevated, and the diagnosis may be confirmed by complement-fixation tests if necessary.

Acute Bacterial Sialadenitis

The clinical setting for acute bacterial sialadenitis involves an aged individual with chronic illness, poor oral hygiene, and dehydration. There is marked tenderness, pain, swelling, and erythema over the involved gland. The parotid gland is most commonly involved, but the submandibular gland may also be affected. Palpation of the gland while observing the duct orifice may reveal purulent material, which can be sent for gram stain and cultures. Frequently, the white blood cell count is elevated, and the patient is febrile. The duct should be palpated for the possible presence of a stone. Sialography should not be performed when an infectious process is suspected in order to avoid spread of the suppurative process.

Parenteral antibiotics are required in the treatment of acute bacterial sialadenitis and are selected based on the results of culture and gram stain. The most common organism is *Staphylococcus aureus*. Correction of dehydration and improvement of oral hygiene are important adjuncts to treatment. If no improvement is observed after 5 days of appropriate antibiotic treatment, the possibility of an abscess should be considered. The fascial covering of the parotid may prevent discovery of the fluctuance by palpation until the abscess breaks into a subcutaneous plane. An abscess requires surgical drainage.

Acute suppurative sialadenitis may be caused by obstruction of the duct by neoplasm or by an infiltrative process, such as Sjögren's disease. Therefore, once the acute inflammatory process has resolved, the possibility of a predisposing disorder should be considered.

Obstructive Salivary-Gland Disease (Strictures and Stones)

Partial obstruction of the ducts of the salivary glands may cause recurrent, often postprandial, painful swelling of the affected gland. Such an obstruction may be caused by stone formation or stricture within the duct. Approximately 90% of all stones occur in Wharton's duct, presumably because of the more mucinous and viscous saliva produced in the submandibular glands. The swelling resolves over minutes or days. Occasionally, a patient will say that he can taste or feel a sandlike material within his mouth.

Between attacks the involved gland will be normal. A stone in Stensen's or Wharton's duct may be detected by manual palpation. The calculi may be sufficiently calcified to render them radiopaque. A dental occlusive view often best demonstrates a stone in the submandibular gland. Contrast sialography is useful in demonstrating the cause of obstruction but should not be performed when the gland is acutely inflamed.

Occasionally a stone can be removed if it lies in the distal salivary duct. In other cases, the stone may be broken up by probing the affected duct. Distal strictures may be corrected by simple surgical procedures.

With significant obstruction of the duct, suppurative complication is almost inevitable. If the obstruction cannot be relieved by removing a stone or correcting a stricture of the duct, removal of the gland is indicated.

CHRONIC PROGRESSIVE INFLAMMATORY DISORDERS

Benign Lymphoepithelial Infiltration of the Salivary Glands

The usual clinical history for benign lymphoepithelial infiltration is diffuse enlargement of one or more of the major salivary glands. Some fluctuation of the size of the gland is common, and the gland may at times be somewhat tender or painful. Superimposed acute suppurative sialadenitis may occur owing to the chronic changes in the ductal system. The terms *Sjögren's syndrome* and *Mikulicz's disease* are the eponyms applied to this disorder. Sjögren's syndrome refers to the triad of keratoconjunctivitis sicca, xerostomia, and a connected tissue disorder, usually rheumatoid arthritis. Systemic lupus erythematosus, scleroderma, and polyarthritis are other associated diseases. Middle-aged women are most commonly affected. Mikulicz's disease refers to the same histological disease but without systemic involvement. The etiology is unknown but may involve an autoimmune basis.

Contrast sialography demonstrates sialectasia and nonobstructive ductal dilatation and delayed emptying of contrast material from the duct structures. In advanced disease, sialectasia may progress to the formation of intraparenchymatous cavitary lesions. Microscopically, the disease is characterized by lymphocytic infiltration of the periductal stroma, hyperplastic ductal elements, and atrophy of salivary acini. In questionable cases, biopsy of minor salivary glands of the lip may be done to confirm the diagnosis.

The treatment for benign lymphoepithelial infiltration of the salivary glands is directed towards preventing the complications of chronic sialectasia. Massage in the direction of the normal salivary flow, good hydration, and sialogogues are helpful in maintaining salivary flow and in preventing obstruction. If recurrent infections occur, removal of the gland may be necessary.

Granulomatous Infiltration of the Salivary Glands

The usual clinical picture for granulomatous infiltration of the salivary glands involves one or more slowly enlarging nodules within the parenchyma of a salivary gland.

The most important aspect of diagnosis is to differentiate these lesions from true neoplasms. A clinical history that includes some other systemic signs of granulomatous disease, such as tuberculosis and sarcoidosis, may suggest the diagnosis, and a skin test will also be useful. Corticosteroid therapy may often result in shrinkage of granulomatous nodules caused by sarcoidosis. The presence of chronic drainage from sinus tracts leading from the skin to the underlying nodules in the parenchyma of the parotid gland suggests actinomycosis, and sulfur granules may be identified upon histological examination of the drainage. Without these clear signs, a biopsy may be necessary to confirm the diagnosis.

Metabolic Disorders

Metabolic disorders show bilateral, symmetrical involvement of salivary glands. There is diffuse, generalized enlargement rather than a discrete mass within the gland. The parotid gland is most severely affected. The salivary glands are commonly affected in alcoholism, with or without cirrhosis, in chronic starvation, in diabetes mellitus, and in thyroid disease.

Symmetrical and diffuse involvement suggests a metabolic disorder. Sialography will demonstrate a normal ductal structure. Biopsy, which is seldom necessary, will show degeneration and fatty replacement of the acini. If the underlying disorder can be reversed, some resolution of the salivary-gland enlargement may occur.

DISCRETE MASS WITHIN A SALIVARY GLAND (SALIVARY NEOPLASM)

A wide variety of benign and malignant neoplasms may arise from the epithelial or stromal components of a salivary gland. Although approximately 80% of all salivary-gland tumors arise in the parotid gland, the incidence of malignancy is much lower in the parotid gland than in the submandibular, sublingual, or minor salivary glands. Only 10% of parotid tumors are malignant, whereas approximately 50% of tumors arising in other major or minor salivary glands are malignant.

A history of a painless mass, slowly enlarging over years, generally suggests the presence of a benign neoplasm. A rapidly progressive painful mass or one that causes facial paresis suggests malignancy. An easily mobile mass with smooth contours suggests the presence of a benign lesion, whereas a poorly mobile, infiltrative lesion suggests malignant disease. Contrast sialography combined with tomography of the salivary gland may be useful in confirming the presence of a mass lesion within the salivary parenchyma.

The presence of a mass just inferior to the angle of the mandible is a frequent differential diagnostic problem. The clinician must decide whether the mass represents a neoplasm within the parotid gland or cervical adenopathy. Because the parotid space lies lateral to the mandible, a mass within the parotid tail, except one that is deeply infiltrative, can be moved superiorly and laterally to the mandible, but because the cervical space is inferior to the mandible, a node in the anterior cervical triangle cannot. Contrast sialography may also delineate an in-

Neoplasms of the Salivary Glands

I. Neoplasms of epithelial origin
    A. Benign
        1. Benign pleomorphic adenoma (mixed tumor)
        2. Papillary cystadenoma lymphomatosum (Warthin's tumor)
        3. Oncocytoma
        4. Clear cell adenoma (acinic cell tumor)
    B. Malignant
        1. Malignant degeneration in a pleomorphic adenoma
        2. Mucoepidermoid carcinoma
        3. Adenocarcinoma
            a. Adenoidcystic carcinoma
            b. Acinic cell carcinoma
        4. Squamous cell carcinoma
        5. Others
II. Neoplasms of stromal origin
    A. Benign
        1. Lipoma
        2. Neuroma
        3. Hemangioma
        4. Lymphangioma
    B. Malignant
        1. Sarcoma

traparenchymal lesion, and Technetium 99 is occasionally useful. For example, a benign Warthin's tumor is almost the only parotid tumor that will incorporate Technetium. Hence, in the aged individual for whom surgical excision is a considerable risk, a positive Technetium scan may be taken as good evidence that the mass represents a Warthin's tumor. However, there is some evidence that on occasions a malignant lesion may demonstrate uptake of Technetium. If a neoplasm is suspected, incisional or needle biopsy is seldom recommended. One exception to this rule is a leukemic infiltrate within the gland. Generally speaking, however, excisional biopsy is carried out if a neoplasm is suspected.

A neoplasm in the superficial or lateral lobe of the parotid gland is removed by superficial parotidectomy. This involves dissection of the main trunk and branches of the peripheral facial nerve, and damage to this nerve is a possible, though infrequent, complication of surgery. If malignancy has been confirmed, the patient should be prepared for the possible sacrifice of part or all of the facial-nerve trunk. Most surgeons will not base decisions concerning the facial nerve on a frozen-section diagnosis. Instead, they prefer to close the wound and await permanent sections before accepting a diagnosis of malignancy. Definitive treatment depends on the histological type and grade of tumor. In some cases, excisional biopsy is sufficient. In other cases primary or supplemental radiotherapy is useful. If neck metastases are clinically palpable, neck dissection is indicated.

Excisional biopsies of suspected neoplasms in the parotid gland are not acceptable practice not only because they carry a higher risk of damage to a branch of the facial nerve, but also because they carry a very significant risk of dissemination of the tumor. Inadequate resection of a benign, mixed tumor of the parotid gland will result in multiple recurrences within the parotid parenchyma and cutaneous incision line. Subsequent removal of recurrences may be extremely difficult and carries a much higher risk of damage to the facial nerve.

The presence of a neoplasm in the submandibular gland requires removal of the gland. Removal of the submandibular gland carries a possible risk of damage to the ramus mandibularis branch of the facial nerve, which innervates the depressor anguli oris. Loss of this nerve will result in elevation of the ipsilateral corner of the mouth and, occasionally, some drooling while drinking liquids. Sacrifice of the ramus division is often necessary if malignancy is suspected or confirmed.

Surgery of the minor salivary glands usually involves a simple biopsy. A benign, mixed tumor originating in the oropharynx, most commonly in the soft palate, requires wide local excision.

11

SORE MOUTH AND THROAT AND HOARSENESS

William R. Wilson

Examination of the mouth and throat
  Varicosities
  Leukoplakia
Sore mouth
  Nonulcerative disorders
    Burning-tongue syndrome
    Vitamin deficiencies
    Dry mouth
    Sjögren's syndrome
  Ulcerative disorders
    Aphthous stomatitis
    Herpetic stomatitis
    Stevens-Johnson syndrome
    Pemphigus and pemphigoid
    Behçet's syndrome
    Acute necrotizing ulcerative gingivitis (Vincent's angina)
    Infectious mononucleosis
    Moniliasis
    Syphilis
    Gonococcal pharyngitis
Pediatric disorders
  Varicella
  Acute herpetic gingivostomatitis
  Herpangina
  Hand-foot-and-mouth disease
  Tonsillitis
    Chronic tonsillitis
    Peritonsillar abscess
    Lingual tonsillitis

Deep pharyngeal pain and discomfort
  Pharyngeal burns
  Foreign body
  Glossopharyngeal neuralgia
  Eagle's syndrome
  Globus hystericus
  Hypopharyngeal diverticulum (Zenker's diverticulum)
  Hiatus hernia and reflux esophagitis
  Irritated throat
Hoarseness
  Hyperkeratosis
  Vocal-cord polyps
  Singer's or screamer's nodules
  Submucosal laryngeal hemorrhage
  Contact ulcers of the larynx
  Laryngeal papillomatosis
  Cysts
  Laryngeal stenosis
  Subacute or chronic laryngitis
    Differential diagnosis
      Trauma
      Reflux laryngopharyngitis
      Occupational and home chemicals
  Respiratory tract infections: subacute and chronic
    Viral laryngotracheal bronchitis
    Diphtheria
    Tuberculosis

Laryngeal trichinosis
Syphilis and leprosy
Mycotic infections of the larynx
  Histoplasmosis
  Coccidioidomycosis
Generalized diseases affecting the
    larynx
  Arthritis
  Hypothyroidism (myxedema)
  Systemic lupus erythematosus
Vocal-cord paralysis
Carcinoma of the larynx
  Carcinoma of the glottis, or true
    vocal cords

  Carcinoma of the supraglottic
    area
  Carcinoma of the subglottic
    area
Laryngeal surgery
  Laryngoscopy
  Tracheotomy and tracheostomy
  Laryngectomy
    Rehabilitative surgery follow-
      ing total laryngectomy
    Supraglottic laryngectomy
    Vertical laryngectomy

EXAMINATION OF THE MOUTH AND THROAT

Examination of the mouth and throat should be done in a purposeful manner. Too often the mouth and pharynx are examined at a glance. A better approach is to examine each structure within the mouth and pharynx quickly and independently. One way to proceed is to examine the structures quickly in the following order: the buccal mucosa on the right, right gums and teeth, palate, right tonsil, posterior pharynx, left tonsil, left buccal mucosa, left gums and teeth, floor of mouth, and, with the patient extending his tongue, the posterior one third of the mobile tongue bilaterally. This last area is the region where carcinoma of the tongue usually arises and therefore requires special consideration. Palpation of the base of the tongue and manual palpation of the floor of the mouth bilaterally complete a thorough oral examination.

Among the normal findings of an examination of the mouth and throat might be a *tight frenulum,* which, if it is of no inconvenience to the patient and does not affect his speech, need not be cut. Another normal finding is *geographic tongue,* in which patients have an area of smooth, red, depilated surface with a smooth margin. The areas of depilation gradually change over time. The cause is unknown, and no treatment is necessary. *Median rhomboid glossitis* is a rather common finding involving a rhomboid area of depilated tongue surface. It is located in the midline, just anterior to the circumvallate papillae. It is asymptomatic, and no treatment is required.

The fissured, or scrotal, tongue is another common variation of the appearance of the glossal surface. Fissured tongue may be responsible for glossitis in patients with poor oral hygiene resulting from debris in the fissures. It has been associated with recurrent facial-nerve palsy in *Melkersson-Rosenthal syndrome,* a triad of facial paralysis, facial edema, and fissured tongue.

The *coated tongue,* common among acutely ill and febrile patients, is due to the accumulation of debris on the dorsum of the tongue secondary to dehydration. It is of no specific diagnostic significance.

The *black hairy tongue* is characterized by marked elongation of filiform papillae, which are probably the result of chronic irritation from smoking or eating heavily spiced foods. Maintenance of good oral hygiene with this disorder is troublesome. The tongue needs to be physically cleaned several times a day with a soft, even-bristled toothbrush and a solution of half-strength hydrogen peroxide and normal saline.

VARICOSITIES

Varicosities are commonly present on the floor of the mouth and the lateral surfaces of the tongue and in the hypopharynx. These are considered normal findings in older patients and are of no clinical significance. They rarely, if ever, bleed.

LEUKOPLAKIA

Leukoplakia is a mucosal disorder found in adult patients. It is usually the result of chronic mucosal irritation, usually secondary to tobacco or alcohol use, poor oral hygiene, or irregular teeth or dental appliances. The lesion that results is sharply demarcated, raised, and white and may be smooth or irregular. Leukoplakia may be premalignant and should be biopsied. Under microscopic examination, hyperkeratosis and acanthosis are common features; dyskeratosis is thought to be an indication of malignancy, and when it is present, the area of leukoplakia should be removed either by surgical excision or, in some instances, cryosurgery. Even with the removal of the irritant, leukoplakia frequently recurs and requires removal once again.

SORE MOUTH

NONULCERATIVE DISORDERS

BURNING-TONGUE SYNDROME

Burning-tongue syndrome occurs most commonly in the middle-aged and elderly, especially postmenopausal women, and is usually of undetermined origin. Local factors include caries, infected gums, and an infected tongue. Treatments such as daily multivitamins plus half-strength milk of magnesia mouthwashes t.i.d. are of some help.

VITAMIN DEFICIENCIES

Vitamin deficiencies, especially of nicotinic acid and riboflavin (ariboflavinosis), result in glossitis (indicated by a red or magenta tongue) and cheilosis. These deficiencies may be due to alcoholism and disorders influencing absorption from the alimentary tract, such as pernicious anemia and Plummer-Vinson syndrome. Treatment consists of bland mouthwashes (antacids and water mixes), vitamins, and, occasionally, anesthetic lozenges.

DRY MOUTH

Dry mouth is commonly caused by chronic nasal obstruction and obligatory mouth breathing. Patients will awaken thirsty several times during the night. Correction of the nasal obstruction, usually done surgically, by straightening the nasal septum and reducing hypertrophied turbinate tissue will correct the dry mouth. Other causes include the chronic use of diuretics, certain antihypertensives, tranquilizers, and antihistamine preparations. Sjögren's syndrome should be kept in mind.

SJÖGREN'S SYNDROME

Sjögren's syndrome is manifested by chronic lacrimal and salivary-gland enlargement (most commonly of the parotid), rheumatoid arthritis, and keratoconjunctivitis sicca. Because it is seen most often in postmenopausal women it is probably an autoimmune disorder.

Although keratoconjunctivitis sicca is the most common symptom of Sjögren's syndrome, xerostomia is the most troubling. With xerostomia, a sialogram demonstrates a characteristic nonobstructive sialectasia. Biopsy of salivary glands, usually of a minor gland from inside the lip, demonstrates ductal dilation, periductal infiltrates of lymphocytes, and atrophy of acini. The erythrocyte sedimentation rate and rheumatoid factor are usually elevated. Carious destruction of teeth is a serious consequence of reduced salivary flow. Treatment of xerostomia is symptomatic and involves the following measures: increased fluid intake; sialagogues, such as tea with lemon and sugarless hard candy, as well as mouth moisturizers;* massage of the glands to keep the saliva flowing and to clear plugs from the ducts; and vigorous dental care.

*For example, MOI-STIR, manufactured by Kinswood Lab.

ULCERATIVE DISORDERS

APHTHOUS STOMATITIS

Aphthous stomatitis is the most common form of mouth lesion. Canker sores may occur anywhere, but they usually occur on the buccal and gingival mucosa or on adjacent surfaces of the tongue. Characterized by a spot of burning pain that begins as one or several small (1 mm to 2 mm in diameter, but occasionally up to 1 cm to 2 cm) gray vesicles, the lesions ulcerate and develop red halos with a yellow gray fibrinous base. The cause is unknown; to date no virus has been identified. Many home remedies exist, none of which significantly alters the 2- to 4-day course of pain, which is followed by several days of healing. The use of anesthetic lozenges is helpful, as is the application of triamcinolone (Kenalog) in Orabase or on cotton to the lesion. Treatment using iontophoresis to draw the triamcinolone into the lesion is under study and has been employed with success. Milk of magnesia and sodium bicarbonate mouth washes are old standbys that are thought to have a preventative effect for patients with frequent recurrences.

HERPETIC STOMATITIS

The vesicles or erosions (cold sores) that occur secondary to herpes simplex type I are usually 1 mm to 3 mm in diameter, and typically occur singly or in groups at the mucocutaneous junction of the lip. They often recur in the same location in response to upper respiratory infections, intense sunlight, and hormonal changes. Intraoral lesions are usually found as a cluster of vesicles or ulcers in association with mucocutaneous-junction lesions or a history of them. The disease is self-limited.

STEVENS-JOHNSON SYNDROME

Stevens-Johnson syndrome is an acute febrile disease of unknown etiology that often presents with vesiculobullous intraoral and lip lesions. There is typically an associated erythema multiforme on the lower extremities. Ocular complications involving the conjunctiva and cornea frequently occur. Some cases have been associated with hypersensitivity to drugs. Treatment includes the administration of corticosteroids and analgesia and hydration.

PEMPHIGUS AND PEMPHIGOID

Pemphigus and pemphigoid often begin as extremely painful oral bullae that quickly burst to form superficial ulcerations with mucosal tags. In pemphigus, oral lesions often precede cutaneous manifestations. Pemphigoid results in predominantly mucosal lesions, occurs in an older age group than pemphigus, and, though it is nonfatal, is capable of marked mucosal scarring. The diagnosis is made by biopsy and immunofluorescent studies. In pemphigus there is an intercellular deposition of antiepithelial autoantibodies. In pemphigoid, autoantibody deposition is found only along the basement membrane.

BEHÇET'S SYNDROME

Behçet's syndrome is rare in the United States; it is seen primarily in the Middle East and Orient. It presents with recurrent ulcerations of the mouth and genitalia and associated inflammatory ocular lesions, and primarily affects young males. It is a disseminated disease frequently associated with joint, vascular, and bowel disease.

ACUTE NECROTIZING ULCERATIVE GINGIVITIS (VINCENT'S ANGINA)

Acute necrotizing ulcerative gingivitis is a disease affecting young adults that results from a combination of poor dental care and decreased resistance to infection. Before it is diagnosed, acute leukemia, agranulocytosis and infectious mononucleosis should be ruled out. The infection occurs secondary to fusiform bacilli and oral spirochetes, generally involving the tonsils, gums, and oral mucous membrane. There is necrosis of the superficial mucosal layers, which leaves a gray, necrotic pseudomembrane and cervical adenopathy. The patient complains of malaise, a moderate temperature elevation, and fetid breath. The infection is very sensitive to penicillin and frequent, half-strength hydrogen peroxide oral irrigations. Occasionally, the hypopharynx and larynx are involved.

INFECTIOUS MONONUCLEOSIS

Infectious mononucleosis is a generalized disease affecting adolescents and young adults that can present as tonsillitis and pharyngitis, often with a white membranous exudate associated with cervical adenopathy, splenomegaly, and malaise. In very young children the Epstein-Barr (EB) virus usually produces a mild tonsillitis that is often indistinguishable from that produced by group A beta streptococci. The amount of atypical lymphocytes among the leukocytes increases to 10% to 25%, and relative lymphocyte counts may reach 70% to 90%. The Monospot test or the heterophil agglutination tests will be positive, but positive serological tests may be delayed beyond the first week; as a result, early negative tests should be repeated. The condition of a patient with extremely severe pharyngitis can be improved by a short course of corticosteroid therapy, in addition to the usual supportive measures. Superimposed bacterial infections do occur and require antibiotic treatment. The acute phase lasts 2 to 3 weeks. Infectious mononucleosis may be less common among persons who have had a tonsillectomy.

MONILIASIS

Moniliasis involves oral or pharyngeal pain and discomfort associated with milky-white, slightly elevated lesions. The curdlike white plaque can be scraped off with a tongue blade, leaving a red, hemorrhagic base. Leukoplakia and lichen planus cannot be removed in this manner. Moniliasis occurs secondary to the fungus *Candida albicans* and can occur at any age. It is usually predisposed by a change in oral flora, for instance, following a course of antibiotics or steroids (especially sprays, such as beclomethasone diproprionate [Vanceril]) in asthmatics or debilitated and elderly patients. Treatment consists of nystatin (Mycostatin oral suspension, 100,000 u/ml) 4 ml to 6 ml q.i.d. or Mycostatin oral tablets (500,000 units per tablet) taken one or two at a time t.i.d.

SYPHILIS

In *primary syphilis,* the lesion may occur wherever the treponeme first enters the body, such as the lip, tongue, or tonsil, approximately 3 weeks after exposure. It usually appears as a single, hard, painless, eroded papule, although occasionally there can be multiple lesions. The "satellite node," an associated large, rubbery, nontender cervical node, is found in the field of lymph drainage. Darkfield examination is of no diagnostic value because of the presence of spirochetes in the oral flora. Serology tests may be positive, but they are often negative until 8 to 12 weeks have passed; therefore, a negative test must be repeated after one month. A history of sexual exposure and a rising titer is sufficient confirmation of the diagnosis. The primary lesion clears with or without treatment.

Secondary syphilis is the more infectious form and is characterized by a macular or macular-papular cutaneous rash. Oral lesions consist of gray, raised, mucinous patches with discrete borders that are found on the tongue and oral mucosa. During secondary syphilis, reagin tests, such as the venereal disease research laboratory (VDRL) test and the rapid plasma reagin card test (RPR-CT) are uniformly positive; a specific treponemal antibody test, such as the fluorescent treponemal antibody-absorption (FTA-ABS) test, is likely to be reactive.

Benzathine penicillin G, 2.4 million units IM, is generally recommended for the treatment of syphilis. For patients with penicillin sensitivity, erythromycin 250 mg q.i.d. for 2 weeks is sufficient.

The oral manifestation of *tertiary syphilis* includes gummatous lesions of the palate. Rhagades, Hutchinson's incisors, and mulberry incisors are seen in *congenital syphilis.*

GONOCOCCAL PHARYNGITIS

Gonococcal pharyngitis is manifested by a bright red, inflammatory reaction in the pharynx and the development of irregular, superficial, whitish gray ulcers with yellowish, fetid exudate 1 to 2 days after exposure. In 50% of patients affected, the infection is a subclinical infection of the oropharynx. A gonococcal focus in the tonsil is not easily eradicated and may lead to disseminated gonorrhea with arthritis. Although the disease is particularly prevalent in homosexuals, it was present in 4% of patients routinely cultured at a prenatal clinic. Cultures require special handling: *Thayer-Martin* chocolate agar plates should be swabbed with a large Z stroke and incubated in a candlejar of CO_2 within 15 minutes. *Transgrow bottles* contain CO_2 and the medium on the side. Bottles must be kept upright when innoculating, and the cap must be returned promptly. These can be transported or mailed to the lab.

PEDIATRIC DISORDERS

VARICELLA

The oral vesicles and ulcers of *varicella* (herpes zoster) are found primarily on the mucosa of the hard and soft palate and are distinguishable from other viral lesions by the appearance of the classical chicken pox vesicles upon the patient's trunk and face. Varicella commonly occurs in epidemics from January to May in children under 10 years of age.

ACUTE HERPETIC GINGIVOSTOMATITIS

Acute herpetic gingivostomatitis results from infection by herpes simplex virus type I in children (ages 1 to 3 most commonly) and, at times, from herpes simplex virus type II in adults. It is characterized by multiple, painful vesicles (rarely seen) and the resulting yellowish gray ulcers (2 mm to 10 mm in diameter), especially on the gingiva; fever; dehydration; and submaxillary adenopathy. Although acute herpetic gingivostomatitis is a self-limited disease, lasting 4 to 10 days, patients may require intravenous hydration as well as fever management.

HERPANGINA

Herpangina is a summertime viral disease affecting children, usually 6 years and younger, that is characterized by the abrupt onset of fever associated with sore throat and dysphagia. There is a characteristic vesicular eruption, 1 mm to 2 mm in diameter, involving multiple, discrete, whitish gray vesicular-ulcerative lesions with a bright red areola located principally on the anterior tonsillar pillars, soft palate, and tonsils. The interior buccal mucosa and gingiva are not involved. Herpangina is self-limited, lasting 1 to 4 days. It occurs secondary to infection by coxsackie-virus, type A or B.

HAND-FOOT-AND-MOUTH DISEASE

Hand-foot-and-mouth disease results from a coxsackie virus A infection and occurs in young children in summer epidemics. On the lips and buccal mucosa, there are painful vesicular-ulcerative lesions plus transient erythematous rash, and characteristic vesicles (up to 30) appear on the palms and soles.

TONSILLITIS

As common as tonsillitis is, it is often poorly understood. Acute tonsillitis is usually (90%) the result of beta streptococcus group A infection. *Staphylococcus aureus* and *Hemophilus influenzae* are also found. In addition, β-hemolytic streptococcus group C and group G, as well as nonhemolytic group A streptococcus have been reported as pathogens. Many physicians use cultures to determine whether or not to treat this disorder with antibiotics, but cultures are a poor way to assess streptococcal tonsillitis because the surface culture of a tonsil is the same as the internal culture only 50% of the time. The decision to treat acute tonsillitis with antibiotics should be based on the presence of tonsillar pain, temperature elevation, elevated polymorphonuclear count (greater than 10,000), negative monospot test, and the presence of enlarged, tender, subdigastric nodes. Patients with these symptoms should be treated with antibiotics, either with penicillin or, in the penicillin-sensitive patient, erythromycin, for 5 to 7 days. Patients who may not be relied upon to take their medication should be treated with benzathine penicillin G (Bicillin) 1.2 million units, IM.

Patients with recurrent streptococcal tonsillitis present a special problem. All the members of the patient's family should be cultured in the hope of locating a carrier. Even if none is found, it may still be worthwhile to treat the entire family simultaneously with antibiotics when the patient has a bout of tonsillitis.

Tonsillectomy should be performed when there are repeated tonsillar infections for 2 years or more despite appropriate antibiotic therapy, especially in a child who is subject to febrile convulsions. Surgery is also indicated in the presence of respiratory obstruction or cor pulmonale, which, though rare, may occur subsequent to obstruction from enlarged tonsils. Some children suffer from poor nutrition and, occasionally, anemia as a result of difficulty in swallowing because of chronic pain and obstruction with deglutition. Other indications are peritonsillar abscess and rheumatic fever. In an adult, halitosis due to chronically infected tonsils is occasionally an indication for surgery. The relationship between tonsillitis and sleep apnea syndrome secondary to hypertrophied tonsils and adenoids is currently under investigation.

Tonsillectomy is a relatively safe, successful operation when done for the proper indications. Studies show that acceptable indications vary widely from physician to physician. In one study of children undergoing adenotonsillectomy, 97% of the parents and 87% of the referring physicians felt the surgery resolved or greatly improved the medical problem for which surgery was performed, a very good statistical record for any operation. On the other hand, however, there is the consideration that in roughly every 20,000 operations there is one death secondary to either hemorrhage or anesthesia. Hemorrhage usually occurs within 24 hours of surgery but can occur up to 8 to 10 days postoperatively.

CHRONIC TONSILLITIS

Chronic tonsillitis is sometimes difficult for the physician to recognize. The tonsils appear smooth and pink and are most often not enlarged or even smaller than normal. Patients complain of sore throat, malaise, and tender subdigastric lymph nodes. In addition, there may be acute exacerbations from time to time.

The tonsils of patients who complain of sore throat should be carefully inspected. The surface of chronically infected tonsils is smooth, pink scar tissue with one or two large crypts instead of the normal velvetlike mucosal surface with multiple small crypts. The examining physician should open the crypts using two long cotton applicators. In most instances this will reveal infected debris. In some cases, removal of the debris by expressing it or by suctioning will clear the patient's symptoms. In some instances, though, the crypts are too deep to keep clear, and a tonsillectomy is required.

Chronic tonsillitis is found in teenagers and adults. Patients who have a minimal gag reflex, and who are not frightened by the proposition, may wish to consider a tonsillectomy under a local anesthetic. In a competent surgeon's hands, the procedure is rapid and safe because the risks of the anesthetic and hemorrhage are kept to a minimum.

PERITONSILLAR ABSCESS

Peritonsillar abscess is an infrequent complication of tonsillitis that can occur unexpectedly even if the patient has been receiving oral penicillin therapy. It is manifested by marked bulging of the tonsil into the oral pharynx and by swelling of the anterior pillars and soft palate, which occurs several days after the onset of tonsillitis. The tonsils may reach the uvula, which is often edematous. There is deep throat pain radiating to the ear and marked spasms of the surrounding musculature, including the pterygoid muscles, resulting in trismus. Because of pain, patients are unable to articulate properly or to swallow even their saliva, and frequently become dehydrated.

The abscess should be immediately incised and drained or aspirated. After anesthetizing the bulging portion of the upper anterior tonsillar pillar with a small amount of Cetacaine spray, an 18-gauge needle can be placed into the abscess, and pus can be aspirated using a 20-ml syringe. Alternately, a No.-15 blade can be used to make a superficial incision through the mucous membrane and superficial musculature of the anterior pillar, and a hemostat can be used to spread the wound until the abscess is entered and drained. The patient experiences an immediate, marked relief of pain. Upon hospitalization, the patient is started on IV antibiotics. It is the practice of many otolaryngologists to proceed with a tonsillectomy at this point. There does not seem to be any increase in surgical difficulty in removing a tonsil with an underlying peritonsillar abscess. Indeed, the dissection is somewhat facilitated by the abscess cavity. Several studies have shown that there is a decreased length of hospital stay and decreased morbidity with the use of this method.

Rarely deaths have occurred secondary to peritonsillar abscess from sudden rupture of the abscess and aspiration or from a gradual progression of the abscess through the deep fascial layers of the neck to the mediastinum.

LINGUAL TONSILLITIS

The lingual tonsils are rarely infected. When they are, the pathogens do not vary from those causing faucial tonsillitis. Pain and swelling can be either unilateral or bilateral, and patients may have difficulty articulating (hot potato voice) and swallowing. In severe cases the airway may be compromised.

Lingual tonsillitis is treated with antibiotics, proper hydration, and management of any airway difficulties. Recurrent infections may require removal of the lingual tonsillar tissue by surgical means, such as electrodissection, cryosurgery, or, recently, laser surgery.

DEEP PHARYNGEAL PAIN AND DISCOMFORT

There are many causes of deep pharyngeal pain and discomfort. Probably the most important is neoplasia involving the posterior tongue, the vallecula, the epiglottis, or the pyriform sinus. Patients may complain of some dysphagia or odynophagia, as well as mild aspiration. In addition, there is localized pain that may at times radiate to the ear. Laryngeal mirror or fiberoptic laryngoscope examination will demonstrate a raised, white, irregular lesion or an irregular ulcer. Biopsy should be arranged at the earliest possible date. Treatment, often a combination of radiotherapy and surgery, should be instituted expeditiously.

PHARYNGEAL BURNS

Occasionally, patients, particularly those with dentures, will develop traumatic pharyngitis secondary to eating hot food. This can result either in a first- or second-degree burn of the posterior pharynx, often in the arytenoid area of the posterior larynx. It is here that hot food is held as the patient decides whether to spit it out, cough, or swallow. Patients with burns complain of pain when swallowing and the sensation of a pharyngeal mass due to local edema. In most cases there is no compromise of the airway. Clear liquids are helpful. Antibiotics and steroids may be necessary for unusually severe burns.

FOREIGN BODY

A small foreign body embedded in a mucosal musculature of the hypopharynx can result in chronic pain generated by swallowing. As with pharyngeal burns, this occurs more commonly in elderly patients who wear dentures. Small foreign bodies, particularly fish bones, may be difficult to see, and the examining physician should look as much for an area of inflammation as for an actual foreign body. Often, the foreign body passes through, leaving an abrasion of the pharynx, but because of residual pain, the patient will complain of a foreign body. If the patient is able to localize a specific point of pain, and if on careful examination the examiner is unable to see a foreign body or area of inflammation, a common-sense approach to the problem would be to ask the patient to return in 12 to 24 hours. If the pain is secondary to an abrasion from a foreign body, it will have cleared. If the foreign body is indeed present, there should be increased inflammation and pain surrounding it, and further diagnostic tests can be undertaken. These tests would include plain films, a barium swallow, particularly for those areas that are poorly visualized directly, or endoscopy for direct examination and removal of the foreign body.

GLOSSOPHARYNGEAL NEURALGIA

Patients with glossopharyngeal neuralgia experience spasms of very severe, unilateral pharyngeal pain that is often triggered by a specific pharyngeal movement, such as yawning or swallowing in a certain way. It occurs most commonly in the middle-aged or elderly, and the cause is unknown. The treatment for persistent cases is sectioning of the glossopharyngeal nerve.

EAGLE'S SYNDROME

Eagle's syndrome is an unusual disorder that is unique to patients who have had a tonsillectomy. It results from an overly long styloid process, caught in a deep scar bed from the tonsillectomy. Pain can be reproduced by palpating the tonsillar fossa, styloid process, and scar. The treatment is resection of the styloid process through the tonsillar bed.

GLOBUS HYSTERICUS

Globus hystericus is a common disorder, usually found in highstrung or nervous patients. The symptom of "having a lump in your throat" is so common that the phrase has become a cliché. On swallowing, one can feel the walls of the hypopharynx come together. This feeling can easily be interpreted as a lump or a mass. Unlike with a true mass, however, when these patients swallow food or liquids the lump disappears and the swallowing is entirely normal. A barium swallow roentgenogram and an explanation of the mechanism causing the sensation are usually sufficient to assuage the patient's fears.

HYPOPHARYNGEAL DIVERTICULUM (ZENKER'S DIVERTICULUM)

Hypopharyngeal diverticulum is usually found in patients 60 years old and older. It occurs primarily on the left side of the pharynx. The predominant symptoms are a sensation of food catching in the throat and discomfort upon swallowing. In addition, the patient will notice a regurgitation of undigested food, particularly at night after lying down, and will tend to aspirate chronically. The diagnosis is made by a barium swallow, which nicely demonstrates the diverticulum. Treatment is by surgical resection. *Cervical osteophytes* commonly appear on x-ray films and rarely, if ever, cause pharyngeal symptoms.

HIATUS HERNIA AND REFLUX ESOPHAGITIS

Pain from the lower esophagus can be referred to the area of the hypopharynx and larynx. For patients complaining of pain in this region who otherwise have no evidence of pharyngeal abnormality, a barium esophagogram should be done in order to determine whether a hiatus hernia is present. The pharyngeal pain will often respond to treatment for the hernia. Be aware that angina pectoris can be responsible for deep throat pain or a strangling sensation.

IRRITATED THROAT

After the possible causes of pharyngeal pain and discomfort listed above have been ruled out, many patients will continue to complain of a chronic sore throat. In some cases, there may be a mild, diffuse edema of the oropharynx with lymph follicular hypertrophy. These patients may be suffering from nicotine stomatitis or from pharyngitis secondary to chemical abuse with alcohol or with mouthwashes, such as Listerine. Other patients may have a chronically dry throat owing to mouth breathing secondary to nasal allergies or other causes of nasal obstruction. In addition to removing the source of irritation, a patient's condition is often improved by painting the throat with Argyrol, a silver-protein solution, and by using Thayer's Slippery Elm lozenges, soothing throat lozenges that contain no sugar.

HOARSENESS

Patients with hoarseness that fails to rapidly resolve within 1 to 2 weeks should have a careful laryngeal mirror examination. The examiner can use either a headlight or a headmirror. The patient should be seated at the same level as the examiner or slightly higher. It is best to explain the whole examination to the patient so that he is put somewhat at ease. He should be told that when he opens his mouth wide and extends his tongue as far as possible, the examiner will gently grasp his tongue and use a warm mirror to look down at his vocal cords. The patient is asked to concentrate on his breathing, which he does in rather rapid, shallow breaths.

The patient should also practice saying "H-E-E" with his tongue extended so he gets the feeling of this maneuver. It is helpful to explain that he will be able to breathe well at all times and that the examination can be accomplished quickly if he does not gag. Patients who are particularly nervous about the examination can be given 5 mg to 10 mg of diazepam (Valium) by mouth one half hour before the examination, and the area of the soft palate where the mirror will be placed can be sprayed with Cetacaine in order to inhibit the gag response. Most patients, including children 5 years old and older, can be guided through an excellent laryngeal examination.

The examiner should look for any pathology involving the true and false cords and should make certain that both cords move well and meet in the midline. The examiner should also make note of the subglottic region when the cords are open, and he should examine the structures surrounding the larynx, particularly the pyriform sinuses, the vallecula, the base of the tongue, and both the lingual and laryngeal surfaces of the epiglottis (Fig. 11-1). Examination of the larynx is relatively easy, and with practice every physician can perform this examination proficiently. Flexible fiberoptic laryngoscopes* can be used to provide a good view of the hypopharynx and larynx. Introduced through the nose, they extend to the hypopharynx, and are well tolerated by most patients.

HYPERKERATOSIS

Hyperkeratosis (leukoplakia) is a white raised area involving one or both of the true vocal cords caused by hyperplasia of the cordal epithelium. This lesion occurs in patients who abuse tobacco and is considered to be a premalignant lesion, particularly when dyskeratosis is present on microscopic examination. The treatment consists of removing the leu-

*Manufactured by Olympus and by Machida.

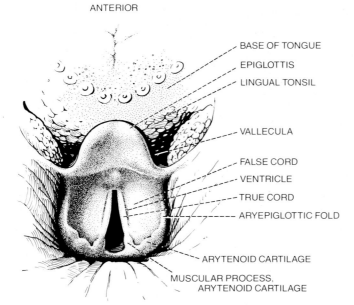

ANTERIOR

BASE OF TONGUE
EPIGLOTTIS
LINGUAL TONSIL

VALLECULA

FALSE CORD
VENTRICLE
TRUE CORD
ARYEPIGLOTTIC FOLD

ARYTENOID CARTILAGE
MUSCULAR PROCESS,
ARYTENOID CARTILAGE

Fig. 11-1. The surface anatomy of a normal larynx viewed from above.

koplakia by microlaryngoscopy. Patients are then examined every 3 months. Leukoplakia can recur, particularly if the patient fails to discontinue smoking.

VOCAL-CORD POLYPS

Vocal-cord polyps represent a thickening of the thin mucosal surface of the vocal cords. The thickening is usually diffuse and presents on both cords, although it may be greater on one side than the other. Polyps result in a lowered vocal pitch and chronic hoarseness. They occasionally become large enough to cause symptoms associated with reduction of the airway size. Unless inflamed, they appear grayish white and have smooth margins. Polyps most often result from vocal abuse, but they may also represent a myxedematous change in patients with hypothyroidism. They occur more commonly in women than in men.

Minor polypoid change will respond to correction of the vocal abuse, either through vocal rest or, if indicated, vocal therapy. Large polyps require surgical removal by microlaryngoscopy. During this procedure, the edematous mucosa, or polyp, is stripped away from the fibrous portion of the true vocal cord. This must be done with precision to prevent excessive scarring, particularly in the area of the anterior commissure. Voice recovery is gradual postoperatively, but for most patients there is a marked improvement in pitch and range. However, a professional, for instance an actor or singer, who relies upon his voice may notice a decrease in his range postoperatively. This is due to unavoidable scarring of the vocal cord, which reduces its natural elasticity.

SINGER'S OR SCREAMER'S NODULES

The most intense vibration of the vocal cords occurs at the junction of the anterior one third and posterior two thirds of the cord. Cheerleaders, teachers who must shout to be heard, children in noisy households, and singers who overuse their voices or who sing with respiratory infections are examples of patients who may develop very small, discrete nodules precisely at the junction of the anterior one third of the vocal cords. These nodules have the effect of holding the vocal cords apart and result in a definite breathiness of voice. They might be compared to calluses, and if discovered early, they may disappear with voice rest. Occasionally, these nodules must be removed to improve the quality of the voice; however, the patient should be warned of the possible vocal-cord scarring that may occur. It is rarely necessary to remove nodules from a child's larynx because he will outgrow the problem.

SUBMUCOSAL LARYNGEAL HEMORRHAGE

Rupture of a mucosal capillary on the vocal cord results in an area of submucosal hematoma and the rapid progression of hoarseness. These hematomas are always small, only several millimeters in size, and therefore never represent an airway hazard. They appear as a small, unilateral, red polyp on the vocal cord. Although the inclination of the examining physician may be to allow the hematomas to resorb, the correct therapy is to remove them immediately. If left alone, the hematomas, rather than resorb, may organize and form a small fibrous nodule on the vocal cord. This fibrous nodule will soon result in the irritation of the apposing surface of the opposite cord and in the development of a second nodule, which will also require removal.

CONTACT ULCERS OF THE LARYNX

Contact ulcers of the larynx cause hoarseness and may also result in discomfort while speaking. They occur in men who are trying to lower the pitch of their voice and also speak loudly. The ulcer develops over the ends of the arytenoid cartilages where the fibrous portions of the vocal cord insert, in other words, slightly posterior to the junction of the anterior two thirds and posterior one third of the vocal cords. The examiner will notice small apposing ulcers, or an ulcer bed filled with granulation tissue. Contact ulcers of the larynx may also occur following endotracheal intubation for surgery, particularly in women, whose smaller larynxes are more subject to pressure from an indwelling endotracheal tube. Occasionally, ulcers may occur secondary to chronic esophageal reflux. Treatment involves the removal of any granulation tissue by means of direct laryngoscopy. The contact ulcers are allowed to heal through voice rest.

LARYNGEAL PAPILLOMATOSIS

Laryngeal papillomatosis is most commonly seen in children; however, papillomas of the larynx now are seen in sexually active adults. While it has not been proven, it is probable that the papillomas are of viral origin and bear a relationship to venereal warts (condylomata acuminata). Children will present within the first few years of life with hoarseness, stridor, and varying degrees of respiratory obstruction. They are occasionally misdiagnosed as having asthma, bronchitis, or recurrent croup. A tracheotomy may be necessary. The papillomas are removed surgically by using microscopic laryngoscopy and cup forceps or by employing laser techniques, which can very precisely burn them away. However, regardless of the method of removal they often recur. Therefore, children may require repeated procedures for papilloma removal over the years, particularly if the disorder extends to the trachea and bronchi. Laryngeal papillomatosis in children is occasionally fatal. Adults should be told they may require several procedures over the ensuing years to completely rid themselves of the problem.

CYSTS

Mucus-containing cysts or those containing mucus and air (a laryngocele) can develop at any age, but if not present at infancy, they usually develop during adulthood. The presence of cysts is indicated by progressive hoarseness and symptoms of airway obstruction, such as stridor and shortness of breath. Small cysts may be removed endoscopically. Larger cysts, in order to prevent their recurrence, should be dissected free in their entirety by way of a formal surgical removal through an external, cervical approach.

LARYNGEAL STENOSIS

Stenosis of the larynx or subglottic region can result from prolonged intubation of the airway. Scarring can occur in the region of the glottis, either near the anterior commissure or in the region of the posterior commissure, or it may occur immediately below the vocal cords inside the circumference of the cricoid ring. If the stenosis is severe enough to impair vocal function or to significantly reduce the airway, surgical correction must be undertaken. In general, this is a complicated task and may require long periods of stenting of the stenotic area and a tracheotomy.

Other causes of laryngeal stenosis include cricothyreotomy or high tracheotomy, chemical or thermal burns, and prolonged granulomatous infections, such as tuberculosis.

SUBACUTE OR CHRONIC LARYNGITIS

Patients with hoarseness that lasts weeks, months, or years and with diffuse thickening and redness of the vocal cords are suffering from subacute or chronic laryngitis. Evaluation includes x-ray films of the chest and sinus and a barium swallow. If sputum is present, a smear and cultures should be obtained. Lab tests might include a complete blood count (CBC), erythrocyte sedimentation rate (ESR), thyroid studies, and an evaluation of the rheumatoid factor. Problem cases in non-smokers as well as smokers may require a laryngeal biopsy and culture of the tissues.

DIFFERENTIAL DIAGNOSIS

Trauma

By far the most common cause of chronic laryngitis in the United States is a combination of smoking and drinking and misuse of the voice. Exposure of the larynx to large amounts of tobacco smoke may result in a disproportionate degree of epithelial thickening from hyperplasia and keratinization, which frequently progress to keratosis and leukoplakia. These changes can be reversed to some degree by the discontinuation of smoking.

Alcohol is able to serve as a laryngeal irritant because it is undoubtedly aspirated in small amounts in the later stages of inebriation. Following the inflammatory response in the larynx, these patients may develop a hyperkeratosis of the laryngeal mucosa, which results in leukoplakia as described above. Leukoplakia may or may not entirely resolve, although it will be improved if the patient stops smoking and drinking. When dyskeratosis is present upon microscopic examination of the biopsy material, leukoplakia is thought to be a premalignant lesion.

Reflux Laryngopharyngitis

Reflux laryngopharyngitis results from an incompetent gastroesophageal sphincter that permits the reflux of gastric juices. At night when the patient is in the recumbent position, gastric juices are able to reflux into the hypopharynx and cause an irritation of the larynx. On examination, the arytenoidal area appears red and swollen, and some patients develop contact ulcers over the vocal process. The patient complains of chronic sore throat and laryngeal pain with hoarseness. The diagnosis is confirmed by x-ray demonstration of reflux esophagitis using an acid barium meal. Treatment includes the administration of antacids before and after meals, and the elevation of the patient's head during sleep. Food should be restricted for at least 3 hours before bedtime.

Occupational and Home Chemicals

Occasionally, a patient will describe the presence of irritating chemical dust or fumes at work, and this of course should be corrected through contact with his employer. Home chemicals, such as oven cleaners and ammonia, can result in laryngeal irritation if not used properly.

RESPIRATORY TRACT INFECTIONS: SUBACUTE AND CHRONIC

VIRAL LARYNGOTRACHEAL BRONCHITIS

Viral laryngotracheal bronchitis is the most common form of laryngeal infection. These infections result in hoarseness, irritation and chronic cough, and, occasionally, pain upon speaking. The treatment consists of voice rest and the use of an effective cough medication. Vocal abuse at the time of infection can result in vocal polyp formation. An occasional case of viral laryngitis will become superinfected with upper respiratory pathogens, such as group A β-hemolytic streptococcus, *Staphylococcus aureus*, and *Hemophilus influenzae*.

DIPHTHERIA

By means of the diphtheria immunization program, diphtheria has been almost eliminated in the United States, but it still may erupt anywhere within the country in miniepidemics involving a few people. Diphtheria pharyngolaryngitis presents as a gray exudate with a characteristic strong fecal odor. The diagnosis is confirmed by the Schick test. Failure to recognize diphtheria accounts for its 10% mortality rate, which has remained unchanged over the years. Treatment includes the administration of diphtheria antitoxin (horse serum) intramuscularly, which prevents the onset of the polyneuritis and myocarditis. Antibiotics, in particular penicillin and erythromycin, are effective.

TUBERCULOSIS

Tuberculosis of the larynx does not occur as a solitary disorder, but always in conjunction with advanced pulmonary tuberculosis. Prior to the availability of effective antitubercular chemotherapy, the incidence of laryngeal tuberculosis among pulmonary tuberculosis patients approached 40%. At this time, however, the incidence of laryngeal tuberculosis is 2% or less in cases of pulmonary tuberculosis. On examination the larynx is red, and there may be granulations and ulcerations, particularly in the area of the posterior commissure. Chronic laryngeal tuberculosis causes scarring and stenosis. The diagnosis can usually be arrived at based on the findings on the chest x-ray films and a positive tuberculin test. Sputum analysis will confirm the diagnosis; however, in some cases laryngeal biopsy may be necessary for confirmation. First-line drugs for treatment include isoniazid, rifampin, ethambutol, and streptomycin.

LARYNGEAL TRICHINOSIS

Laryngeal trichinosis, which usually clears spontaneously in 2 or 3 weeks, is suggested by an increased eosinophil count. Other diagnostic maneuvers may be employed if necessary. These include an intradermal skin test with *Trichinella* antigen and serodiagnostic tests for anti-*Trichinella* antibody titers. A muscle biopsy is confirmatory.

SYPHILIS AND LEPROSY

Syphilis and leprosy have been reported to involve the larynx, but such cases are very unusual.

MYCOTIC INFECTIONS OF THE LARYNX

As with tuberculosis, mycotic infections of the larynx are usually associated with rather severe, pulmonary mycotic infections. Although previously confined to certain regions of the country, because of travel mycotic infections are now found in patients from any region. Mycotic infections of the larynx may present in a variety of ways, ranging from a small granuloma of the vocal cord, to an inflammatory laryngeal disease, to cicatricial deformities.

HISTOPLASMOSIS

Histoplasmosis is usually a benign, self-limited disease that results from the histoplasma capsillatum, which is found particularly in soil in the Midwest that has been contaminated with poultry droppings. The diagnosis is made by chest x-ray films. The histoplasmin test is not recommended for diagnosis because there are many false-negative and false-positive results owing to frequent anergy and cross reactions respectively. In fact, the test itself can initiate antibody titers. The diagnosis is best confirmed by rising titers of histoplasma antibody. Because the disorder in general is self-limited, no treatment is used. At this time, amphotericin B is the only useful drug, and it is not employed routinely because of its toxicity.

COCCIDIOIDOMYCOSIS

Coccidioidomycosis is endemic to the southwestern United States. One week to one month after exposure, the patient notices a primary pulmonary lesion and complains of fever, cough, and malaise. This disorder is self-limited in 95% of patients, but occasionally a patient will develop a pulmonary abscess or cavitary pulmonary disease. Skin tests for coccidioidomycosis are useful because they are specific and do not stimulate the manufacture of antibodies. The diagnosis can also be made through serological techniques by the measurement of rising antibodies against coccidioidomycosis. Most patients require no treatment. As with histoplasmosis, amphotericin B is the only effective drug.

Other mycotic infections reported to affect the larynx are North American blastomycosis, moniliasis, actinomycosis, and nocardiosis and infections caused by *Aspergillus fumigatus* and *Cryptococcus*. These infections would not cause laryngeal disease without extensive pulmonary disease.

GENERALIZED DISEASES AFFECTING THE LARYNX

ARTHRITIS

Both rheumatoid and gouty arthritis can affect the larynx, but laryngeal symptoms are seen more frequently secondary to rheumatoid arthritis. The cricoarytenoid joints are frequently involved. Although autopsy studies indicate that there is laryngeal involvement in 80% to 90% of patients with arthritis, only 25% of these patients develop laryngeal symptoms. In general, symptomatic laryngeal rheumatoid arthritis occurs only in patients with marked degenerative joint disease. The patients initially note hoarseness associated with some pain, or they note a full sensation in the throat. Examination demonstrates arytenoid swelling or redness. In time, the vocal cords may become fixed and bowed, and the airway may become compromised. Occasionally a patient will require a tracheotomy or laryngeal surgery, such as an arytenoidectomy, in order to maintain an adequate airway. Medical treatment of laryngeal arthritis is directed against the systemic condition. Pathology includes synovial thickening and destruction of the cricoarytenoid joint with panus formation.

HYPOTHYROIDISM (MYXEDEMA)

Hypothyroidism can result in the thickening of the vocal cords and the development of mild to extensive polypoid changes on the vocal cords. These developments, combined with the results of appropriate thyroid studies (resin T_3 uptake, T_4, and TSH level) establish the diagnosis. Treatment includes thyroid replacement therapy and vocal-cord stripping (polyp removal) if required.

SYSTEMIC LUPUS ERYTHEMATOSUS

Systemic lupus erythematosus is a rare cause of acute or subacute laryngitis, in which there is hoarseness associated with edema and hyperemia. In an occasional case there may be mucosal ulcerations or hemorrhagic bullae involving the larynx. Other manifestations during the chronic stage include chronic hypertrophic laryngitis, cricoarytenoid arthritis, and transient vocal-cord paralysis. Laboratory tests to establish the diagnosis of systemic lupus erythematosus include an ESR and an antinuclear antibody study, and treatment is directed against the primary condition.

VOCAL-CORD PARALYSIS

Hoarseness may represent a partial or complete paralysis of the vocal cords. There are various causes for unilateral vocal-cord paralysis, but among these three are most common. The first is an idiopathic loss of function that in most cases represents a viral inflammation of the recurrent nerve. These losses are usually self-limited, and cord function will gradually return over a period of months up to one year.

The second common cause of vocal-cord paralysis is injury of the recurrent nerve or nerves during surgery. Thyroid surgery can result in injury to the recurrent nerves in the neck; cardiac surgery can result in injury to the recurrent nerve as it passes around the aorta. Patients in whom the recurrent nerve is injured awaken from surgery with a very breathy, weak voice. If the nerve has been traumatized but not cut, function might return over time. In our experience, injury to the superior laryngeal nerve occurs most commonly following carotid endarterectomy. The findings from this injury are more subtle, because this nerve ennervates only the cricothyroid muscle, which functions to tense the cord. The remaining adductors and abductors are unimpaired. Because the superior laryngeal nerve also serves to provide sensation to the ipsilateral superior larynx, the patient may notice some aspiration, particularly of clear liquids, in addition to a weakened voice with limited vocal range.

Finally, bronchogenic carcinoma of the left lung involving the recurrent nerve on the left side can present as hoarseness.

CARCINOMA OF THE LARYNX

Approximately 98% of the malignant tumors of the larynx are squamous cell carcinoma, which has the potential to metastasize to regional cervical lymph nodes. The 5-year cure rate for small lesions is 90% or greater with preservation of the larynx and voice. Early detection is mandatory because once the tumor has enlarged and begun to metastasize the rate of cure falls and the rate of morbidity climbs.

For purposes of cancer staging and prognostication, the larynx is divided into three regions. The *supraglottic* region is that portion of the larynx that includes the epiglottis, aryepiglottic fold, and the false vocal cords. The *subglottic* region is the area extending approximately 1 cm below the vocal cords. The final region is the *glottis*, or true vocal cords.

CARCINOMA OF THE GLOTTIS, OR TRUE VOCAL CORDS

Over 75% of the carcinomas of the larynx arise on the true vocal cords. This is fortunate because in these instances, hoarseness is an early and persistent symptom, and indirect examination of the larynx will readily demonstrate a small lesion involving one or both vocal cords. The tumor will therefore be discovered before it has invaded the deep musculature of the larynx or metastasized. The treatment of choice is radiation therapy. A common radiotherapeutic course might involve 6500 rad given over 6 weeks. In general, patients tolerate radiation therapy of this type very well. After the resolution of the initial pharyngitis and laryngitis secondary to radiation, the patient's voice returns to near normal.

Patients with early recurrence of glottic carcinoma can be treated by removal of the affected vocal cord. A variety of surgical techniques are available in addition to standard resection techniques. These include cryosurgical removal, laser resection methods or, at times, a vertical laryngectomy (Fig. 11-2).

CARCINOMA OF THE SUPRAGLOTTIC AREA

Approximately 25% of carcinomas of the larynx involve the supraglottis. Squamous cell carcinomas evolving in this area represent a greater hazard to the patient than those that develop in the glottis because tumors arising here do not cause hoarseness until a very late stage of development and, for this reason, may remain undetected until the tumor has become bulky enough to be felt as a mass or to cause pain, generally referred to the ipsilateral ear. Also, these tumors will metastasize very easily, and if they are located toward the center of the supraglottis, they can result in metastases to both sides of the neck.

Small tumors, 1 cm to 2 cm in size, can be treated through radiation therapy to the supraglottic larynx and to the site of cervical lymph-node spread in the neck. In some centers, this lesion is treated surgically, that is, by resection of the supraglottic larynx. This surgery is reserved

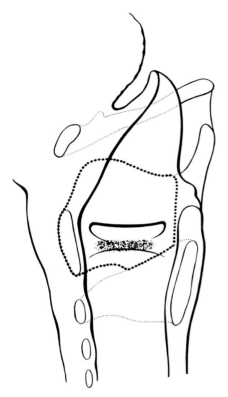

Fig. 11-2. The dotted lines mark the resection margins of a vertical laryngectomy.

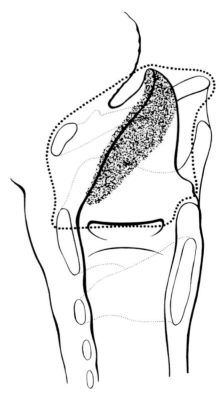

Fig. 11-3. The supraglottic laryngectomy is used for tumors that do not involve the glottis (vocal cords). These patients must be in good health with good pulmonary function. The dotted lines indicate the typical resection margins for a tumor involving the stippled area. This operation can be combined with a neck dissection.

for younger patients who are in good general health and have good pulmonary reserve. Unfortunately, most patients with carcinoma of the supraglottis are not seen by a physician until the disease has become rather extensive. The treatment in this case involves preoperative or postoperative radiation, supraglottic laryngectomy (Fig. 11-3), or total laryngectomy, plus ipsilateral or bilateral neck dissections.

CARCINOMA OF THE SUBGLOTTIC AREA

Carcinoma of the subglottic larynx tends to be a silent tumor and causes little or no symptomatology until symptoms of respiratory obstruction become apparent. The principal modes of therapy are radiation and surgery. Unfortunately, the failure rate due to local recurrence is high.

LARYNGEAL SURGERY

LARYNGOSCOPY

Direct laryngoscopy is the most common surgical procedure performed on the larynx. It is used for examination and biopsy as well as for the removal of leukoplakia polyps, nodules, and papillomas of the vocal cords. These procedures are done through a laryngoscope that is fixed into position, and an operating microscope is used to improve visualization of the internal laryngeal structures. Microlaryngeal instruments have been developed that greatly facilitate the removal of small lesions of the vocal cords with a minimum of injury. Recently, the carbon dioxide laser has been used to remove small lesions of the larynx with enhanced precision.

TRACHEOTOMY AND TRACHEOSTOMY

In general, endolaryngeal procedures do not require a tracheotomy, but when there is a compromised airway secondary to tumor, edema, or hemorrhage, a tracheotomy is necessary. Tracheotomies are temporary and are generally removed after a few days when the immediate airway problem has resolved.

There is some confusion in the literature regarding the terms *tracheotomy* and *tracheostomy*. *Tracheotomy* is a temporary opening made through the skin of the neck and carried through the anterior wall of

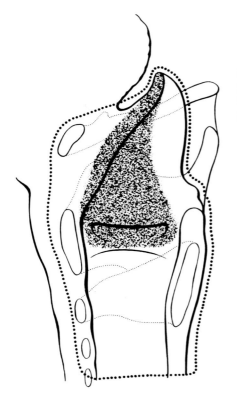

Fig. 11-4. The total laryngectomy encompasses the entire larynx, including the hyoid bone, down to the second or third tracheal ring. A permanent tracheostomy is required.

the trachea. *Tracheostomy* is a permanent stoma created by sewing the margins of the trachea to the cervical skin; it is commonly done after the transecting of the trachea during a laryngectomy.

LARYNGECTOMY

After laryngoscopy, laryngectomy is the second most common procedure performed on the larynx (Fig. 11-4). The most frequently employed laryngectomy is a wide-field, or total, laryngectomy. This procedure is done for extensive glottic, supraglottic, or infraglottic tumors of the larynx; if there is metastatic neck disease, it is combined with a neck dissection. Because of the propensity of supraglottic tumors to metastasize, some surgeons will perform a prophylactic neck dissection on the side of an extensive supraglottic tumor.

The ramifications of this type of surgery for the patient are in general poorly understood. Care must be taken to ensure that the patient understands the changes that are going to occur in his life. Although laryngectomy is a very significant occurrence, the loss of the larynx is not the end of the world. Most patients learn to adapt, although loss of the voice coupled with disfigurement and the presence of a stoma in the neck may affect their self-image. The patient also loses the ability to blow his nose, whistle, and to converse while eating. Because the larynx serves to stabilize the chest during the Valsalva maneuver, the loss of this function causes an inability to lift heavy objects. There is an increased tendency towards constipation, and, finally, embarrassment about breathing through the neck may result in a loss of intimacies for some patients. All of these problems need to be thoroughly discussed preoperatively with each patient and his family. Many laryngectomy patients are reformed alcoholics, and the stress of this postlaryngectomy syndrome will often result in a resumption of old drinking patterns.

With good training, approximately half the patients that undergo a laryngectomy will develop esophageal speech satisfactorily enough to converse with strangers without embarrassment. Some patients, though, because of the anatomical structure of the remaining cervical esophagus, are incapable of developing esophageal speech. One alternative is the use of a vibrator placed against the hypopharyngeal wall so that the patient can articulate the buzzing sound into discernible speech. The tone of this speech is monotonous and tends to be so loud and irritating that it draws attention to the laryngectomee. As a result, many patients feel uncomfortable with this device. A second device, the Cooper Rand, is much better accepted by most laryngectomy patients. This instrument has a small plastic tube that the patient inserts in the corner of his mouth, and the vibrations produced by this machine are much softer and more pleasing.

REHABILITATIVE SURGERY FOLLOWING TOTAL LARYNGECTOMY

Many surgical procedures have been developed that attempt to reestablish the ability to speak in the laryngectomy patient. Basically, they all work by the same principle: they create a fistula between the trachea and esophagus, so that if the trachea is occluded air is forced through the fistula into the esophagus, causing the upper esophagus to vibrate and allowing the patient to produce speech by articulation. These procedures all have one major pitfall; it is very difficult to create a fistula between the esophagus and trachea that permits the free flow of air from the trachea to the esophagus, but at the same time prevents the flow of liquids from the esophagus to the trachea, which causes aspiration. A recent technique that is enjoying some success is the placement of a Silastic flutter valve between the trachea and esophagus through a very small fistula.

Supraglottic Laryngectomy

Supraglottic laryngectomy is a procedure that removes the structures of the larynx down to the true vocal cords. This type of conservation surgery is possible because the lymphatic flow from the supraglottic portion of the larynx does not extend to the glottis. Resection margins, though close along the glottic margin, are generally secure.

Patients must be carefully evaluated before undergoing this surgery. They must have good pulmonary function in order to allow them to withstand the initial aspiration and to permit them to forcefully cough material free from the tracheobronchial tree. They must also be willing to endure 2 or 3 weeks of relearning to swallow without the benefit of the supraglottis to protect the lower airway. Once this is accomplished, these patients regain their voice and do not have a stoma, thus avoiding many of the difficulties associated with total laryngectomy.

Vertical Laryngectomy

Vertical laryngectomy is reserved for patients with a glottic tumor, usually a postradiation recurrence, that is limited to one side of the glottis. The patients are left with a weak and breathy voice, but they have no particular difficulty in swallowing and can make themselves well understood. There is only a temporary tracheotomy.

12
AIRWAY EMERGENCIES

William R. Wilson

Acute airway emergencies
  Foreign body in the larynx
  Acute spasmodic croup
  Acute viral laryngitis
  Epiglottitis
  Tracheobronchial foreign bodies
Chronic respiratory obstruction in
    a child
  Laryngomalacia
  Congenital laryngeal webs
  Subglottic stenosis
  Subglottic hemangioma

Laryngeal cysts and laryngo-
    celes
Neural lesions of the larynx
Vascular compression of the tra-
    chea
Respiratory obstruction in the
    newborn infant
Other causes of acute laryngeal
    obstruction
  Acute allergic laryngeal edema
  Hereditary angioneurotic edema
    (HANE)

ACUTE AIRWAY EMERGENCIES

All physicians, especially those in primary care, should be prepared to deal with acute airway obstruction on a moment's notice in order to relieve hypoxia or anoxia before irreversible cerebral injury occurs.

When dealing with a comatose patient whose tongue partially obstructs the upper airway, the physician should bring the patient's jaw and lax tongue forward by placing his fingers behind the angle of the jaw and lifting forward. Secretions are suctioned, and if the airway is not easily maintained by placing the patient in a lateral Trendelenburg position with his jaw thrust forward, a pharyngeal airway can be inserted.

FOREIGN BODY IN THE LARYNX

A patient with a foreign body, usually food, in the larynx (cafe coronary) will not reach the emergency room for treatment. The Heimlich maneuver should be tried in the restaurant once or twice. If this fails to clear the airway, the patient should be placed supine, and the physician should make a quick attempt to remove the foreign body with his fingers or, if they are available in the restaurant, with forceps. If the airway remains obstructed, a cricothyreotomy can be accomplished with a quick stab into the larynx through the cricothyroid membrane, followed by insertion of a stiff, hollow tube, such as the plastic barrel of a ball-point pen. Cricothyreotomy is an emergency procedure only and should not be used on an elective basis because it can result in laryngeal injury.

ACUTE SPASMODIC CROUP

Acute spasmodic croup occurs in small children between the ages of 1 and 3 years old. It seems to occur most frequently in children with allergies or in nonallergic children following an emotional upset. It is manifested by a croupy, barking cough; a stridulous respiration; chest retractions; and, occasionally, intermittent cyanosis. The attack occurs without any prodromata, often in the middle of the night. The child is afebrile and has no signs of infection. In the vast majority of cases, only moderate respiratory distress occurs. The most effective treatment is humidification; at home this is best achieved by running a shower. Another remedy is to break the spasm by inducing vomiting with syrup of ipecac.

Occasionally a child will develop marked retractions with cyanosis and a depressed sensorium and will require hospitalization. In the hospital, the child is placed in a cool mist tent, and an intravenous is begun for hydration. Oxygen administration is helpful but obscures cyanosis as a finding. Racemic epinephrine 2.25% diluted 1:25 or 1:10 in normal saline is administered by an intermittent positive pressure breathing (IPPB) machine capable of delivering liquid particles 0.5 microns to 4 microns in size. Treatments can be given for 5 to 10 minutes hourly over 3 to 4 hours until symptoms improve. The efficacy of steroids is controversial in the treatment of acute spasmodic croup and is being investigated by double-blind studies. Respiratory depressants, such as sedatives and opiates, are contraindicated.

Children who fail to improve on the regimen described above will require the insertion of a nasotracheal tube, which should be put in place in the operating room. Following oxygenation by mask, the child is anesthetized with oxygen and halothane, and an oral endotracheal tube is passed. Once this is accomplished and the airway is secured, a pediatric laryngoscope is used to examine the larynx and upper trachea. Patients with croup manifest a swelling of the larynx, particularly in the subglottic area. Once other pathologies, particularly foreign bodies, have been ruled out, the orotracheal tube is then replaced by a nasotracheal tube, which is carefully taped into position at the nares. The child is returned to a floor on which nurses skilled in the care of patients with respiratory obstruction are available. With light sedation, children tolerate the nasotracheal tube for the necessary 2 to 3 days without difficulty. If the tube becomes dislodged shortly after its insertion, it must be replaced. After several days, the tube should be removed in the operating room. The larynx is again examined by direct laryngoscopy to make certain there has been sufficient resolution of the intralaryngeal swelling. Treatment with nasotracheal intubation has greatly reduced the morbidity and mortality secondary to emergency pediatric tracheotomy. If nasotracheal intubation is not possible, then of course tracheotomy must be used.

ACUTE VIRAL LARYNGITIS

Viral laryngitis is not a life-threatening disease except in small children, in whom laryngeal edema, particularly in the subglottic area, can result in a marked reduction of the airway. The condition is manifested by a low-grade fever, a cough, and throat discomfort. The vocal cords are red and thickened. The repsonsible agents are most commonly parainfluenza viruses 1, 2, and 3, but other viruses may be responsible, including respiratory syncytial virus, adenovirus, *Mycoplasma pneumoniae* (Eaton agent), and, occasionally, measles.

Although many physicians use ampicillin routinely to treat acute viral laryngitis, the incidence of complicating pneumonia is unchanged by the antibiotic coverage. Therefore, as a general rule, antibiotics are contraindicated, although there is some basis for the use of erythromycin if there are *M. pneumoniae* infections present in the community. Patients with long-term laryngotracheal bronchitis can develop a secondary bacterial infection after 5 or 6 days. The proper antibiotic, based on sputum culture, should be selected at that time. Other supportive measures, such as cool mist, hydration, and oxygenation can be employed. Nasotracheal intubation or tracheotomy is used if necessary.

EPIGLOTTITIS

Epiglottitis is denoted by a painful throat that over a matter of hours becomes associated with a characteristic muffled (hot potato) voice, but not hoarseness, and gradual airway obstruction. Children will assume an erect sitting position with their neck hyperextended in order to keep the airway open. Drooling is common because of pain on swallowing. This clinical picture is associated with an elevated temperature, pulse, and respiratory rate, and dehydration and exhaustion often follow shortly thereafter.

In the case of a severely ill and obtunded child, examination of the pharynx and larynx should be made only in the operating room. For patients who are less acutely ill, a clinical suspicion of acute epiglottitis can best be confirmed by a lateral x-ray film. Examination of the pharynx should be done only when emergency airway equipment is available. The most common organism associated with epiglottitis is *Hemophilus influenzae,* although other respiratory pathogens are sometimes involved. The drug and dosage of choice for treatment has been ampicillin 250 mg to 500 mg IV q.6 hr. However, resistant *H. influenzae* has begun to emerge, and chloramphenicol (25 mg to 50 mg/kg/24 hr) is now suggested. Steroids are probably beneficial in reducing epiglottic edema, and one popular schedule of steroid administration is dexamethasone given intravenously 1 mg/kg up to a total of 5 milligrams, and then 1 milligram for every 5 kilograms. This dose is repeated b.i.d. or q.i.d. until after the nasotracheal tube has been removed.

The establishment of a nasotracheal airway or tracheotomy should not be delayed in children with epiglottitis. Respiratory arrest due to sudden obstruction of the laryngeal introitus by the enlarged epiglottis can occur very unexpectedly. Nasotracheal intubation should be established almost without exception in all children under 5 years of age who have epiglottitis. Adults with acute epiglottitis often do not require a tracheotomy (nasotracheal intubation is not tolerated by alert adults) because their airway is sufficiently large to permit respiration around the enlarged epiglottis. In general, they respond well to corticosteroids and antibiotic therapy while under observation for respiratory distress in a hospital situation.

TRACHEOBRONCHIAL FOREIGN BODIES

Aspiration of a foreign body into the lower respiratory tract is characterized by the sudden onset of coughing, choking, and wheezing. It occurs most commonly in young children ranging in age from 6 months old to four years old. Not infrequently, the initial symptomatic period is short and is followed by a relatively symptom-free period in which the child may be fine except for intermittent periods of croupy cough and wheezing. If the foreign body is undiscovered for a long period of time, it may result in focal atelectasis and pneumonitis, fever, cough, and, occasionally, hemoptysis. Foreign bodies of vegetable origin, such as nuts, peas, and beans, will swell and have a tendency to cause a greater inflammatory response than inert foreign bodies.

A child with croup should be considered to have a foreign body in his lower respiratory tract until proven otherwise. In addition to auscultation and inspiratory and expiratory chest roentgenograms, fluoroscopy may be required to make a proper assessment for foreign bodies.

CHRONIC RESPIRATORY OBSTRUCTION IN A CHILD

LARYNGOMALACIA

Laryngomalacia is by far the most common laryngeal anomaly in small children, and it is the most common cause of chronic respiratory obstruction. It is not a disease; rather, it is due to an anatomical variation in the structure of the larynx in children up to 2 years of age. Children with laryngomalacia have a folded, omega-shaped epiglottis with excessive floppiness of the aryepiglottic folds. During inspiration, the folds are pulled into the introitus of the larynx. The stridor in these children is intermittent and will improve or clear if the child is turned from his back onto his abdomen. However, no matter how certain the diagnosis may appear, these children should have an x-ray study of the larynx and chest, as well as direct laryngoscopy. The latter is done with the child sedated and bundled, but without a topical or general anesthetic.

CONGENITAL LARYNGEAL WEBS

The majority of laryngeal webs are partial and are located between the true vocal cords. They result in a weak, hoarse cry and stridor with crying.

Occasionally, laryngeal webs can occur more superiorly between the false vocal cords. In these cases, children are stridulous but have a normal cry. The treatment is division of the web and frequent dilatations of the larynx until the vocal cords are well healed in a separated position.

SUBGLOTTIC STENOSIS

The subglottic region is the narrowest region of the pediatric airway and is therefore the most critical. Stenosis may result in this area from several causes. In certain children, the cricoid cartilage, which forms a complete ring immediately above the first ring of the trachea, may not develop satisfactorily, resulting in a narrowed airway. Other children may develop tissue thickening on a congenital basis or perhaps, if they were premature, secondary to scarring from prolonged endotracheal intubation. Still others may have some narrowing of the subglottic airway owing to a prolonged use of a high tracheotomy. When subglottic stenosis is present to a minor degree, it predisposes the child to frequent episodes of croup. When the subglottic airway is sufficiently narrowed to produce respiratory embarrassment, a tracheotomy should be placed. In patients who do not respond spontaneously, surgical correction consists of widening the internal lumen of the cricoid cartilage, usually by a cartilage-implant technique.

SUBGLOTTIC HEMANGIOMA

For reasons unknown, hemangiomas occur in the lower respiratory tract in the immediate subglottic area. Children with hemangiomas have stridor, and x-ray films will show the subglottic tumor mass. Direct laryngoscopy reveals the presence of a vascular tumor. The diagnosis should be made by visual examination, not by biopsy. A further clue to the diagnosis of hemangioma is the presence of cutaneous hemangiomas elsewhere on the body.

Most subglottic hemangiomas regress spontaneously, and one satisfactory method of treatment is to perform a tracheotomy and wait for the hemangiomas to regress on their own. Electrodesiccation of the tumor using a carbon dioxide laser has also been performed with success. A previously accepted treatment method, namely, radiation therapy using approximately 300 rad to 500 rad, has been abandoned because of the risk of the delayed development of radiation-induced thyroid carcinoma.

LARYNGEAL CYSTS AND LARYNGOCELES

Laryngeal cysts and laryngoceles result from the invagination of the mucous membrane of the larynx, usually from the ventricular area. They produce a mass effect in the false cord and the aryepiglottic fold. Rarely, internal thyroglossal-duct cysts in the base of the tongue are responsible for chronic respiratory obstruction. The diagnosis is made by x-ray studies and direct laryngoscopy. In children these cysts are usually marsupialized endoscopically and followed.

NEURAL LESIONS OF THE LARYNX

Unilateral vocal-cord paralysis results in a hoarse and breathy cry and a weakened cough, but there is little or no respiratory distress. In children, left paralysis is often associated with anomalies of the heart and great vessels, while right-cord paralysis may be due to birth trauma. *Bilateral laryngeal paralysis* is manifested by stridulous inspirations, but a normal cry. The vocal cords are in close approximation, and they vibrate well when air is passed through them, but they do not adduct on inspiration. Bilateral laryngeal paralysis is associated with cerebral retardation and meningomyelocele, or it can result from birth trauma.

VASCULAR COMPRESSION OF THE TRACHEA

Vascular compression of the trachea is a not uncommon cause of stridor in an infant. It is usually caused by an anomalous right innominate artery or, much less commonly, a double aortic arch. Other causes of vascular compression are unusual. The symptoms usually begin very early in life and range from mild stridor and wheezing to severe bouts of dyspnea. Feeding problems are associated with respiratory complaints. Differential diagnosis includes consideration of tracheomalacia and compression owing to thymus enlargement. Diagnosis is made by a combination of x-ray and endoscopic studies. Surgical correction of the vascular anomaly is the treatment of choice.

RESPIRATORY OBSTRUCTION IN THE NEWBORN INFANT

A newborn child is an obligate nasal breather and obstruction of his nose will result in apnea. Causes of nasal obstruction include bilateral choanal atresia, encephalocele, tumors of the nose and nasopharynx, and nasal stenosis. Respiratory obstruction in the infant that originates in the oropharynx may be due to macroglossia, a small mandible (Pierre Robin syndrome), or the presence of a tumor, such as in cystic hygroma. Laryngeal obstruction of the airway in the newborn child may be due to a large congenital web of the larynx or congenital atresia of the larynx. The latter is almost invariably fatal unless there is a very alert obstetrical crew available to perform an immediate tracheotomy. Tracheoesophageal fistulas, because they are associated with puddling of secretions in the hypopharynx and aspiration, may also result in respiratory obstruction in the newborn infant.

OTHER CAUSES OF ACUTE LARYNGEAL OBSTRUCTION

ACUTE ALLERGIC LARYNGEAL EDEMA

Acute allergic laryngeal edema is most frequently the result of a food allergy, such as a sensitivity to shellfish. Laryngeal edema is also part of the anaphylactic response to marked insect-sting allergy. The immediate treatment for these disorders is the injection of 0.3 ml to 0.5 ml of epinephrine 1:1000 subcutaneously for adults and 0.01 ml/kg for children, and the administration of appropriate corticosteroids and antihistamines, which serve to prevent the reformation of the edema. Epinephrine may be repeated in 10 minutes. The use of oxygen and procedures to establish an emergency airway may be necessary.

HEREDITARY ANGIONEUROTIC EDEMA

Hereditary angioneurotic edema (HANE) can produce cutaneous urticaria as the result of a hereditary absence of C-1-esterase inhibitor, which allows the complement reaction to progress after only a slight provocation, such as minor trauma, infection, or emotional stress. In addition, laryngeal edema can occur after manipulation of the larynx during intubation for surgery or following dental extractions. The complement reaction results in the release of histamine followed by swelling and edema secondary to increased vascular permeability. The treatment for an acute attack is to establish an airway; epinephrine, antihistamines, and corticosteroids are of no benefit.

In the United States, there are approximately 1200 people afflicted with this autosomal-dominant genetic disorder. Among these persons the mortality rate runs as high as 20% to 30%. Physicians should be alerted to patients who develop episodes of submucosal or subdermal edema for no apparent reason during their late teens and early twenties. Swelling episodes that occur in the gastrointestinal tract cause abdominal cramping, pain, and vomiting; in the respiratory tract, swelling causes vague episodes of coughing followed by atelectasis or pleural effusion. Diagnosis is made by studies of the C4 and C-1-esterase inhibitor serum levels.

Treatment for HANE involves prophylaxis and the avoidance of unnecessary trauma and stress. Prophylaxis prior to mandatory surgical procedures includes the transfusion of 2 units of fresh plasma 24 hours prior to surgery and the use of epsilon aminocaproic acid and other antifibrinolytic agents.

A more recent method of treatment includes the administration of hormones that are variations of androgens found effective in the long-term control of HANE.

13

EVALUATION OF NECK MASSES

Joseph B. Nadol, Jr.

Anatomical considerations
  Triangles of the neck
    Anterior triangles of the neck
    Posterior triangles of the neck
  Contents of the cervical triangles
  Skeletal landmarks in the neck
  Lymph nodes of the head and neck
    Occipital nodes
    Retroauricular (mastoid) nodes
    Preauricular nodes
    Parotid nodes
    Facial nodes
    Submandibular nodes
    Submental nodes
    Superficial cervical nodes
    Deep cervical chain
    Anterior cervical nodes
Techniques for physical examination

Diagnostic strategy for the evaluation of a neck mass
Lymphadenomegaly
Congenital or developmental cysts and masses
  Branchial-cleft cysts
  Thyroglossal-duct cysts
  Cystic hygroma and hemangioma
Masses attached to normal structures of the neck
  Masses within the skin
  Masses derived from nerve tissue
  Tumors attached to or derived from blood vessels or associated structures
  Masses within the thyroid gland
  Lesions within the esophagus
  Tumors arising from cartilaginous structures

The differential diagnosis of a neck mass involves literally all classes of disease processes, including metastatic disease from practically any part of the body, neurogenic and vascular disorders, and a variety of cysts and neoplasms of normal organs or structures of the neck (see Differential Diagnosis of Neck Masses under Diagnostic Strategy for the Evaluation of a Neck Mass). Therefore, the examiner must follow a strategy that is designed to reduce diagnostic possibilities to a minimum and allow intelligent selection of further diagnostic procedures, such as skin tests, radiography, or biopsy. Assessing a neck mass requires a working knowledge of both the regional anatomy of the neck and the disorders likely to occur in the area of the neck in which the mass is found. Although theoretically any of the disorders listed under Differential Diagnoses of Neck Masses can be found in many areas of the neck, practically the physician can reduce the diagnostic possibilities to one or a few of them based on the location and other characteristics of the mass.

ANATOMICAL CONSIDERATIONS

For the purposes of evaluating a mass, the neck is best understood by dividing it into triangles. In addition, there are a few landmarks that will help the examiner remember the relative position of relevant structures of the neck.

TRIANGLES OF THE NECK

The neck can be divided into anterior and posterior triangles. These are further subdivided into four anterior subtriangles and two posterior subtriangles (Fig. 13-1).

ANTERIOR TRIANGLES OF THE NECK

The anterior triangle is delineated by the body of the mandible superiorly, the midline of the neck anteriorly, and the sternocleidomastoid muscle posteriorly. It is subdivided into the submandibular (digastric), carotid, submental (suprahyoid), and muscular triangles.

The *submandibular* (digastric) triangle is bounded superiorly by the body of the mandible, anteriorly by the belly of the digastric muscle, and posteriorly by the posterior belly of the digastric muscle. The *carotid* triangle is bounded superiorly by the posterior belly of the digastric

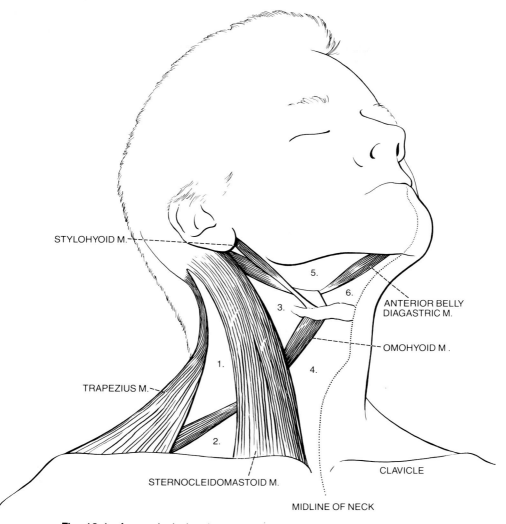

STYLOHYOID M.

ANTERIOR BELLY
DIAGASTRIC M.

OMOHYOID M .

TRAPEZIUS M.

CLAVICLE

STERNOCLEIDOMASTOID M.

MIDLINE OF NECK

Fig. 13-1. Anatomical triangles of the neck. (*1*) occipital; (*2*) subclavian; (*3*) carotid; (*4*) muscular; (*5*) submandibular; (*6*) submental.

muscle, anteriorly by the superior belly of the omohyoid muscle, and posteriorly by the sternocleidomastoid muscle. The *submental* (suprahyoid) triangle is bounded anteriorly by the midline of the neck, posteriorly by the anterior belly of the digastric muscle, and inferiorly by the body of hyoid bone. And the *muscular* triangle is bounded anteriorly by the midline of the neck, posteriorly by the anterior of the omohyoid muscle, and posteroinferiorly by the sternocleidomastoid muscle.

POSTERIOR TRIANGLES OF THE NECK

The posterior triangle of the neck is bounded anteriorly by the sternocleidomastoid muscle, posteriorly by the trapezius muscle, and inferiorly by the body of the clavicle. It is further subdivided into the occipital
and the subclavian (omoclavicular) triangles. The *occipital* triangle is
bounded anteriorly by the sternocleidomastoid muscle, posteriorly by
the trapezius muscle, and inferiorly by the posterior belly of the omohyoid muscle; the *subclavian* (omoclavicular) triangle is bounded superiorly
by the posterior belly of the omohyoid muscle, anteriorly by the sternocleidomastoid muscle, and inferiorly by the body of the clavicle.

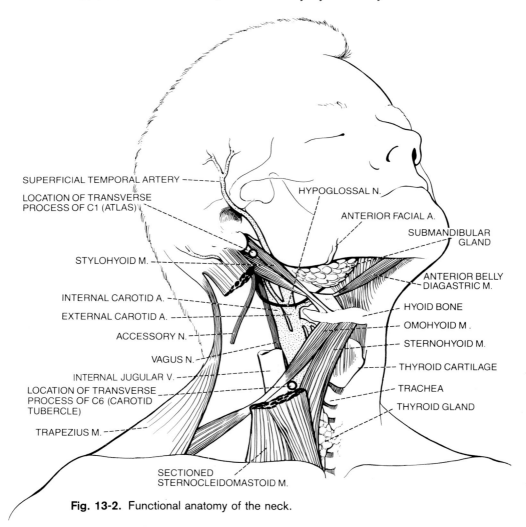

SUPERFICIAL TEMPORAL ARTERY

LOCATION OF TRANSVERSE
PROCESS OF C1 (ATLAS)

HYPOGLOSSAL N.

ANTERIOR FACIAL A.

SUBMANDIBULAR
GLAND

STYLOHYOID M.

ANTERIOR BELLY
DIAGASTRIC M.

INTERNAL CAROTID A.

HYOID BONE

EXTERNAL CAROTID A.

OMOHYOID M .

ACCESSORY N.

STERNOHYOID M.

VAGUS N.

THYROID CARTILAGE

INTERNAL JUGULAR V.

LOCATION OF TRANSVERSE
PROCESS OF C6 (CAROTID
TUBERCLE)

TRACHEA

THYROID GLAND

TRAPEZIUS M.

SECTIONED
STERNOCLEIDOMASTOID M.

Fig. 13-2. Functional anatomy of the neck.

CONTENTS OF THE CERVICAL TRIANGLES

The most significant anatomical structures located in the triangles are listed under Contents of the Triangles of the Neck and are demonstrated in Figure 13-2.

Contents of the Triangles of the Neck

A. Anterior triangles
   1. Submandibular (digastric) triangle
     a. Glands and organs
       (1) Submandibular gland
     b. Vasculature
       (1) Anterior facial artery and vein
     c. Nerves
       (1) Hypoglossal nerve
     d. Muscles
       (1) Mylohyoid muscle
       (2) Hyoglossus muscle
     e. Lymph nodes
       (1) Submandibular node
   2. Carotid triangle
     a. Glands and organs
       (1) Carotid body
     b. Vasculature
       (1) Internal and external carotid artery
       (2) Superior thyroid artery
       (3) Internal jugular vein
     c. Nerves
       (1) Vagus nerve
       (2) Hypoglossal nerve
       (3) Accessory nerve
       (4) Laryngeal and superior laryngeal nerves
     d. Muscles
       (1) Thyrohyoid muscle
       (2) Inferior constrictor muscle
     e. Skeleton
       (1) Greater cornu of hyoid bone
       (2) Ala of thyroid cartilage
     f. Lymph nodes
       (1) Superficial cervical node
       (2) Deep cervical node

(Continued)

Contents of the Triangles of the Neck *(Continued)*

    3. Submental triangle
        a. Muscles
            (1) Mylohyoid muscle
        b. Lymph nodes
            (1) Submental node
    4. Muscular triangle
        a. Glands and organs
            (1) Larynx and trachea
            (2) Thyroid gland
        b. Vasculature
            (1) Common carotid artery
            (2) Inferior thyroid artery
            (3) Internal jugular vein
        c. Nerves
            (1) Vagus nerve
            (2) Cervical sympathetic chain
            (3) Descendens hypoglossi
        d. Muscles
            (1) Sternohyoid muscle
            (2) Sternothyroid muscle
        e. Skeleton
            (1) Thyroid cartilage
            (2) Cricoid cartilage
            (3) Tracheal rings
            (4) Transverse process of sixth cervical vertebra (carotid
                tubercle)
        f. Lymph nodes
            (1) Superficial and deep cervical nodes
 B. Posterior triangles
    1. Occipital triangle
        a. Nerves
            (1) Greater occipital nerve
            (2) C3 and C4
            (3) Accessory nerve
            (4) Brachial plexus
        b. Muscles
            (1) Levator scapulae
            (2) Splenius capitis
            (3) Scalenus anterior, scalenus medius, and scalenus
                posterior

(Continued)

Contents of the Triangles of the Neck (*Continued*)

    c. Lymph nodes
      (1) Occipital node
      (2) Accessory node
      (3) Superficial cervical node
      (4) Transverse cervical node
  2. Subclavian triangle
    a. Vasculature
      (1) Subclavian artery and vein
      (2) Thyrocervical trunk
    b. Nerves
      (1) Phrenic nerve
    c. Muscles
      (1) Scalenus medius and scalenus anterior
    d. Lymph nodes
      (1) Transverse cervical node
      (2) Superficial cervical node

SKELETAL LANDMARKS IN THE NECK

The greater cornu of the hyoid bone is in close proximity to several important structures of the neck, including the carotid bifurcation, the internal jugular vein, the vagus nerve, the hypoglossal nerve, the superior thyroid artery, and the superior laryngeal nerve.

The transverse process of the first cervical vertebra (atlas) is located a fingerbreadth anterior and inferior to the mastoid process. The internal jugular vein and lower cranial nerves (nerves IX, X, XI, and XII) are located just anterior to this bony process.

The transverse process of the sixth cervical vertebra (carotid tubercle) is located at the level of the arch of the cricoid cartilage and approximately at the anterior border of the sternocleidomastoid muscle. Just anterior to this bony prominence is the common carotid artery, which can be compressed against the carotid tubercle to control hemorrhage. Also, the vertebral artery enters its foramen at this level.

LYMPH NODES OF THE HEAD AND NECK

Lymph nodes of the head and neck include the occipital, retroauricular (mastoid), preauricular, parotid, facial, submandibular, and submental nodes and the superficial, deep, and anterior cervical nodes (Fig. 13-3).

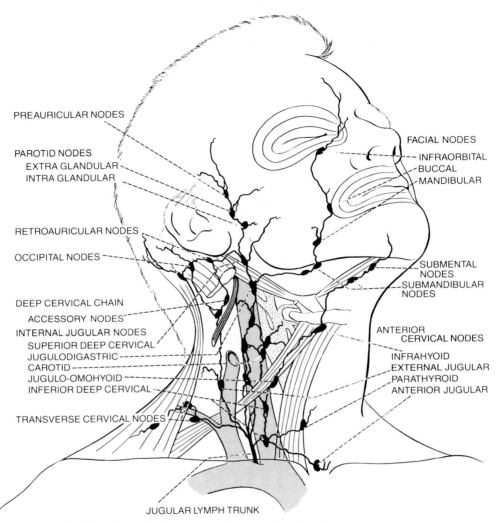

Fig. 13-3. Lymphatic drainage of the head and neck.

Occipital Nodes

Occipital nodes are located near the anterior attachment of the trapezius muscle to the skull. They receive afferent lymphatics from the posterolateral scalp and drain into the deep cervical chain.

Retroauricular (Mastoid) Nodes

The retroauricular (mastoid) nodes are located at the insertion of the sternocleidomastoid muscle to the mastoid bone. They receive afferent lymphatics from the posterior temporal and parietal areas and drain into the deep cervical chain.

Preauricular Nodes

The preauricular nodes are located just anterior to the tragus of the auricle and receive afferent lymphatics from the pinna and temporal regions of the scalp. They drain into the deep cervical nodes.

Parotid Nodes

The parotid nodes are divided into two groups, the extraglandular and intraglandular nodes. The extraglandular nodes are located deep (medial) to the parotid fascia near the preauricular nodes, which lie more superficially. The intraglandular nodes are deep within the parotid gland near the junction of the superficial and deep lobes. The parotid nodes receive afferent lymphatics from the anterior temporal scalp, external auditory canal, eyelids, and root of the nose and drain into the deep cervical chain.

Facial Nodes

The facial nodes are divided into the infraorbital, buccal, and supramandibular nodes. The infraorbital nodes overlie the orbicularis oculi. The buccal node is in a subcutaneous plane near the junction of the buccinator and orbicularis oris muscles. The supramandibular nodes lie lateral to the mandible near the anterior facial artery. The facial nodes receive afferent lymphatics from the eyelids, conjunctiva, nasal skin and mucosa, and cheek and drain into the submandibular nodes.

Submandibular Nodes

The submandibular nodes are located under the body of the mandible in close proximity to the submandibular gland. They are further subdivided into preglandular, retroglandular, and intracapsular nodes. These nodes receive afferent lymphatics from the cheek, nose, upper and lower lips, anterior nasal mucosa, gums, teeth, soft and hard palates, anterior aspect of the tongue, submandibular and sublingual glands, and the floor of the mouth. They drain into the deep cervical chain.

Submental Nodes

The submental nodes lie between the paired anterior bellies of the digastric muscle in the submental triangle and receive afferent lymphatics from the lip, the floor of the mouth, the cheeks, the incisor region of the gingiva, and the anterior tongue. They drain into the submaxillary node and then into the ipsilateral deep cervical chain and, occasionally, into the contralateral deep cervical chain.

Superficial Cervical Nodes

The superficial cervical nodes are located along the course of the external jugular vein. They receive afferent lymphatics from the ear and parotid area and drain into the deep cervical chain.

Deep Cervical Chain

The deep cervical chain is usually divided into the internal jugular, accessory, and transverse cervical chains. The internal jugular chain lies anterior to the internal jugular vein high in the neck and posterior to it lower in the neck. This chain includes the jugulodigastric node at the level of the posterior belly of the digastric muscle; carotid nodes at the carotid bifurcation; the jugulo-omohyoid node at the level of the crossing of the omohyoid muscle and the internal jugular vein; and supraclavicular or inferior deep cervical nodes superior to the level of the clavicle. The accessory chain is located along the course of the accessory nerve and receives afferent lymphatics from the posterior aspect of the scalp and the mastoid areas. The transverse cervical (supraclavicular) chain is located along the course of the transverse cervical artery and vein. It receives afferent lymphatics from the spinal accessory chain, the pectoral area, part of the arm, and the viscera and drains into the inferior deep cervical nodes and the jugular trunk.

Anterior Cervical Nodes

The anterior cervical nodes lie between the two carotid sheaths below the level of the hyoid bone. The superficial anterior jugular nodes lie along the course of the anterior jugular vein and drain into the deep cervical chain. The deep anterior cervical nodes consist of the prelaryngeal, pretracheal nodes along the course of the recurrent laryngeal nerve. They receive afferent lymphatics from the thyroid gland and infraglottic larynx, and they drain into the deep jugular chain and also communicate with anterior mediastinal nodes. The jugular trunk is formed by the superficial, deep, and anterior cervical chains. On the right, this empties into the right lymphatic duct, and on the left, into the thoracic duct.

TECHNIQUES FOR PHYSICAL EXAMINATION

During examination, the physician should mentally divide the patient's neck into its triangles by delineating the sternocleidomastoid and trapezius muscles. The neck is then examined in a rostral to caudal direction in a systematic fashion with reference to cervical triangles and cartilaginous and bony landmarks. There are several maneuvers the physician can perform that will help ensure a thorough examination of this area:

1. The hyoid, thyroid, and cricoid cartilages and tracheal rings should be delineated and checked for displacement and mobility.
2. The submental and submandibular triangles should be examined bimanually with one of the physician's forefingers in the anterior and lateral floor of the mouth.
3. The thyroid gland and its underlying cartilaginous structures should be displaced to one side, to be examined with the physician's opposite hand. Also, asking the patient to swallow during palpation of the gland may help to delineate masses and determine mobility.
4. The structures deep to the sternocleidomastoid muscle should be palpated by displacing the muscle both anteriorly and posteriorly.
5. The patient's neck should be placed in a neutral or slightly flexed position to allow relaxation of the cervical musculature and to allow the physician's fingers to probe deep within the triangles of the neck.

DIAGNOSTIC STRATEGY FOR THE EVALUATION OF A NECK MASS

When a mass is discovered, its characteristics are evaluated and recorded.

1. Location in a cervical triangle and proximity to known major structures: Does the mass feel attached to known structures, such as the thyroid gland or the carotid artery?
2. Consistency: Is the mass soft, fluctuant, easily mobile, well-encapsulated, and smooth, or is it firm, poorly mobile and fixed to surrounding structures? Does it pulsate? Is there a bruit? Does it appear to be superficial or attached to the skin, or is it in deeper areas of the neck? Is it tender or nontender?
3. Concomitant pathology: Is there any other evidence of significant disease in the head and neck? To answer this question, the physician must thoroughly examine the patient's scalp, face, external ear, tympanic membrane, parotid, oropharynx, nose,

nasal pharynx, laryngopharynx, and tongue by techniques already described.

Based on this initial evaluation of the mass, which provides knowledge of its consistency, its location in the cervical triangles, and its association with adjacent structures, as well as of the presence or absence of concomitant pathology in the head-and-neck structures, a working diagnosis is formulated that assigns the mass to as few as possible of the diagnostic categories listed under Differential Diagnosis of Neck Masses.

Differential Diagnosis of Neck Masses

A. Lymphadenomegaly
  1. Inflammatory disorders
      a. Bacterial and viral illnesses
      b. Cat-scratch fever
      c. Actinomycosis
      d. Sarcoidosis
      e. Toxoplasmosis
      f. Mononucleosis
  2. Neoplastic disorders
      a. Primary lymphoma
      b. Metastatic tumors
          (1) Head and neck primary (90%)
          (2) Distant primary (10%)
B. Congenital or developmental cysts and masses
  1. Branchial-cleft cysts
  2. Thyroglossal-duct cyst
  3. Cystic hygroma
  4. Hemangioma
  5. Laryngocele
C. Neoplasm or other enlargement of a structure or organ contained in the neck
  1. Skin
      a. Sebaceous cyst
      b. Lipoma
  2. Muscle
      a. Torticollis
  3. Nerve
      a. Neurofibroma
      b. Neurinoma
  4. Blood vessel
      a. Aneurysm
      b. Carotid-body tumor

(Continued)

Differential Diagnosis of Neck Masses (*Continued*)

      c. Hemangiopericytoma
      d. Glomus jugulare
   5. Thyroid
   6. Esophagus
   7. Larynx
      a. Chondroma

LYMPHADENOMEGALY

Lympadenomegaly may consist of either inflammatory or neoplastic disorders. In both, knowledge of the afferent supply of the involved lymph node is critical for further evaluation. In the presence of acute infectious diseases, such as pharyngitis, tonsillitis, dental infection, and URI, and infection of the skin, no further diagnostic maneuvers may be necessary to formulate a diagnosis of the cause of lymph node enlargement. Acute inflammatory nodes usually are tender, mobile, and doughy.

Neoplastic nodes may be primary or metastatic. In 90% of the lymph nodes of the neck containing metastases, the primary tumor is in the head and neck; the other 10% are derived from primary tumors in distant structures, including the viscera.

A frequent diagnostic problem involves the identification of a probable lymph node and the inability to determine whether the node represents a chronic inflammatory disorder, such as toxoplasmosis or sarcoidosis, or a primary or metastatic neoplastic process. All nodes should be considered metastatic until proven otherwise, and several steps should be undertaken before an open biopsy of the neck is done. Although it would seem that biopsy of a node would save time in the diagnostic work-up, there is evidence that premature open biopsy of a neoplastic node, later identified as having metastasized from a head-and-neck primary tumor, results in a poorer prognosis than if the primary node and metastasis are treated in an orderly fashion. Proper evaluation of a node requires a careful history of dysfunction, such as dysphagia, hemoptysis, hematemesis, hoarseness, or a sensation of a mass in the mouth or throat, and a history of drinking and smoking habits. A thorough head-and-neck examination, including mirror examinations of internal cavities, is also performed.

There are differences of opinion as to how many additional diagnostic steps should be undertaken in the absence of evidence of a primary tumor in the head and neck prior to open biopsy. Certainly, any suggestive symptoms should be thoroughly investigated by any available means, including the use of radiography. If a patient complains of dysphagia, a barium swallow should be done; however, a barium swallow is not a substitute for a thorough examination of the oropharynx and hypopharynx. A chest x-ray film may indicate primary lung disease, involvement of mediastinal nodes, or other metastases to pulmonary parenchyma. If indicated, a lateral plain film of the nasopharynx or tomography in the submental-vertex plane will provide additional information concerning tumors of the nasopharynx and skull base. Plain films of the paranasal sinuses may give evidence of an otherwise occult lesion. Sialography is not usually performed unless there is a suggestive clinical history or findings. X-ray films of the structures of the ear are not indicated unless there is clinical evidence of significant ear disease. Any suggestive thoracic or abdominal symptoms are appropriately evaluated.

The age of the patient must also be considered before open biopsy because benign cervical adenopathy is common in the first and second decades of life. Even if the node is subsequently determined to be a neoplastic process, it is rare that waiting a few weeks to reevaluate a suspected node after careful evaluation and measurement will adversely affect the prognosis of a patient. The test of time, if performed intelligently, may save the patient considerable unnecessary work-up and surgery.

Depending on the systemic findings, history of the node enlargement, and exposure of the patient, certain skin tests or serological tests may be helpful in arriving at a diagnosis. These include tests for tuberculosis, syphilis, sarcoidosis, toxoplasmosis, lupus erythematosus, mononucleosis, and cat-scratch fever.

If these efforts do not result in the identification of the cause of lymphadenomegaly, open biopsy is indicated. In very large or multiply enlarged nodes, a needle biopsy may be performed. In a smaller node, excisional biopsy is usually preferred.

CONGENITAL OR DEVELOPMENTAL CYSTS AND MASSES

BRANCHIAL-CLEFT CYSTS

Branchial-cleft cysts are located just anterior to the sternocleidomastoid muscle in the carotid triangle. A cystic mass with or without an external sinus tract is present. The diagnosis is more obvious in the presence of an external fistulous tract and a history of intermittent discharge, and often there is a history of fluctuating size and intermittent tenderness. Branchial-cleft cysts may become symptomatic at any age, but most are diagnosed in the first two decades of life. For final diagnosis and treatment, surgical excision is performed.

THYROGLOSSAL-DUCT CYSTS

The thyroglossal-duct cyst is a remnant of the tract of descent of the thyroid gland into the neck from the tongue base. It is therefore almost always found in the midline, either in the submental or muscular triangles. Thyroglossal-duct cysts may be found at any age, but most are found in the first decade of life. It is not uncommon for them to present slightly lateral to the midline, and an external fistula to the skin of the anterior neck may or may not be present. A thyroglossal-duct cyst must be differentiated from dermoid cysts, lymphadenomegaly in the anterior jugular chain, and cutaneous lesions, such as lipomas and sebaceous cysts. The cyst is often ballotable. It may be located above or below the hyoid bone and moves with it. Surgery is almost always required not only because of cosmetic considerations but also because of the high incidence of recurrent infection, including abscess formation.

CYSTIC HYGROMA AND HEMANGIOMA

Cystic hygromas are almost always first seen by the second year of life, although a few may be first diagnosed in adult life. Clinically, they are diffuse, soft, doughy, irregular masses. They may compromise the airway, depending on their location and size. Because spontaneous regression occurs in some patients, surgery is postponed unless the airway is compromised.

Superficial cutaneous hemangiomas are easily diagnosed by their appearance. Deeper hemangiomas may be more difficult to diagnose. In three quarters of the patients afflicted with the condition, it is present at birth, and in nearly 90% of these, it is diagnosed in the first year of life. There is a female predominance. Larger hemangiomas, especially cavernous hemangiomas, may have a palpable thrill. Because of the spontaneous regression of a high proportion of hemangiomas in the first 2 years of life, expectant observation is usually practiced.

MASSES ATTACHED TO NORMAL STRUCTURES OF THE NECK

MASSES WITHIN THE SKIN

Superficial intracutaneous or subcutaneous masses may be sebaceous cysts or lipomas, and the final diagnosis and treatment usually involves simple surgical excision, often done as an office procedure under a local anesthetic.

MASSES DERIVED FROM NERVE TISSUE

With masses derived from nerve tissue, a definitive diagnosis is rarely made preoperatively. Neurofibromas most commonly originate from the cervical sympathetic trunk and may produce a Horner's syndrome. They may arise from the glossopharyngeal, vagus, hypoglossal, or spinal accessory nerves, causing associated dysfunction. Occasionally, they may also arise from the trunks of the trigeminal or facial nerves. Small neuromas or neurofibromas may be difficult to differentiate from lymph nodes, and often the final diagnosis is made by excisional biopsy.

TUMORS ATTACHED TO OR DERIVED FROM BLOOD VESSELS OR ASSOCIATED STRUCTURES

Tumors attached to or derived from blood vessels or associated structures include aneurysms of the common carotid artery or subclavian artery and chemodectomas (glomus tumors or nonchromaffin paragangliomas) arising from chemoreceptor bodies. Carotid-body tumors present as a painless, slowly growing mass at the carotid bifurcation. Occasionally, a bruit may be present. The tumor is not separable from the carotid artery by palpation. The differential diagnosis includes consideration of an aneurysm of the carotid, a branchial-cleft cyst, a neurogenic tumor, or nodal metastases fixed to the carotid sheath. In the head and neck the most common chemodectomas arise from the tympanic bodies in the middle ear, the glomus jugulare at the skull base, the vagal body near the skull base along the inferior ganglion of the vagus, and the carotid body at the carotid bifurcation. Glomus tympanicum tumors and glomus jugulare tumors are usually first diagnosed by an appearance of a vascular mass behind the tympanic membrane. Glomus intravagale tumors often grow to substantial size at the skull base before diagnosis.

Other than the glomus tympanicum type, these tumors require carotid angiography for evaluation, which should usually be done by a transfemoral route so that the opposite neck may be surveyed, because there is a low incidence of bilateral and multiple chemodectomas as a heredofamilial tendency. The radiologist should be asked to record the venous phase of arteriography, especially with glomus jugulare tumors. The treatment of these tumors is surgical, if possible. Larger, unresectable tumors may be controlled for many years with radiotherapy.

MASSES WITHIN THE THYROID GLAND

Masses within the thyroid gland can be evaluated chemically and by radionuclide scanning, needle biopsy, or open biopsy.

LESIONS WITHIN THE ESOPHAGUS

Occasionally a Zenker's diverticulum will be large enough to present as a ballotable mass within the neck. Associated symptoms include dysphagia, food retention, and regurgitation. A barium swallow is diagnostic.

TUMORS ARISING FROM CARTILAGINOUS STRUCTURES

Chondromas or chondrosarcomas may rarely arise from the thyroid or cricoid cartilages. They are firmly fixed to these structures and may present as a mass in the neck or as the cause of a compromised airway.

14

RADIOLOGY OF THE EARS, NOSE, AND THROAT FOR THE PRIMARY-CARE PHYSICIAN

Alfred L. Weber
Chief of Radiology
Massachusetts Eye and Ear Infirmary
Associate Professor of Radiology
Harvard Medical School

William R. Wilson

Sinus x-ray series
  Water's view
  Caldwell view
  Base, or submentovertical, view
  Lateral view
Tomography of the paranasal
      sinuses
Radiologic interpretation of sinus
      disease
  Normal appearance of the sinus
  Acute sinus disease
  Chronic sinus disease
  Fluid in the sinuses
  Retention cysts
  Polyps
  Mucoceles
Benign tumors of the paranasal
      sinuses
  Osteomas
  Fibrous dysplasia (ossifying fi-
      broma)
Malignant lesions of the paranasal
      sinuses
Facial trauma
  Trimalar fractures
  Le Fort fractures
  Trauma of the orbits
  Nasal fractures
  Fractures of the mandible

Radiology of the salivary glands
  Contraindications
  Complications
  Radiographic findings
Radiology of the larynx
Benign lesions of the larynx
  Laryngotracheal bronchitis (croup)
  Acute supraglottitis (epiglottitis)
  Retropharyngeal abscesses
  Foreign bodies
  Papillomatosis
  Subglottic hemangioma
  Cysts
  Laryngoceles
  Polyps
Malignant lesions of the larynx
Plain-film evaluation of the tem-
      poral bone
  Radiologic findings
    Acute mastoiditis
    Chronic mastoiditis
    Cholesteatoma
    Acoustic neuromas
      Computed tomography
        evaluation of acoustic
        neuromas
    Trauma of the temporal bone

255

The purpose of this chapter is to provide the primary-care physician with practical information regarding radiology of the head and neck for ear, nose, and throat disorders. A discussion of the radiologic views necessary for diagnosis as well as practical instructions for interpreting the films will be provided.

SINUS X-RAY SERIES

The sinus x-ray series consists of an upright Water's view, a Caldwell view, and lateral and base views. This set of films has proved to be very useful for the assessment of acute and chronic sinus disease; tumors of the sinuses, nose, nasopharynx, and orbit; and facial trauma. The primary-care physician should be familiar with the correct positioning of the patient for the various views (Fig. 14-1) and the fundamentals of radiologic interpretation that follow.

THE WATER'S VIEW

The Water's view (Fig. 14-2) shows the maxillary antrum better than any other view of the skull. This view is easily recognized by remembering that the positioning is roughly approximate to placing the patient's chin and nose on the x-ray plate. The roof of the maxillary antrum is the floor of the orbit, and the inferior orbital rim is seen as a thick, bony rim above the orbital floor, which is projected approximately 2 mm below it; therefore, there are two lines to be evaluated in assessing the inferior bony orbit. The ethmomaxillary plate and the ethmoid air cells are also demonstrated. In the Water's view, the anterior ethmoid air cells are projected superiorly, and the posterior ethmoid air cells are projected inferiorly. The anterior portion of the medial wall of the maxillary antrum, which is the lateral wall of the nasal fossa, is also seen. Other structures demonstrated by the Water's view are the zygomatic arch, the frontozygomatic suture, the zygomatic bone, the maxillary bone, the linea innominata (cortex of the temporal surface of the greater wing of sphenoid) and the mandibular condyles. The open-mouth Water's view affords a reasonable visualization of the sphenoid sinus as well as of the odontoid process.

CALDWELL VIEW

The Caldwell view best demonstrates the size and shape of the orbits (Fig. 14-3). In this view the patient is positioned with his nose and

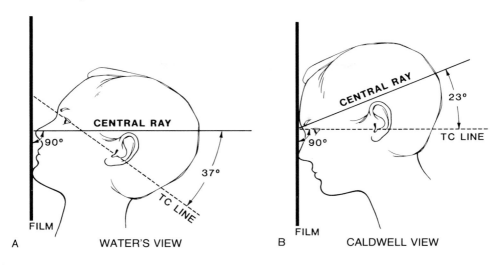

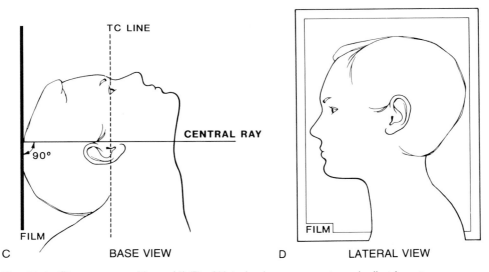

Fig. 14-1. Sinus x-ray positions. (*A*) The Water's view represents an inclined postero-anterior view with the tragocanthal line (TC line) forming a 37° angle with the central ray. (*B*) In the Caldwell view, or posteroanterior projection, the TC line is perpendicular to the plane of the film, and the central ray is directed caudally at 23°. (*C*) In the base, or submentovertical, view, the TC line is placed parallel to the x-ray plate, and the central ray passes submentally and perpendicular to the TC line and x-ray plate. (*D*) In the lateral view, the sagittal plane is parallel to the x-ray plate.

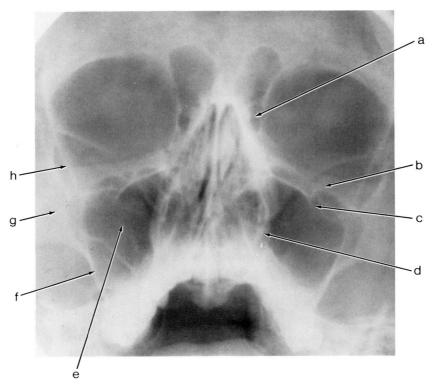

Fig. 14-2. Water's view of the sinuses shows (*a*) anterior ethmoid air cells; (*b*) rim of orbit; (*c*) floor of orbit; (*d*) medial anterior wall of the antrum; (*e*) antral cavity; (*f*) lateral wall of the antrum; (*g*) body of zygoma; and (*h*) innominate line made by a tangential view of the cortex of the greater wing of sphenoid.

forehead on the x-ray plate. The structures demonstrated on this view are the linea innominata, the superior orbital fissure, the lesser and greater wings of the sphenoid bone, and the anterior and posterior portions of the lamina papyracea (medial wall of the orbit). In addition to the orbital structures seen in this view, the frontal and ethmoid sinuses, the planum sphenoidale, and the floor of the sella turcica are also visualized. The medial wall of the maxillary antrum and the ethmomaxillary plate are also seen. If there is a decrease in the bony density of the medial wall of the antrum in comparison with the other side, bone destruction from a tumor should be considered, and further investigation with polytomography would be suggested.

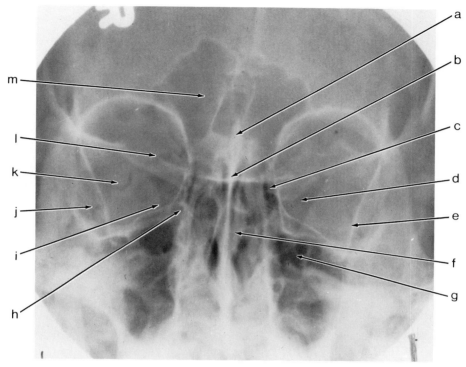

Fig. 14-3. Caldwell view of the paranasal sinuses reveals (*a*) crista galli; (*b*) planum sphenoidale; (*c*) ethmoid sinuses; (*d*) superior orbital fissure; (*e*) innominate line; (*f*) floor of sella turcica; (*g*) foramen rotundum; (*h*) medial wall of orbit, anteriorly; (*i*) medial wall and floor of orbit, posteriorly; (*j*) lambdoid suture projected through orbit; (*k*) greater wing of sphenoid; (*l*) lesser wing of sphenoid; and (*m*) frontal sinus.

BASE VIEW

The base, or submentovertical, view best demonstrates the anatomy of the base of the skull, the anterior wall of the middle cranial fossa, the posterior wall of the orbit, and the posterior wall of the maxillary antrum (Fig. 14-4). The posterior wall of the orbit is continuous with the middle cranial fossa, and both are formed by the greater wing of the sphenoid. On this view, the posterior wall of the maxillary antrum has an S-shaped curve. The foramen ovale and foramen spinosum, the medial and lateral pterygoid plates, and the pterygopalatine fossa (immediately anterior to the pterygoid bones) are also demonstrated. The sphenoid sinus and intersphenoidal septum are seen in the midportion of the skull base.

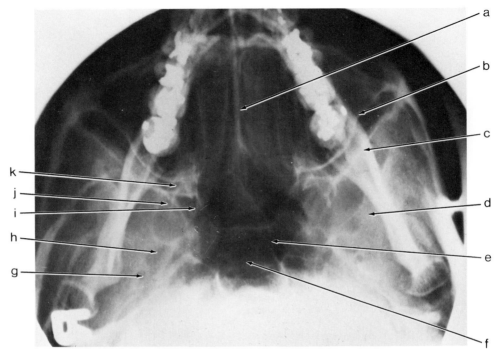

Fig. 14-4. Base view of the skull domonstrates (a) nasal septum; (b) posterior wall of the maxillary antrum; (c) posterior wall of the orbit (note S shape); (d) middle cranial fossa; (e) intersphenoidal septum; (f) sphenoid sinus; (g) foramen spinosum; (h) foramen ovale; (i) medial pterygoid plates; (j) lateral pterygoid plates; and (k) pterygopalatine fossa.

Although the sphenoid sinus can be seen on the lateral view, only the base view shows each sphenoid sinus as a separate entity.

LATERAL VIEW

The lateral view demonstrates the sella turcica, the anterior and posterior clinoids, the nasopharyngeal soft tissues, the anterior and posterior walls of the frontal sinus, the pterygopalatine fossa, and the hard palate (Fig. 14-5). The sphenoid sinus, clivus, and odontoid processes are also well visualized. This view is useful for the evaluation of nasopharyngeal masses, for example, for examining adenoids in children or the question of benign and malignant masses in adults (Fig. 14-6).

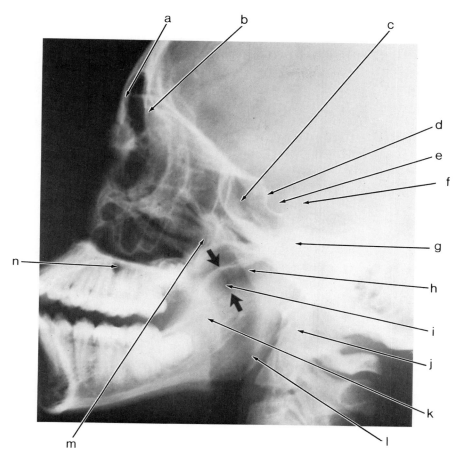

Fig. 14-5. Lateral sinus view demonstrates (*a*) anterior wall of the frontal sinus; (*b*) posterior wall of the frontal sinus; (*c*) sphenoid sinus; (*d*) anterior clinoid processes; (*e*) sella turcica; (*f*) posterior clinoid processes; (*g*) clivus; (*h*) roof of the nasopharynx; (*i*) opening of the eustachian tubes (indicated by arrows); (*j*) odontoid process; (*k*) uvula; (*l*) posterior wall of the oropharynx; (*m*) pterygopalatine fossa; and (*n*) hard palate.

TOMOGRAPHY OF THE PARANASAL SINUSES

Tomographic examination of the sinuses is best carried out by taking images at every 5 mm in the coronal, lateral, and, in some cases, basal projections. Usually eight sections are needed to demonstrate the an-

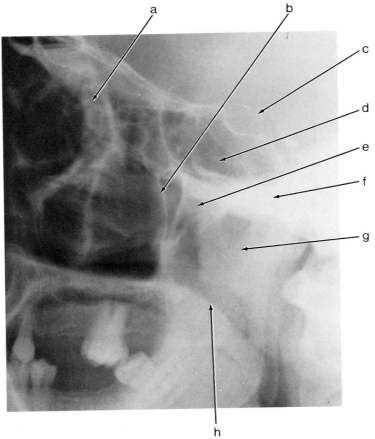

Fig. 14-6. The lateral view demonstrates (a) cribriform plate area; (b) posterior wall of the maxillary antrum; (c) sella turcica; (d) sphenoid sinus; (e) pterygoid bone; (f) clivus; (g) a hemispherical, sharply defined nasopharyngeal mass caused by hypertrophied adenoid tissue; and (h) soft palate.

teroposterior extent of the sinuses. Further cuts posteriorly can be obtained to demonstrate the nasopharynx and oropharynx.

Tomography in the coronal plane is helpful for demonstrating inflammatory and neoplastic processes in the nasal cavities and sinuses, tumors of the nasopharynx, fractures involving the orbit and sinuses, erosion of the lacrimal bone, and enlargement or destruction of the lacrimal fossa by lacrimal-gland tumors and for assessing the alveolar ridge of the maxilla and hard palate (Fig. 14-7A).

CORONAL VIEW　　　　　　　　　LATERAL VIEW

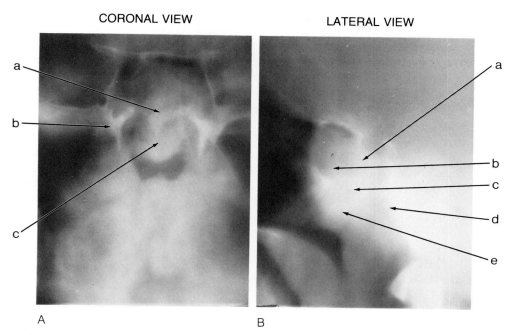

A　　　　　　　　　　　　　B

Fig. 14-7. Patient with carcinoma of the nasopharynx. (*A*) Coronal view reveals (*a*) destruction of the floor of the sphenoid sinus, and tumor within the sphenoid sinus; (*b*) sclerosis in the pterygoid bone; and (*c*) mass in the midportion of the nasopharynx. (*B*) A lateral polytome demonstrates (*a*) erosion of the floor of the sella; (*b*) extension of mass into the cavity of the sphenoid sinus; (*c*) destruction of the floor of the sphenoid sinus; (*d*) destruction of the anterior border of the clivus; and (*e*) mass in the nasopharynx.

Lateral tomograms of the sinuses encompass the paranasal sinuses and the nasal cavity in the anteroposterior dimension. These are often obtained in order to demonstrate the sphenoid sinus and nasopharynx to best advantage (Fig. 14-7B). The orbital rim and floor are seen particularly well; therefore, lateral tomograms are particularly helpful in evaluating fractures involving the floor of the orbit.

Basal-projection tomography is used to visualize displacement, bone destruction, or hyperostosis in the medial and lateral walls of the maxillary antrum and ethmoid sinus. This view is indicated for assessing destruction of the posterior wall of the maxillary antrum and of the anterior, posterior, and lateral walls of the sphenoid sinus. This view also best demonstrates the posterior wall of both orbits and the base of the skull, including the foramen ovale and foramen spinosum and the middle cranial fossa.

RADIOLOGIC INTERPRETATION OF SINUS DISEASE

NORMAL APPEARANCE OF THE SINUS

In a normal sinus study, the mucosa is not demonstrated on the radiograph, and the bony walls are clear-cut and distinct. The walls of the sinuses vary considerably in thickness in different individuals, and they may also vary in thickness in different parts of the same sinus. Variation in the thickness of the bony outline, which is most common on the anterior wall of the frontal sinus, causes a loss of translucency if the wall is slightly thicker than normal. The sinuses are lucent in proportion to the size of the air-filled cavity and the relative thickness of the bony wall. A small sinus with a thick, bony wall will appear less translucent than a large, well-developed sinus with a thin, bony wall.

ACUTE SINUS DISEASE

If a sinus becomes diseased, swelling of the mucosa will impart increased density to the sinus cavity. This may be associated with an air-fluid level, best demonstrated in the upright projection of the Water's (Fig. 14-8) or lateral view. The swelling of the mucosa may also be recognized as a hazy, thick, white line around the periphery of the sinus cavity. This thickened mucosal outline may parallel the bony wall of the sinus or may project as an undulating, wavy density along the bony wall. The thickness of the sinus mucosa may be gauged by observing it along the medial wall of the antrum in the Water's or Caldwell view. If the mucosal swelling is associated with the secretion of fluid or pus, the entire sinus becomes opacified. Persistent opacity of one sinus or unilateral opacity of several sinus chambers suggests the possibility of a malignant process.

Demineralization of the bony walls may be associated with acute infection and is most frequently seen in the ethmoid sinuses. In rare instances, considerable loss of bone secondary to infection may occur in the outline of the sinuses, simulating malignant disease.

CHRONIC SINUS DISEASE

Chronic sinus disease is recognized on x-ray film as a combination of membrane thickening and increased radiodensity of the bone (bony sclerosis) of the sinus walls. In advanced cases, there may be complete opacification of the sinus cavity. A hallmark of chronic sinusitis is scle-

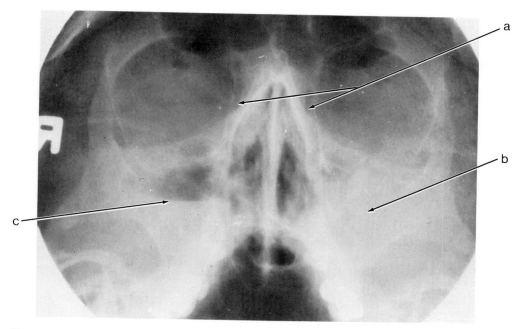

Fig. 14-8. Patient with acute sinusitis. Water's view reveals (a) increased density in both ethmoid sinuses; (b) completely opacified left antrum; and (c) air-fluid level in the midportion of the right maxillary antrum.

rosis of the outline of the bony wall (Fig. 14-9). Thickening of the bone is often associated with contraction of the sinus cavity, which is particularly obvious in the maxillary antra after Caldwell-Luc surgery. Increased density in the paranasal sinus with sclerosis may also be caused by chronic granulomatous disease of various etiologies. Sclerosis in the maxillary antrum is best demonstrated in the posterior wall of the antral cavity.

FLUID IN THE SINUSES

It is not possible to evaluate the nature of the fluid within a sinus cavity radiologically, but air-fluid levels are apparent on x-ray film. They are best demonstrated with the patient erect because it is in this position that the air and fluid separate to form an air-fluid level (see Fig. 14-8). The boundary between the air and the fluid remains horizontal whichever way the cavity is tilted, but it is lost if the patient is placed in the

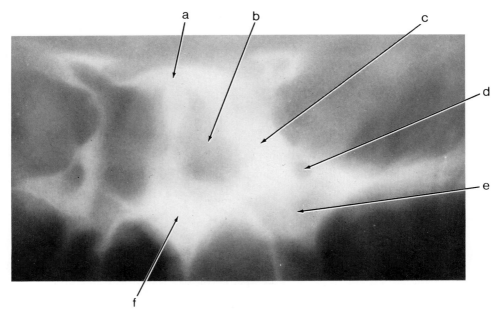

Fig. 14-9. Coronal tomographic section of a patient with chronic sphenoid sinusitis demonstrates (*a*) sclerosis in the planum sphenoidale; (*b*) mucosal thickening within the sphenoid sinus cavity; (*c*) sclerosis in the lateral wall of the sphenoid sinus; (*d*) the well-seen foramen rotundum surrounded by sclerosis in the pterygoid bone; (*e*) pterygoid bone; and (*f*) floor of the sphenoid sinus.

recumbent position. Most patients with an air-fluid level have associated thickening of the mucosal membrane.

RETENTION CYSTS

Retention cysts are most commonly encountered in the maxillary sinuses. They appear as smooth-walled, dome-shaped densities and are found most often in the floor of the maxillary sinus (Fig. 14-10). The mucosal lining of the remainder of the affected sinus is usually normal in appearance. Retention cysts may also be found in other sinuses; in any case they are clinically insignificant.

POLYPS

Nasal polyps arise primarily in the ethmoid labyrinth. As the polyps expand, the bony partitions of the ethmoid become decalcified and are

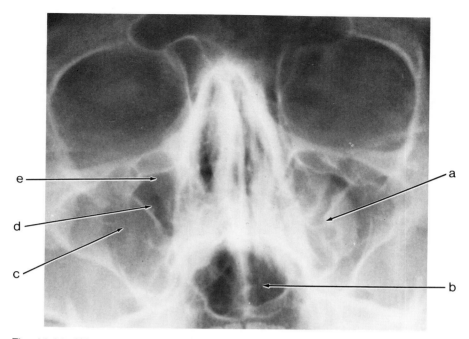

Fig. 14-10. Water's view reveals (*a*) a hemispherical, homogenous, sharply defined retention cyst arising from the medial wall of the antrum; (*b*) sphenoid sinus projected through the oral cavity in the open-mouth view; (*c*) greater wing of the sphenoid; (*d*) superior orbital fissure; and (*e*) lesser wing of the sphenoid.

no longer visible on x-ray film. When large enough, the polyps prolapse into the nose, and in advanced cases the nasal cavities may become completely obstructed. Polyps that are large enough to extend through the posterior choanae (choanal polyps) into the nasopharynx appear as a soft-tissue mass on the lateral or basal projections. Most choanal polyps have their origin in the maxillary antrum. In chronic polypoid panrhinosinusitis, all the sinus cavities are involved, leading to complete sinus opacification (Fig. 14-11).

MUCOCELES

Mucoceles represent a collection of mucous secretions and desquamated epithelium enclosed in the mucous-secreting respiratory membrane of a sinus cavity or compartment. An enlarging mucocele will cause the adjacent bony structures to expand and become thinner, a process that will continue until the structures are destroyed. Mucoceles may extend

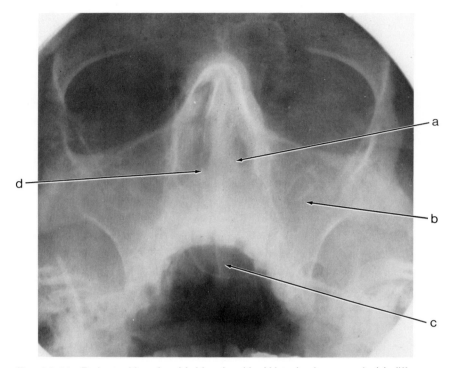

Fig. 14-11. Patient with polypoid rhinosinusitis. Water's view reveals (*a*) diffuse increase in density of the nasal cavities; (*b*) complete opacification of the maxillary antrum; and (*c*) marked increase in density in the sphenoid sinus. Note at (*d*) deviation of the nasal septum to the right.

by contiguity to adjacent sinuses, for example, from the frontal sinus to the ethmoid sinus and *vice versa,* and from the sphenoid sinus to the posterior ethmoid sinuses. Mucoceles occur most often in the frontal and ethmoid sinuses, less frequently in the sphenoid sinus, and only rarely in the maxillary sinuses. Multiple sinus involvement is unusual but has been reported. The majority of mucoceles occur in adults, but they are also seen in the pediatric age group, particularly in children with cystic fibrosis. The radiologic findings consist of a well-demarcated, homogenous soft-tissue mass in a sinus cavity and opacification of a sinus cavity with expansion, thinning, or interruption of the bony wall. Calcification of the mucocele has been reported in about 5% of cases.

In the frontal sinus, a mucocele will cause the loss of the scalloped margin of the normal sinus wall (Fig. 14-12). In some patients, the sinus may be more opaque than normal because of fluid accumulation within its cavity. In others, the sinus may appear more radiolucent if the bone

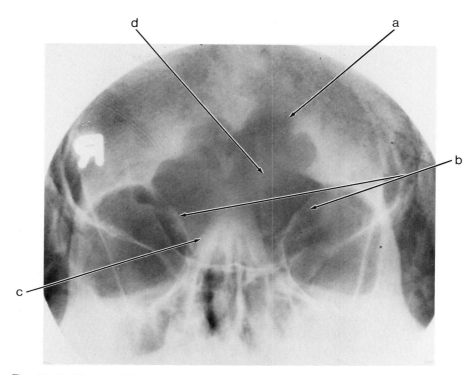

Fig. 14-12. Patient with frontal mucocele that extends into the upper ethmoid sinuses. The Caldwell view shows (*a*) loss of scalloping of the frontal sinus wall with sclerosis; (*b*) inferior displacement of the upper medial wall of the orbit on both sides; (*c*) slight expansion of the upper ethmoid sinus; and (*d*) slight increase in density of the expanded frontal sinus cavity.

loss is great enough to more than compensate for the increased density caused by the fluid content of the sinus. Large frontal-ethmoid mucoceles may displace the supraorbital ridge and adjacent roof of the orbit.

BENIGN TUMORS OF THE PARANASAL SINUSES

Among the lesions that may extend into the paranasal sinuses are benign tumors and cysts that may arise from dental structures, such as ameloblastomas, dentigerous cysts, and various benign odontogenic tua

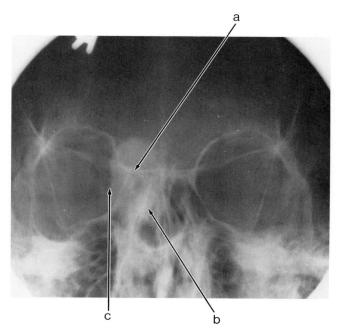

c   b

Fig. 14-13. Patient with an osteoma of the right ethmoid sinus. Caldwell view reveals (*a*) a homogenous, sharply defined bony mass within the right ethmoid sinus, extending at (*b*) into the nasal cavity and at (*c*) the medial aspect of the right orbit.

mors. Also, angiofibromas of the nasopharynx may invade the sphenoid sinus, and large pituitary adenomas can involve the sphenoid sinus and simulate primary sphenoid-sinus lesions.

A large variety of other benign tumors may affect the paranasal sinuses as well. The most commonly encountered are osteoma, fibrous dysplasia (ossifying fibroma), and a large variety of rare lesions, such as neurogenic tumors, hemangioma, and so forth.

OSTEOMAS

Osteomas are manifested radiologically as dense, rounded masses with clear-cut outlines (Fig. 14-13). They may be very dense (ivory osteomas) or may have lucent centers (cancellous osteomas). They occur most commonly in the frontal and ethmoid sinuses.

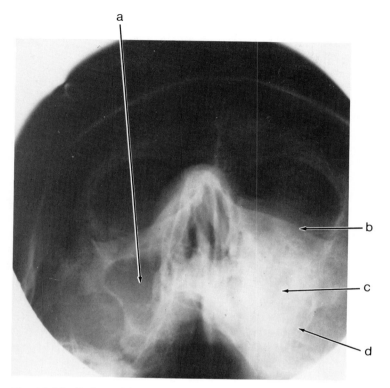

Fig. 14-14. Patient with fibrous dysplasia of the left antrum and adjacent facial bones. Water's view shows (*a*) normal right antrum; (*b*) thickening and superior displacement of the inferior orbital rim; (*c*) diffuse new bone formation with expansion in the left maxillary antrum; and (*d*) expansion and inferior displacement of the lateral wall of the left maxillary antrum.

FIBROUS DYSPLASIA (OSSIFYING FIBROMA)

The roentgen appearance of these benign tumors depends on the amount of fibrous tissue that develops relative to the newly formed osteoid and calcified matrix (Fig. 14-14). The sinus cavity may reveal complete, uniform opacification with masses of calcified matrix and bone. Most often, there is expansion of the involved sinus cavity with considerable thinning or loss of the bony sinus wall. Also, there is often extension into neighboring structures, such as the orbits, the nasal cavity, the oral cavity, and the adjacent skull.

MALIGNANT LESIONS OF THE PARANASAL SINUSES

By far the most common malignant lesion encountered in the paranasal sinuses is carcinoma (Fig. 14-15). A large variety of other lesions, such as melanomas, lymphomas, fibrosarcomas, esthesioneuroblastomas, plasmacytomas, hemangiopericytomas, and various other sarcomas, has also been encountered. There are no distinguishing radiologic features among these various lesions, other than the fact that calcium is encountered in chondrogenic and osteogenic sarcomas.

The most common radiographic finding of sinus malignancy is an indistinct mass in the sinus cavity. Another finding that identifies malignant tumors is lytic bone destruction of the outline of the sinus cavities and, at times, of the adjacent facial bones and orbits. Bony sclerosis may be encountered in the sinus walls, the sphenoid bone, and the pterygoid bone as a nonspecific finding resulting from associated inflammation.

Malignant lesions of the paranasal sinuses may extend into the nasal cavity, oral cavity, orbit, intracranial cavity, pterygopalatine fossa, and infratemporal fossa (see Fig. 14-7 *A* and *B*). Extension of the tumor is best evaluated by computed tomography (CT).

FACIAL TRAUMA

The most common fractures of the maxillofacial regions are zygomatic-arch fractures, trimalar fractures, and Le Fort fractures. A sinus x-ray series, namely Caldwell, Water's, lateral, and basal views of the facial bones, is used to assess a patient with maxillofacial trauma. If a zygomatic-arch fracture is suspected or present and needs to be analyzed in detail, a specific zygomatic-arch view should be obtained. If a more detailed assessment of facial-bone fractures is required, particularly when associated with orbital fractures and fractures in the naso-orbital complex, anteroposterior (AP) and lateral tomographic studies are indicated.

Facial fractures can be divided into three categories: isolated fractures, such as those occurring in the sinuses, orbital rim, alveolar process of the maxilla, and zygomatic arch; zygomaticomaxillary complex, or trimalar, fractures, which are frequently encountered; and midfacial fractures, such as Le Fort fractures, types I, II and III.

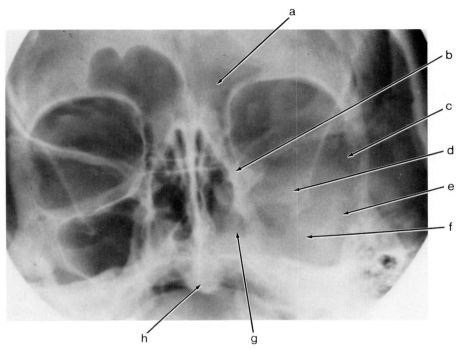

Fig. 14-15. Patient with carcinoma of the left maxillary antrum. Water's view reveals (*a*) increased density in the frontal sinus; (*b*) increased density in the left ethmoid sinus with destruction of the ethmomaxillary plate; (*c*) erosion of the inferior lateral wall of the orbit; (*d*) erosion of the inferior orbital rim and floor; (*e*) destruction in the left maxillary bone; (*f*) mass in the left antrum; (*g*) destruction of the medial wall of the left antrum (compare with normal right side); and (*h*) incidental finding of a torus palatinus.

TRIMALAR FRACTURES

Trimalar, or tripod, fractures are fractures of the face that result in malar-eminence displacement (Fig. 14-16). The malar eminence is usually displaced downward and medially. Fractures are present in the lateral wall of the orbit, usually at the frontozygomatic suture, through the zygomatic arch, and through the rim of the orbit and the lateral wall of the maxillary antrum. Trimalar fractures may be associated with an orbital-floor fracture; in such cases, the degree of deformity and depression of the orbital floor can vary widely. There may be herniation of orbital tissue in the upper portion of the antrum. The fractures through the zygomatic arch may be single or multiple with different degrees of depression or, in some instances, outward buckling (Figs. 14-17 and 14-18).

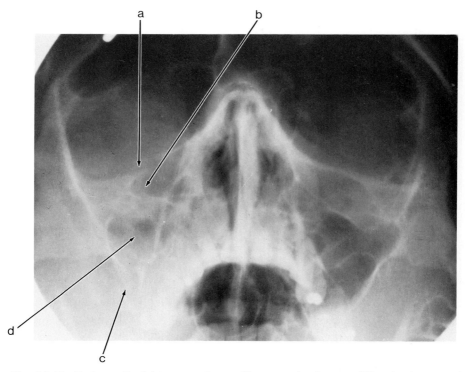

Fig. 14-16. Patient with right zygomaticomaxillary complex fracture. Water's view reveals (*a*) fracture of inferior orbital rim; (*b*) fracture of adjacent floor; (*c*) fracture of lateral wall of maxillary antrum; and (*d*) complete opacification of the right antrum, probably secondary to blood.

LE FORT FRACTURES

The three types of Le Fort fractures have the following characteristics in common: They are all bilateral; some portion of the face is mobile; and all of them extend through the pterygoid plates bilaterally. The Le Fort I fracture (Fig. 14-19) extends through the lateral and medial walls of the maxillary antra immediately above the alveolar ridge, with posterior extension through the pterygoid plates. The maxillary alveolar ridge is bilaterally mobile. The Le Fort II fracture (Fig. 14-20), also called a pyramidal fracture, is characterized by increased mobility of the mid-pyramid of the face. These fractures extend through the lateral walls of the maxillary antra and the rims of the orbits and across the base of the nose bilaterally, with the plane of fracture extending posteroinferiorly through the pterygoid plates.

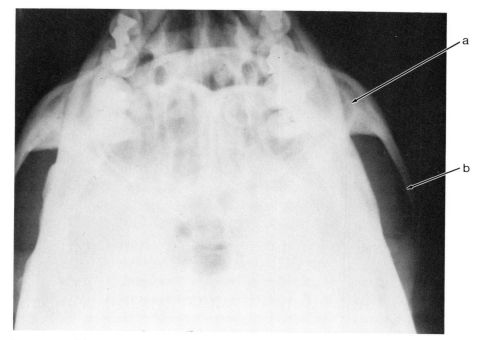

Fig. 14-17. (*a*) Normal zygomatic bone and (*b*) normal zygomatic arch.

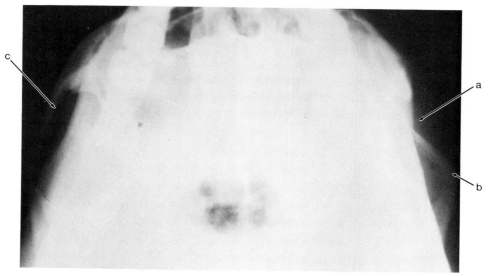

Fig. 14-18. Patient with left zygomaticomaxillary complex fracture. Zygomatic arch view demonstrates (*a*) depression of the anterior portion of the left zygomatic arch; (*b*) second fracture of the posterior zygomatic arch; and (*c*) normal right zygomatic arch.

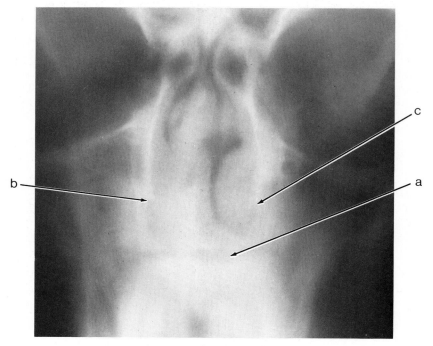

Fig. 14-19. Patient with Le Fort I fracture. Anteroposterior (AP) tomographic section of the facial bones reveals (*a*) linear fracture through the maxilla and (*b* and *c*) fractures through the medial wall of both maxillary antra.

In the Le Fort III fracture, also known as craniofacial disassociation, the fracture extends through the lateral walls of the orbits across the base of the nose and ethmoids, with the plane of the fracture extending posteroinferiorly through the pterygoid plates.

TRAUMA OF THE ORBITS

Fractures that may occur in the orbit include fractures of the floor of the orbit, which in such cases is usually depressed (blowout fractures); medial-wall fractures; fractures of the roof of the orbit; lateral-wall fractures involving the superior orbital fissures; and optic-canal fractures. Fractures of the orbital floor are the most common.

The radiographic signs of an orbital-floor fracture consist of the following: On the Water's view, there is an increase in distance from the palpable margin of the rim of the orbit to the floor of the orbit more posterior, and there is a polypoid mass in the superior portion of the maxillary antrum (Fig. 14-21). This polypoid mass is particularly significant when there are associated spicules of bone. The Water's film should not be overextended for visualization of the floor of the orbit. The ideal view for visualizing depression of the floor of the orbit is a Water's view in which the petrous pyramids are superimposed on the lower third of the maxillary sinus. For detailed assessment of orbital-floor fractures, particularly if surgery is contemplated, tomograms in the coronal and sagittal planes should be obtained.

NASAL FRACTURES

The paired nasal bones constitute the upper portion of the nasal framework. The nasal bones articulate with the frontal processes of the maxilla laterally and with the nasal spine of the frontal bone superiorly. The nasal bones are thick at their superior articulation, and the upper two thirds of the bones becomes thinner towards the tip. The bony nasal septum articulates with the undersurface of the nasal bones and lends additional support to the dorsum of the nose. The roentgenographic examination of the nasal bones consists of a lateral view (Fig. 14-22), Water's and hyperextended Water's projection, and a superoinferior projection of the nasal bones with an occlusal film.

A blow from direct frontal forces results in a smash fracture of the nasal bones with comminution. The comminuted fragments may be driven into the orbit or ethmoidal region, and there is lateral splaying of the left and right nasal bones. In this type of injury, there may be damage to the nasolacrimal ducts, the perpendicular plate of the ethmoid, the ethmoid sinuses, and the cribriform-plate area. In severe cases, there may be broadening and widening of the inner orbital space. If the force of impact is applied to the side of the nasal bones, only one nasal bone shows displacement, but more frequently both nasal bones are fractured along with the nasal septum, resulting in lateral shifting of the entire bony framework. The bone on the side of the injury is displaced medially, the one on the opposite side laterally. The septal cartilage or alar cartilages may be fractured in conjunction with the bone. Not uncommonly, there may be isolated fractures of the anterior portion of the nose, and there may be a variable degree of superoinferior displacement of the nasal bones, best demonstrated in the lateral projection. Depending upon the location of impact, an associated fracture of the nasal spine may occur in all types of nasal fractures and may be demonstrated radiographically. In the lateral projection, fracture lines are oblique or perpendicular to the normal lucent lines of the nose,

(Text continues on p. 280)

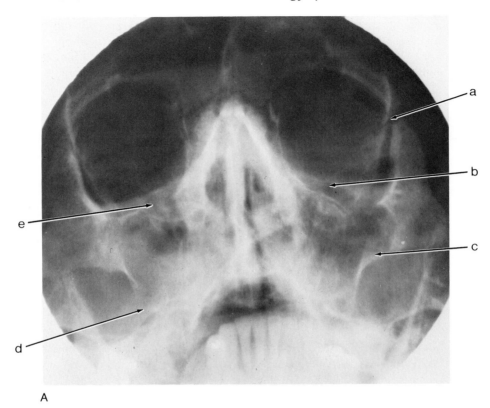

A

Fig. 14-20. (*A*) This patient sustained trauma to the facial bones. Multiple views reveal a Le Fort II fracture. Water's projection reveals (*a*) widening of the left zygomaticofrontal suture; (*b*) fracture in the inferior orbital rim and floor; (*c*) fracture through the lateral wall of the left maxillary antrum; (*d*) fracture in the inferior lateral wall of the right antrum; and (*e*) fracture in the inferior rim and floor of the right orbit. (*B*) Caldwell view of the orbits and facial bones reveals (*a*) fracture through the root of the nasal bones; (*b*) fracture in the inferior orbital rim and floor of the left orbit; and (*c*) fracture in the right inferior orbital rim and floor. (*C*) Coronal tomographic section of the orbits and facial bones reveals (*a*) fracture in the cribriform plate and the roof of the ethmoid sinuses; (*b*) fracture in the floor of the left orbit; (*c*) fracture in the lateral wall of the left antrum; (*d*) fracture in the lateral wall of the right antrum; and (*e*) fracture in the floor of the right orbit. (*D*) Coronal tomographic section reveals (*a*) fracture in the lateral and medial plate of the left pterygoid bone and (*b*) fracture in the medial and lateral plate of the right pterygoid bone.

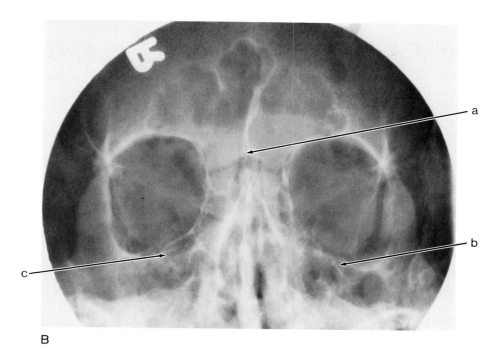

B

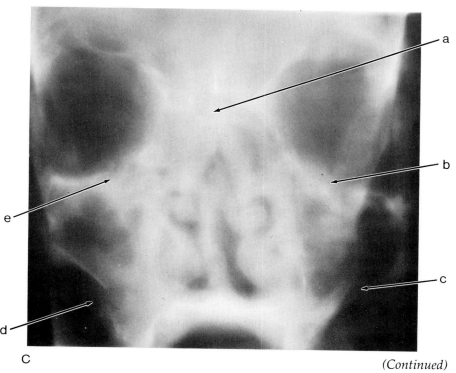

C

(Continued)

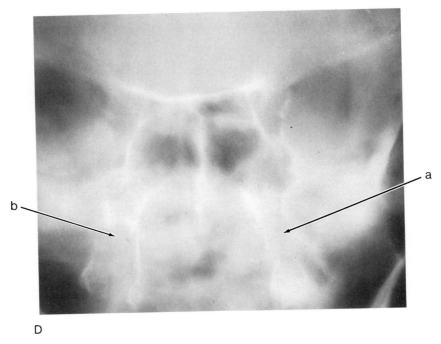

D

Fig. 14-20. *(Continued)*

which are caused by sutures, nerves, and blood vessels within the groove of the nasal bones. These sharply defined, longitudinal lucent lines course along the nasal bones from anterior to posterior.

For detailed assessment of nasal fractures, AP tomography in the hyperextended Water's projection can be carried out.

Nasal fractures may be encountered singly or in combination with other facial-bone fractures. Figure 14-23 shows a lateral view of a fractured nose.

FRACTURES OF THE MANDIBLE

Roentgenographic studies are used to determine the extent, direction, and location of a fracture within the mandible. For routine evaluation of the mandible, a posteroanterior (PA), left and right oblique views, and lateral views are obtained. These can be supplemented by an occlusal view of the mouth, which outlines the fractures of the symphysis to better advantage. Panorex views of the mandible are helpful for evaluation of the condylar and coronoid processes. In some cases, tomo-

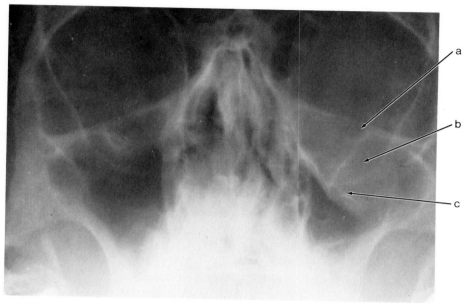

Fig. 14-21. Blowout fracture of the left orbit. Water's view shows (*a*) normal inferior orbital rim; (*b*) hemispherical soft-tissue density in the upper half of the left maxillary antrum; and (*c*) linear bony density representing the depressed and fractured orbital floor.

grams of the mandible, particularly the ascending ramus, coronoid process, and mandibular condyle, are helpful for detailed assessment. Postoperative roentgenograms should be obtained for evaluating the effectiveness of reduction and the position of the fragments after treatment.

Mandibular fractures are classified according to location and may be described as follows:

1. Fractures of the symphysis, located in the region between the lower canine teeth.
2. Fractures of the canine region.
3. Fractures in the body of the mandible, located between the canine teeth and the angle of the mandible.
4. Fractures of the angle of the mandible: those fractures occurring through the angle of the mandible behind the second or third molar (Fig. 14-24).
5. Fractures of the ramus of the mandible: those fractures occurring between the angle of the mandible and the sigmoid notch.
6. Fractures of the coronoid process.

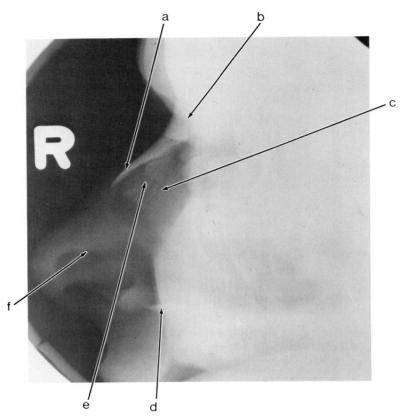

Fig. 14-22. Lateral view of the nasal bones reveals (*a*) normal nasal bones; (*b*) nasofrontal suture; (*c*) nasomaxillary suture; (*d*) nasal spine; (*e*) normal grooves for vessels and nerves; and (*f*) cartilaginous structures of the nose.

   7. Fractures of the condylar process (Fig. 14-25): these include all fractures of the neck above the level of the sigmoid notch of the mandible.

RADIOLOGY OF THE SALIVARY GLANDS

In addition to plain films of the salivary glands, radiographic sialography has become an important diagnostic procedure for the evaluation of salivary calculi, sialectasia, strictures, fistulae, and tumors. Sialo-

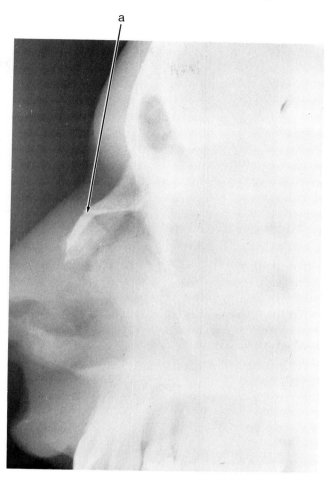

Fig. 14-23. Patient with fracture in the midnasal bones. Lateral view shows a linear fracture (a) with slight anterior buckling of the nasal bones.

graphic procedures using the injection of a contrast material should be carried out with fluoroscopy. Recently, CT has been combined with sialography to provide better definition and differentiation of soft-tissue detail.

The examination technique generally requires the dilation and cannulation of either Stensen's or Wharton's ducts with small catheters. In general, it is not necessary to use premedication or a local anesthetic for sialography because neither cannulation nor the injection of contrast material is painful to the patient if done carefully. The contrast materials used in sialography are of two general categories; Ethiodol (ethiodized poppy seed oil) is the contrast medium of choice in most cases. It con-

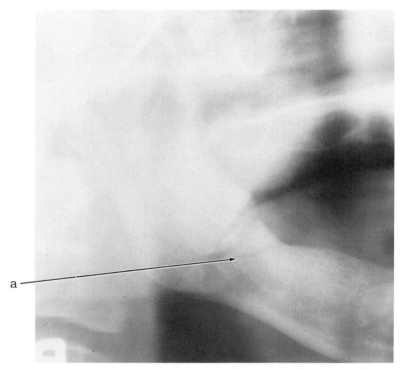

Fig. 14-24. Panorex view of the mandible reveals (*a*) a linear, slightly comminuted fracture through the angle of the right mandible.

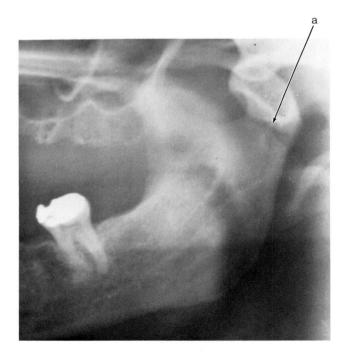

Fig. 14-25. Patient with left condylar fracture. Panorex view shows (*a*) fracture through the neck of the left mandible.

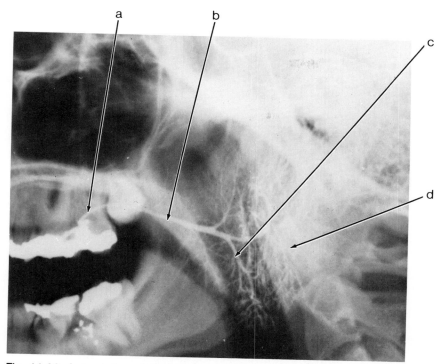

Fig. 14-26. Lateral view of the parotid sialogram reveals (*a*) normal duct orifice opposite the second molar; (*b*) normal main duct (Stensen's duct); (*c*) normal primary branches within the gland; and (*d*) normal secondary and tertiary branches within the gland. The size and shape of the parotid gland varies among individuals.

tains 37% iodine and has a high radiographic density, and it therefore produces excellent opacification of both ducts and parenchyma. It does not cause serious reactions even if extravasated into the tissues. Water-soluble contrast material, such as Hypaque Sodium 50% or Renografin-60, should be used if it is anticipated that the contrast material may be retained, as in inflammatory disease secondary to stones.

Preliminary films of the salivary glands are obtained in order to avoid confusion because of the calcification that may occur in many structures, including lymph nodes, tonsils, blood vessels, and ligaments, as well as in the salivary ducts or glands. Sialograms of normal parotid and submandibular glands are shown in Figures 14-26 and 14-27.

Calculi in the submandibular salivary ducts may be demonstrated best by an intraoral film of the floor of the mouth or by oblique films of the mandibular area (Fig. 14-28). Parotid-duct stones are best dem-

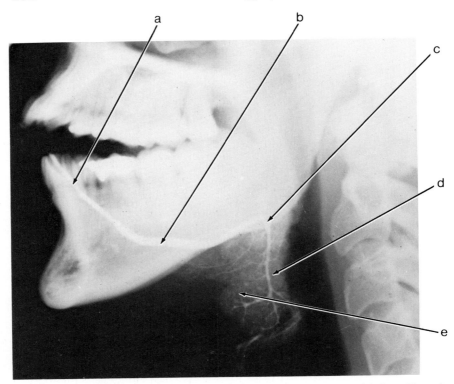

Fig. 14-27. Lateral view of normal submandibular sialogram shows (*a*) the orifice of the submandibular duct behind the lingual surface of the mandible; (*b*) normal duct; (*c*) normal curvature of the duct; (*d*) major branches within the gland; and (*e*) parenchyma of the gland. Note inferior position of the submandibular gland with respect to the adjacent mandible. Also, the gland varies in size and shape among individuals.

onstrated by anteroposterior views taken with the patient's cheek puffed out, supplemented by lateral oblique and base views. Eighty percent of salivary calculi are opaque on plain films. However, they are often less dense than contrast material, so on sialography they may appear as a radiolucent filling defect within the contrast material.

Sialography is indicated when there is recurrent, acute swelling in the region of a salivary gland during eating, which suggests intermittent obstruction of the salivary duct from a calculus, stricture, mucous impaction, or inflammation of the gland. Recurrent swelling of a gland that lasts a few days or weeks suggests a chronic inflammatory process. In Sjögren's disease, sialography demonstrates various degrees of sialectasia (Fig. 14-29). Sialography is also used to determine whether a

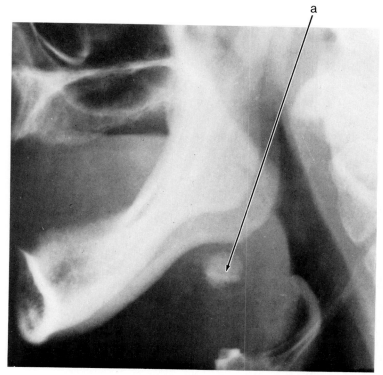

Fig. 14-28. Patient with calcified stone. Lateral view shows (*a*) a radiopaque calculus in the hilus of the submandibular gland below the mandible.

suspected or definitely palpable mass is intrinsic or extrinsic to a gland and, if within the gland, whether it is inflammatory, encapsulated, or infiltrative. Usually it is not possible with sialography to distinguish a benign from a malignant lesion or a cyst from a tumor, and often it is not possible to distinguish a neoplastic mass from an inflammatory one.

CONTRAINDICATIONS

Sialography should not be performed in an acutely infected gland because it may exacerbate symptoms.

Sensitivity to contrast material does not contraindicate the examination. Reactions to the contrast material are rare. If thyroid-function

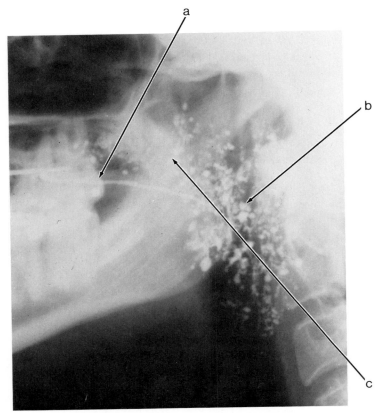

Fig. 14-29. Patient with Sjögren's disease. Lateral view of the parotid sialogram shows (*a*) normal main parotid duct; (*b*) sialectasia, which is evenly distributed throughout the entire parotid gland; and (*c*) some aberrant parotid tissue above the main duct, anterior to the main gland.

tests are to be done, they should be performed before sialography because retained iodinated contrast material may interfere with them.

COMPLICATIONS

If the acini have been distended with dye, the affected gland will usually be considerably enlarged at the completion of the study. The enlargement and pain may take the next few hours or days to diminish. Following sialography, an infection may rarely occur in the gland, or a previously existing infection may be exacerbated.

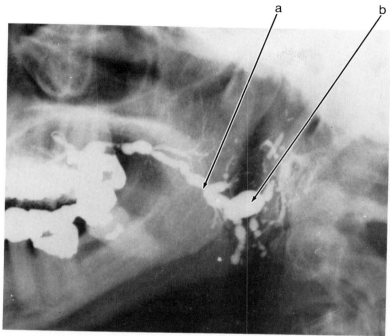

Fig. 14-30. Patient with recurrent parotitis. Lateral view of the parotid gland reveals (*a*) strictures in the main duct and (*b*) intervening dilatation of the main duct and the branches within the parotid gland.

RADIOGRAPHIC FINDINGS

In inflammatory disease, the intraparenchymal ducts reveal a pruned-tree appearance secondary to nonfilling of the smaller ducts. The main duct and intraparenchymal ducts may be irregular in caliber, and single or multiple strictures may be visible (Fig. 14-30). There is localized or diffuse dilation of ducts, often interspersed with areas of narrowing. There may be extravasation of contrast material into abscess cavities within the gland or outside of it.

Whether stones are radiolucent or not, sialography will help determine their location and size. The status of the gland proximal to the stone can be assessed in order to decide whether to remove the stone only or to excise the entire gland. Stones near the orifice of the duct may not be seen during the introduction of contrast material and are visualized on postevacuation films because of the retention of contrast material proximal to the stone.

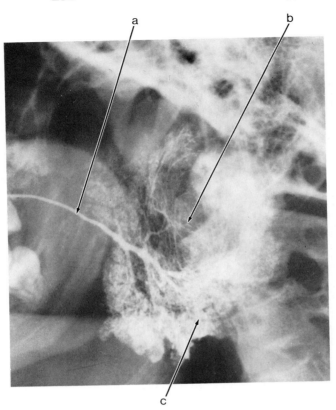

Fig. 14-31. Patient with pleomorphic adenoma of the parotid gland. Lateral view of the parotid gland following introduction of Ethiodol shows (*a*) a normal main parotid duct and (*b*) a filling defect in the mid- to superior portion of the parotid gland. Note draping of ducts around mass and (*c*) a normal parenchymogram of the parotid gland.

For the demonstration of salivary masses, optimal parenchymal opacification by the use of Ethiodol is required. Large masses are demonstrated on conventional fluoroscopic films or on overhead films (Fig. 14-31). Tomography has greatly enhanced the identification of tumors that are small, at the periphery of a gland, or in the deep lobe of the parotid (Fig. 14-32). In most instances, differentiation among benign tumors, malignant tumors, and cysts is not possible. However, occasionally a sialogram will reveal a large, irregular mass with poorly defined margins, displacement and invasion of the ducts, and pooling of contrast material. In the context of a patient with a palpable hard mass, pain, and rapid growth, a malignant tumor should be suspected.

RADIOLOGY OF THE LARYNX

The initial study of the larynx should involve a *lateral view* of the patient's neck. His head should be in the neutral or slightly hyperextended position, and he should be breathing quietly. This lateral film demon-

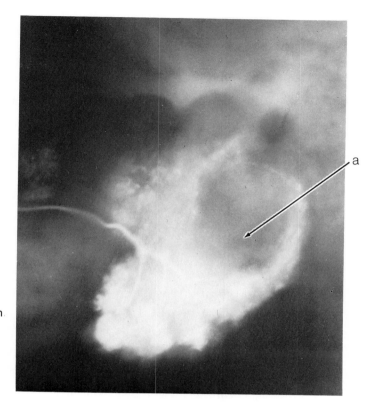

Fig. 14-32. Lateral tomogram of the parotid in the parenchymal phase shows (*a*) a well-defined filling defect in the superior–posterior portion of the parotid gland.

strates to best advantage the larynx, upper trachea, posterior portion of the tongue, vallecular area, precervical soft tissues, and cervical spine (Fig. 14-33). It can be supplemented by a xeroradiogram, which shows some of the laryngeal structures in slightly greater detail, particularly in the evaluation of cartilaginous structures, foreign bodies, and soft-tissue abnormalities caused by edge enhancement.

Following the lateral view, an *AP view* of the larynx and trachea is obtained using the high-KV technique (120 kilovolts [KV]) and a 1-mm copper filter attached to the x-ray tube (Fig. 14-34). The filter will obliterate some of the overlying cervical spine and will enhance the interface between the soft-tissue structures of the larynx and the air in the larynx and trachea.

To study the dynamics of the larynx, particularly the motion of the cords, *fluoroscopy* is often used in conjunction with spot films. A *barium swallow* is part of the fluoroscopic examination of the larynx and hypopharynx when a patient has difficulty swallowing or if a tumor is suspected.

If the presence of a laryngeal mass is indicated by the conventional

(Text continues on p. 294)

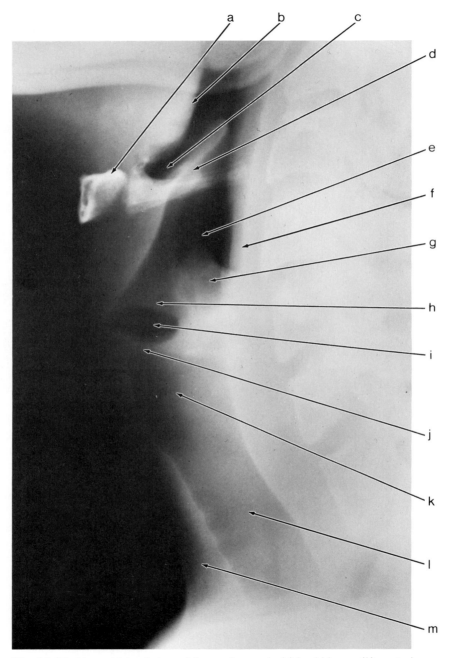

Fig. 14-33. Normal lateral view of the neck reveals (*a*) hyoid bone; (*b*) posterior tongue; (*c*) vallecular area; (*d*) epiglottis; (*e*) aryepiglottic folds; (*f*) precervical soft tissues; (*g*) arytenoid area; (*h*) false cord; (*i*) laryngeal ventricles; (*j*) true cord; (*k*) subglottic space; (*l*) trachea; (*m*) soft tissues anterior to trachea.

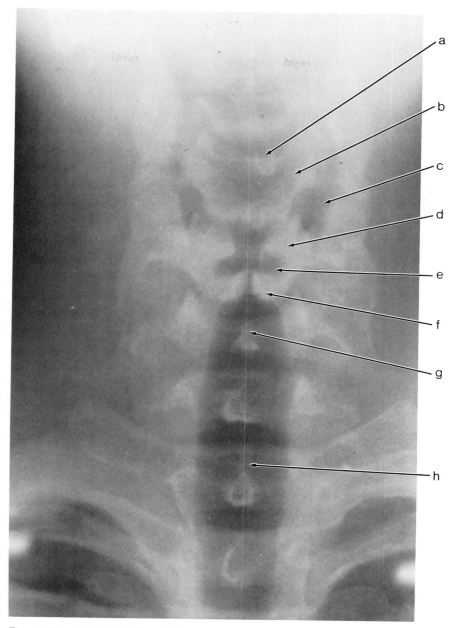

Fig. 14-34. AP high-KV film of the neck. (*a*) laryngeal vestibule; (*b*) aryepiglottic fold; (*c*) pyriform sinus; (*d*) false cords; (*e*) laryngeal ventricle; (*f*) true cord; (*g*) subglottic space; and (*h*) trachea.

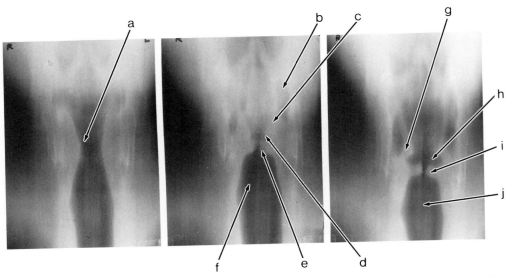

Fig. 14-35. Normal AP tomographic section of the neck. (*a*) glottic space at inspiration; (*b*) aryepiglottic fold at phonation of "e"; (*c*) false cord; (*d*) laryngeal ventricle; (*e*) true cord; (*f*) subglottic space at inspiration of "e"; (*g*) false cord; (*h*) laryngeal ventricle; (*i*) true cord, and (*j*) subglottic space. Note normal "shoulders" of the upper portion of the subglottic space formed by the undersurface of the vocal cords and adjacent lateral wall of the larynx.

films, *tomography* is usually the next step in the evaluation. With the patient phonating the sound indicated by the letter "e," a series of AP views of the larynx is made in sequence, from the anterior portion of the cervical spine to the anterior part of the thyroid cartilage. During inspiration, a single film of the larynx is made through the vocal cords. Additional films are taken as the patient inspires "e" and performs a modified Valsalva maneuver (Fig. 14-35).

    Laryngography is another valuable radiologic procedure in the investigation of laryngeal disease. It has an advantage over tomography in that fluoroscopy can be used with it for assessing laryngeal anatomy and laryngeal movements. For laryngography, the patient is premedicated with 0.4 mg of atropine to control salivary secretion. The larynx is anesthetized with 1% Xylocaine, using a soft rubber catheter (French 8, 10, or 12) that is introduced through the nose and positioned into the vallecular area or to the level of the tip of the epiglottis. Once adequate anesthesia is achieved, oily Dionosil is introduced through the catheter to coat the intralaryngeal structures and upper trachea. Following adequate coating of the laryngeal structures, spot films are obtained in varying positions. Laryngography will provide information about the staging of malignant tumors and is also very useful in the assessment of laryngeal stenosis.

CT scans have also been used in the evaluation of laryngeal abnormalities and metastatic lymph nodes in the neck.

BENIGN LESIONS OF THE LARYNX

LARYNGOTRACHEAL BRONCHITIS (CROUP)

Laryngotracheal bronchitis, also known to many as croup, is a common cause of acute upper-airway obstruction in infants. The entire airway may be involved in the inflammatory process, but the glottis and the subglottic regions are usually most critically involved. On the frontal view of the larynx, the subglottic airway is tapered up to the cords, appearing funnel shaped (Fig. 14-36). In the lateral projection, there is a general increase in density in the subglottic airway. These radiographic features are the result of the inflammatory edema affecting the subglottic portion of the larynx. The hypopharynx is often distended with air, secondary to the laryngeal obstruction. Croup should be differentiated from congenital subglottic stenosis, subglottic hemangioma, or subglottic mucosal cysts.

ACUTE SUPRAGLOTTITIS (EPIGLOTTITIS)

In acute supraglottitis, airway obstruction is most often severe, and the infection is almost always caused by *Hemophilus influenzae*. Radiographically, the diagnosis is made from the lateral view, which shows the swollen epiglottis, aryepiglottic folds, and arytenoid area (Fig. 14-37). This swelling may almost completely obliterate the normal airway. There is often associated dilation of the hypopharynx and pyriform sinuses. In most cases the glottic and subglottic portion of the larynx are not involved.

RETROPHARYNGEAL ABSCESSES

The normal thickness of the retropharyngeal space is about one third of the anteroposterior diameter of a cervical body. A retropharyngeal abscess is indicated by bulging of the posterior pharyngeal soft tissues

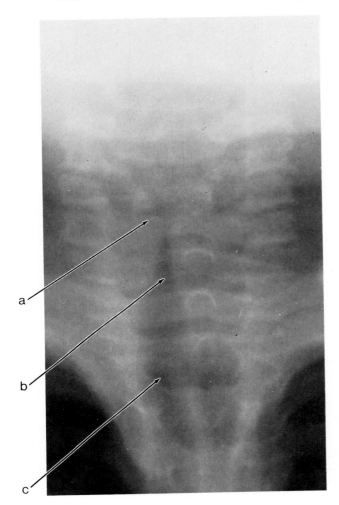

Fig. 14-36. Patient with croup. AP high-KV view of the larynx reveals (*a*) vocal cords; (*b*) funnel shape of the narrowed subglottic space produced by subglottic swelling (compare with Fig. 14-35); and (*c*) normal trachea.

and loss of normal cervical lordosis; in other words, the neck appears to be abnormally straight (Fig. 14-38). The amount of widening of the retropharyngeal space depends on the stage and severity of the infection. Air pockets secondary to abscess formation with or without fluid levels may be demonstrated, and there may be associated swelling of laryngeal structures.

FOREIGN BODIES

Foreign bodies (Fig. 14-39) in the air and food passages commonly present symptoms of stridor, dyspnea, dysphagia, coughing, and chronic pneu-

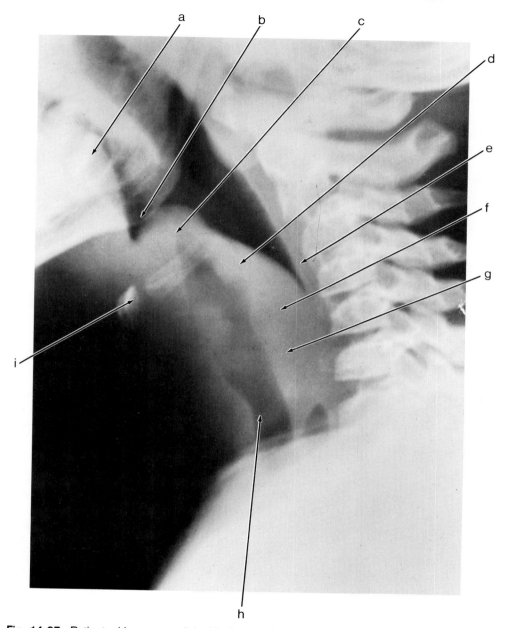

Fig. 14-37. Patient with severe epiglottitis. Lateral view of neck reveals (*a*) posterior tongue; (*b*) vallecular area; (*c*) markedly swollen epiglottis; (*d*) markedly swollen aryepiglottic folds; (*e*) posterior pharyngeal wall; (*f*) markedly thickened arytenoid area; and (*g*) markedly thickened postcricoid portion of larynx. Note (*h*) normal trachea and (*i*) hyoid bone.

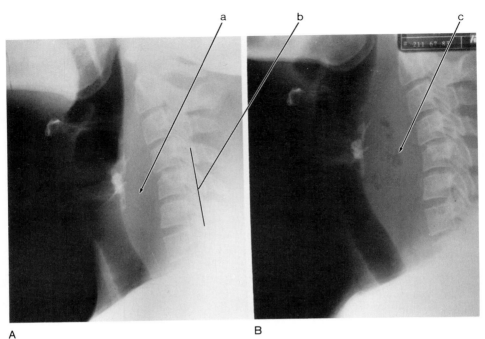

Fig. 14-38. Patient with retropharyngeal abscess. Lateral view of the neck. (*A*) At (*a*) there is widening of the retropharyngeal space. Normal space is about one third of the width of the anteroposterior diameter of a cervical vertebral body (compare with Fig. 14-37*e*). (*b*) Note the straightening of the cervical spine secondary to muscle spasm (compare to Figs. 14-33 and 14-37). (*B*) At (*c*) there is anterior displacement of the larynx and trachea. This view demonstrates a more advanced retropharyngeal abscess with lucencies secondary to gas bubbles.

monia. It is not uncommon, especially in pediatric cases, for the presence of these obstructions to be overlooked for periods ranging from 1 month to 2 years. Misdiagnosis may result from the age of the patient (as in cases where children are unable to communicate adequate histories and parents are unaware of foreign-body ingestion), from the attribution of symptoms to other respiratory disorders (especially when x-ray procedures are not ordered or in the presence of nonradiopaque obstruction), or from the patient's belief that the foreign body has been expelled, in which case his complaints are considered to be the result of residual irritation. Also, selected eating habits, that is, if the patient is on a soft or liquid diet, can account for a lack of symptoms in food-passage obstruction.

Any suspicion of foreign-body ingestion warrants radiologic evaluation, and the lateral neck film is the most important part of the ex-

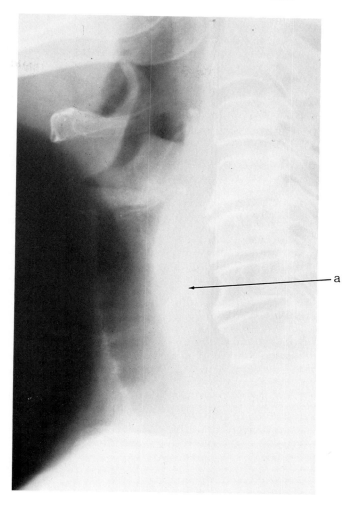

Fig. 14-39. Lateral view of the neck of a patient with the wishbone of a chicken (*a*) in the cervical esophagus.

amination. Radiopaque foreign bodies, such as bones, coins, or other metallic objects, are clearly defined on this film. Most bones, such as chicken, pork, and fish bones, lodge in the hypopharynx. Occasionally, these bones may be seen in the vallecular area. If the bone is very thin, radiographic evaluation may be difficult, particularly if there is extensive calcification of the cartilaginous structures of the larynx. There may be associated soft-tissue swelling, as indicated by the increase in distance from the larynx and trachea to the cervical spine.

If the foreign body is not clearly defined on conventional films, a barium swallow is indicated. In this study, a filling defect, secondary to the foreign body and adjacent edema, may be seen in the pharynx and esophagus. A coin, a metallic object, or a large piece of meat lodged in the esophagus may completely obstruct the flow of barium.

If a foreign body is suspected in the air passages, anteroposterior and lateral chest films, as well as fluoroscopy, are indicated. A foreign body in the bronchi may cause air trapping of the involved portion of the lung with a mediastinal shift on inspiration and expiration. If the obstruction in the bronchus becomes complete, there may be drowning of the lung or atelectasis in the respective lobe. Failure to remove a foreign body may result in superimposed pneumonia with bronchiectasis or abscess formation. Foreign bodies are rare in the larynx. The majority of air-passage foreign bodies are located in the bronchi, and only a small percentage are found in the trachea. Most air-passage foreign bodies occur in pediatric age groups, especially in children between the ages of 1 and 5 years old.

The more common obstructing objects in the air passages are vegetables, nuts, and pointed metallic objects, such as safety pins. Bones and meat are the foreign bodies that commonly lodge in food passages.

PAPILLOMATOSIS

Papillomas present as irregular soft-tissue excrescences, most commonly around the glottis of the larynx. They may be small or may involve a significant portion of the larynx and lead to airway obstruction. They may extend into the trachea and bronchi. These masses are shaggy and irregular in appearance, and they may lead to airway obstruction in the trachea or to atelectasis with chronic inflammation in the lung. Extension into the lung has been reported and is characterized by cystic areas.

SUBGLOTTIC HEMANGIOMAS

In the presence of subglottic hemangiomas, the radiologic findings consist of a distinctive, homogenous, sharply defined, asymmetric soft-tissue density in the subglottic portion of the larynx. Symptoms, such as stridor and hoarseness, may resemble those of croup; however, in most instances, the symptoms commence before 6 months of age, whereas laryngotracheal bronchitis (croup) usually occurs after this age. Symptoms may be minimal, but they may be exacerbated when the infant has an upper respiratory infection.

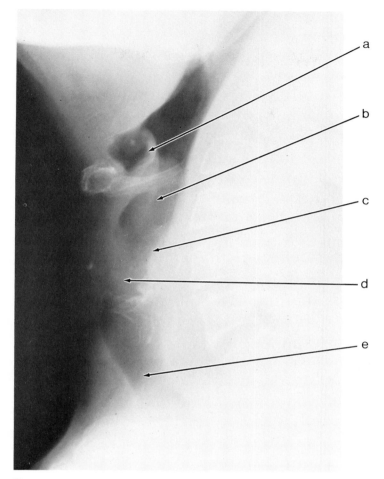

Fig. 14-40. Patient with a cyst arising from the aryepiglottic fold of the larynx. Lateral view of the neck reveals (*a*) normal epiglottis; (*b*) a homogenous, sharply defined, oval-shaped density in the region of the aryepiglottic fold; (*c*) artyenoid area; (*d*) glottic portion of the larynx; and (*e*) normal trachea.

CYSTS

Cysts of the larynx may occur in the region of the epiglottis, the ary-epiglottic folds, and, to a lesser extent, the false and true vocal cords (Fig. 14-40). These cysts are homogenous and sharply defined and project as a hemispherical soft-tissue density in the air-filled larynx. They may cause airway obstruction if they are large.

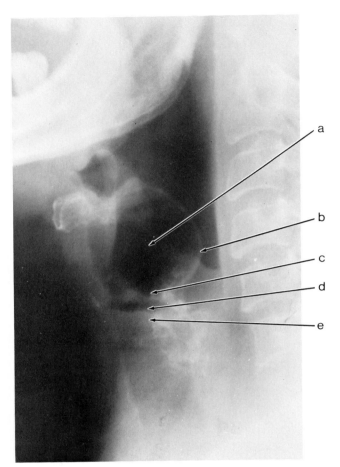

Fig. 14-41. Patient with a laryngocele of the larynx. Lateral view of the neck shows (*a*) a large, oval-shaped cyst; (*b*) posterior displacement of the aryepiglottic fold; (*c*) false cord; (*d*) laryngeal ventricle; and (*e*) true vocal cord.

LARYNGOCELES

Laryngoceles are air-filled cysts or sacs that arise as elongations and expansions of the ventricular appendage or saccule. The saccule elongates upwards and expands into the laryngeal vestibule and pyriform sinus. If the cyst remains within the larynx, it is called an *internal laryngocele*. However, it may also expand laterally and break through the weak zone of the thyrohyoid membrane to present as a localized bulge or mass in the side of the neck (Fig. 14-41) that varies in size with changes in intralaryngeal pressures. In such instances, the cyst is known as an *external laryngocele*. Combined types are common, and indeed all external laryngoceles are really combined, since they originate from the ventricle.

Laryngoceles are seen radiographically as circumscribed air spaces that may, on occasion, contain an air-fluid level or polypoid tissue within the wall. On occasion, a laryngocele may extend into the pre-epiglottic space.

POLYPS

Benign polyps arise from the vocal cords or false vocal cords, causing the cords to appear floppy and thick. Less commonly, the polyps are pedunculated and hang by a stalk with a bulbus. This latter form of polyp can move within the larynx on deep inspiration and expiration.

MALIGNANT LESIONS OF THE LARYNX

On radiologic examination, laryngeal carcinomas are manifested by an irregular mass. Exophytic lesions are bulky with ulcerations and air collections within the tumor (Fig. 14-42). Infiltrative tumors cause en-

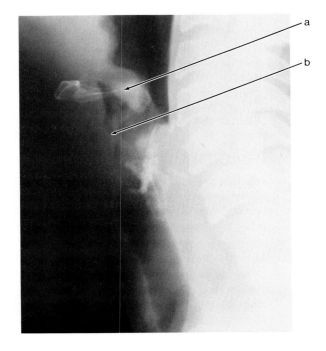

Fig. 14-42. Patient with squamous cell carcinoma of the supraglottic portion of the larynx. Lateral view of the neck shows (*a*) tumor involving the soft tissue on the supraglottic area obliterating the outline of the vallecula, epiglottis, and aryepiglottic folds and (*b*) marked compromise of the supraglottic laryngeal air space with considerable irregularity in its outline.

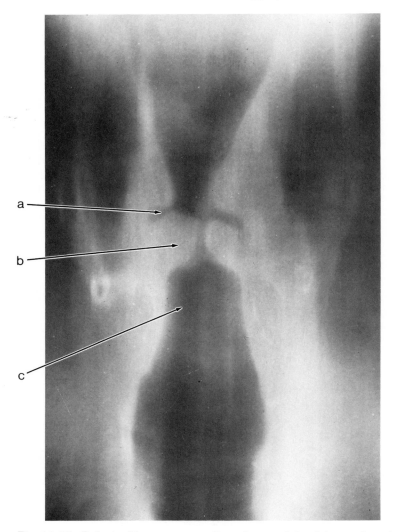

Fig. 14-43. Patient with squamous cell carcinoma of the right vocal cord. AP tomographic section of the larynx shows (*a*) normal, but smaller right laryngeal ventricle; (*b*) marked thickening of the right cord (see normal left side for comparison); and (*c*) normal subglottic space.

largement and distortion of the involved larynx and limitation of movement of the vocal cords (Fig. 14-43). Advanced lesions may extend beyond the larynx. During radiologic evaluation of lesions of the larynx, it is important to determine the size and margins of the lesion. Also, the mobility of the vocal cords, aryepiglottic folds, and epiglottis and the distensibility of the pyriform sinuses and valleculae should be assessed by phonation maneuvers (see Fig. 14-35). Extension of a tumor into the postcricoid portion of the hypopharynx is best assessed with a barium swallow, and CT will provide increased accuracy in evaluating the extent of the tumor.

Although it is useful in determining the extent of a laryngeal or hypopharyngeal lesion, x-ray evaluation alone is not sufficient to rule out tumors of this area, and it is best used only as a complement to direct or indirect laryngoscopy.

PLAIN-FILM EVALUATION OF THE TEMPORAL BONE

The structures of the middle and inner ear are poorly shown in the regular anteroposterior and lateral projections of the skull. In order to bring out specific regions of the ear, such as the ossicles, aditus ad antrum, attic, or mastoid antrum, special views are needed. The special views of the temporal bone routinely indicated include a well-coned Towne, basal, Law's, Schüller's, and modified Owen's views. These are supplemented by transorbital and Stenver's views for detailed assessment of the internal auditory canal. These special films of the temporal bone are usually obtained prior to the use of special radiographic studies, such as polytomography, CT, and angiography. When a polytomographic study is to be done, only two or three of these plain films will be obtained.

RADIOLOGIC FINDINGS

For the primary-care physician, familiarity with radiologic positioning (Fig. 14-44) and interpretation of the Schüller's (Fig. 14-45), Towne (Fig. 14-46), and transorbital views (Fig. 14-47) will be most useful. These three views should answer basic questions regarding the presence of acute and chronic mastoiditis and temporal-bone tumors and fractures, in addition to serving as preliminary films when further studies are indicated.

ACUTE MASTOIDITIS

In acute mastoiditis, the earliest change noticeable radiologically is a loss of translucency of the cells, particularly around the mastoid antrum

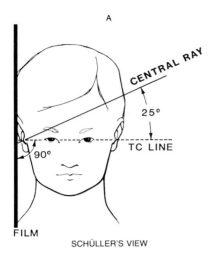

SCHÜLLER'S VIEW

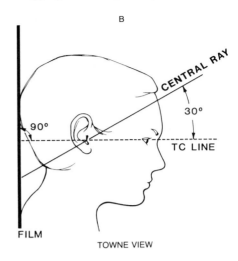

TOWNE VIEW

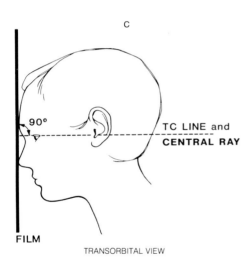

TRANSORBITAL VIEW

Fig. 14-44. (*A*) In the Schüller's view the midsagittal plane of the head is parallel to the table top. The tube is angled caudally 25°. (*B*) In the Towne view the patient is supine, with the TC line perpendicular to the table top and the tube angled caudally approximately 30°. (*C*) For the transorbital view, the patient lies face down, and both the TC line and tube are perpendicular to the table top.

(Fig. 14-48). This rapidly spreads throughout the entire mastoid air system. If the infection is not arrested, the bony cell walls decalcify and disappear from view, usually in 2 to 3 weeks. If the infection and edema subside, recalcification of the cell walls may take place. In many cases, radiographs indicate that the cell walls have apparently disappeared, although during surgery distinct cell walls can be seen.

Cell breakdown within the mastoid with abscess formation is characterized by a single, large cavity or by multiple cavities, which show

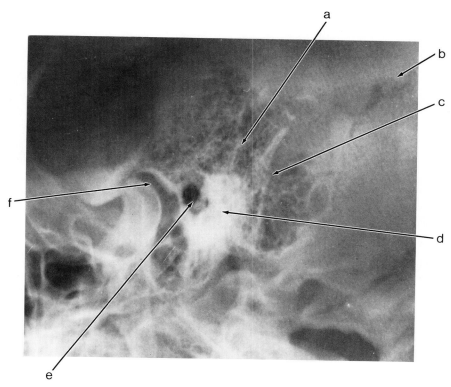

Fig. 14-45. Normal Schüller's projection of the mastoid demonstrates (*a*) mastoid air cells; (*b*) lambdoid suture; (*c*) sigmoid sinus plate; (*d*) labyrinth; (*e*) bony external ear superimposed on middle ear cavity; and (*f*) temporomandibular joint.

up on the radiograph as lucent areas within the mastoid. The tegmen or sigmoid sinus plate may be interrupted secondary to bone erosion. If the abscess involves the tip of the mastoid, it may erode the cortex of bone and spread into the soft tissues of the neck (Bezold's abscess). Occasionally, giant mastoid cells may be interpreted as an abscess cavity. In such cases, a careful examination will reveal a well-defined bony cortex, which may, however, be paper thin.

CHRONIC MASTOIDITIS

Chronic infection of the mastoid is characterized by new bone formation and sclerosis involving the mastoid in varying degrees (Fig. 14-49). The extent of sclerosis is dependent on the infecting organism and the duration of the disease. On tomographic study there may be minimal ero-

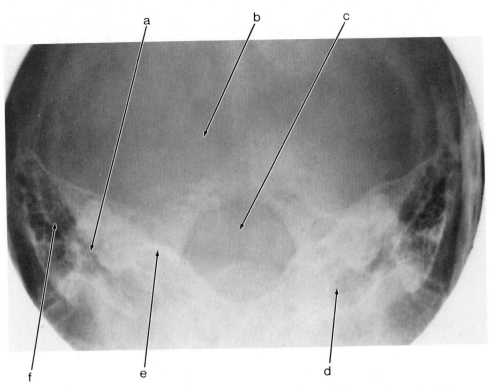

Fig. 14-46. Normal Towne view of the temporal bones shows (*a*) tympanic cavity; (*b*) occipital bone; (*c*) foramen magnum; (*d*) jugular fossa; (*e*) apex of petrous pyramid; and (*f*) mastoid.

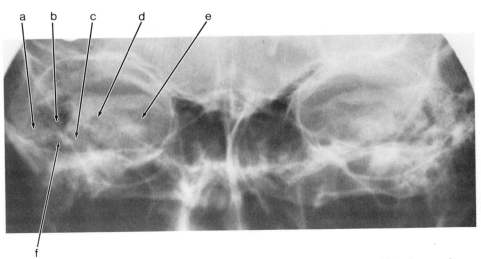

Fig. 14-47. Transorbital view of the temporal bones shows (*a*) mastoid; (*b*) epitympanic recess; (*c*) tympanic cavity; (*d*) vestibule; (*e*) internal auditory canal; and (*f*) spur.

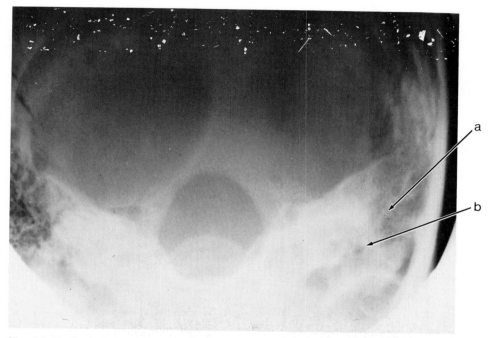

Fig. 14-48. Patient with acute, left mastoiditis. Towne view of the temporal bone shows (*a*) diffuse increase in density in the left mastoid with no cell breakdown (see right side for comparison) and (*b*) increased density in the left tympanic cavity.

sion of the spur or partial erosion of the ossicles, predominantly of the long process of the incus. Chronic mastoiditis may also be complicated by abscess formation within the mastoid process. The condition has then to be differentiated from destruction resulting from other causes, such as cholesteatoma or a postsurgical cavity.

CHOLESTEATOMA

The vast majority of cholesteatomas arise in the middle ear or attic. Cholesteatomas do not produce a distinct outline within these structures, and, as a result, their presence can only be inferred from the secondary bone erosion it produces. Consequently, a cholesteatoma that does not produce bone erosion cannot be diagnosed radiologically. The area of bone erosion in cholesteatoma has a clear-cut outline, often with marginal sclerosis surrounding the bone defect.

The earliest change in cholesteatoma of the epitympanic recess is a variable degree of erosion of the spur of the adjacent lateral epitympanic wall. If the erosion progresses, there is concomitant enlargement

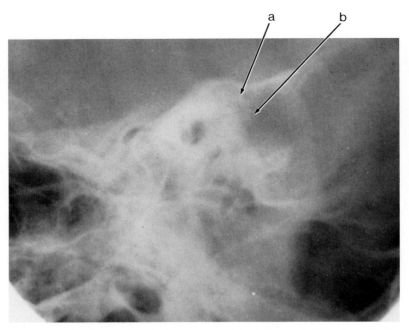

Fig. 14-49. Patient with a cholesteatoma of the left ear. Schüller's projection shows (*a*) sclerosis in the left mastoid; (*b*) ill-defined lucent area representing destruction by cholesteatoma.

of the epitympanic recess. There often is associated ossicular destruction, and the long process of the incus demonstrates the most frequent and earliest involvement. From the epitympanic recess, the cholesteatoma may extend into the central mastoid tract or into the petrous pyramid (Fig. 14-50). Complications from cholesteatoma secondary to bone erosion include fistula formation, most commonly of the lateral semicircular canal; erosion of the facial-nerve canal with partial paresis of the facial nerve; erosion of the tegmen tympani with intracranial complications; and erosion into the labyrinthine portion of the petrous bone. In end-stage cholesteatoma, there is complete or marked destruction of the ossicular chain.

ACOUSTIC NEUROMAS

Acoustic neuromas account for approximately 10% of unilateral sensorineural hearing losses combined with marked loss of vestibular function of unknown origin. They usually originate within the internal auditory canal and, therefore, produce osseous changes that are detectable by a proper radiographic study. Whenever conventional radiography is used,

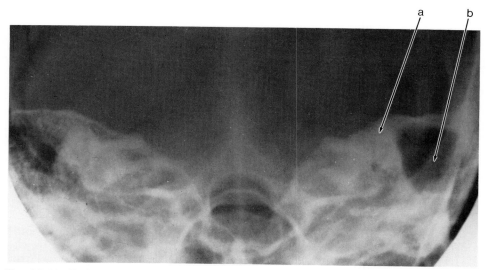

Fig. 14-50. Patient with large cholesteatoma. Towne view of the temporal bone reveals (*a*) sclerosis in the remaining mastoid and (*b*) large cholesteotoma cavity, which is sharply marginated (see right side for comparison).

two projections are indispensable for the study of the internal auditory canal: the transorbital view, which shows the canal at its full length, and the Stenver's view, which shows the opening or porus of the canal en face, although the canal is quite foreshortened.

A more precise study of the internal auditory canal can be obtained by tomography (Fig. 14-51), particularly when the petrous pyramids are extensively or asymmetrically pneumatized. Tomography most frequently is performed in the coronal projection, which is the most satisfactory projection for the study of the shape and size of the internal auditory canal and of the length of its posterior wall. Both sides should always be examined for comparison purposes. The following four parameters should always be examined in order to detect changes indicative of an acoustic neuroma:

1. Vertical diameter: The height of the internal auditory canal normally ranges between 2 mm and 9 mm, with an average of 4.9 mm. An enlargement of 1 mm to 2 mm of any portion of the internal auditory canal under investigation in comparison to the corresponding segment of the opposite side should arouse suspicion, and an enlargement of 2 mm or more should be considered definitely abnormal.

2. Length of the posterior wall: This normally ranges between 4 mm and 12 mm, with an average of 8 mm. Shortening of the

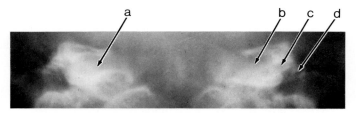

Fig. 14-51. Patient with left acoustic neuroma. AP tomographic section of the temporal bone demonstrates (*a*) normal right internal auditory canal; (*b*) marked enlargement of the left internal auditory canal with erosion of the superior and inferior walls; (*c*) vestibule; and (*d*) middle ear cavity with spur and ossicles.

posterior wall of one canal from between 2 mm to 3 mm should be considered suggestive of a tumor. Shortening by 3 mm or more is definitely abnormal.

3. Outline of the canal: The lumen of the normal internal auditory canal is surrounded by a well-defined white line, which is made up of cortical bone that is denser than the surrounding bone of the petrosa. Destruction or demineralization of this cortical outline is respectively a positive or suggestive indication of a space-occupying lesion within the canal.

4. Crista falciformis: This divides the canal into two compartments, but is always located at or above the midpoint of the vertical diameter of the internal auditory canal. A reverse of this ratio or an asymmetry of at least 2 mm in the position of the crista is strongly suggestive of an intracanalicular mass.

Computed Tomography Evaluation of Acoustic Neuromas

Almost all medium-sized (2 cm to 3 cm) and large acoustic neuromas will be visualized on CT scans. Although scans done without contrast enhancement do not detect as many tumors as those done after the injection of a contrast medium, they sometimes permit differentiation of artifact from tumor and differentiation of meningioma and other lesions from acoustic neuroma. Depending on the size of the tumor, there may be displacement of the fourth ventricle, enlargement of the ipsilateral cerebellopontine angle, ambient cisterns adjacent to the mass, and hydrocephalus.

CT scans following intravenous injection of a contrast medium show a much higher percentage of tumors than unenhanced scans. Immediately after the injection of contrast material, an acoustic neuroma usually appears as a uniform, homogenous, high-density lesion. Small acoustic neuromas (less than 1 cm) at the porus or within the internal auditory canal may be demonstrated on CT scan following the introduction of metrizamide (Amipaque) or air into the cerebellopontine-angle cistern. These tumors are demonstrated on the CT scan by filling defects within the air or metrizamide shadow outside of the internal auditory canal or by nonfilling of the internal auditory canal by the contrast agents.

Pantopaque cisternography is an additional procedure performed for evaluation of acoustic neuromas. About 5 ml to 6 ml of Pantopaque (iophendylate) are injected into the subarachnoid space of the lumbar spine. The patient is placed in the prone position, and under fluoroscopic control, the Pantopaque is advanced into the cerebellopontine-angle cistern. With the patient's head at different degrees of rotation, from straight lateral to PA, multiple spot films are obtained of the internal auditory canals. A tumor is indicated by a filling defect in the Pantopaque column within the cerebellopontine-angle cistern or by nonfilling of the internal auditory canal.

TRAUMA OF THE TEMPORAL BONE

Fractures of the temporal bone are best evaluated by preliminary mastoid films (Fig. 14-52) followed by AP, lateral tomography, and Stenver's polytomography. There are two different types of fractures: longitudinal fractures, which occur along the long axis of the petrous bone, and transverse fractures, which occur across the axis of the petrous bone. Seventy-five percent of temporal-bone fractures are longitudinal. These fractures usually begin in the parietal and temporal bones. The fracture line is often seen through the anterior walls of the external auditory canal and tympanic cavity just below the petrotympanic fissure and, superiorly, through the tegmen. Eighty to ninety percent of longitudinal fractures are associated with fracture and dislocation of the ossicles. The most common ossicular abnormality is displacement and joint separation (82%), often with dislocation of the incus (57%). Less commonly, ossicular injuries involve fractures of the stapedial arch (30%) and of the malleus (11%).

Although less common (25% of all temporal-bone fractures), transverse fractures are potentially more serious than longitudinal ones. For instance, they may be associated with fractures of the occipital bone and skull base. Also, medial fractures transverse the internal auditory canal, damaging the cochlea and the vestibular and facial nerves. Total hearing loss, marked vestibular upset, and facial weakness or paralysis occur frequently. Lateral fractures more often may pass through the labyrinth (from the cochlea to the round window) and result in a cerebrospinal fluid leak with the risk of subsequent meningitis. Facial-nerve paresis

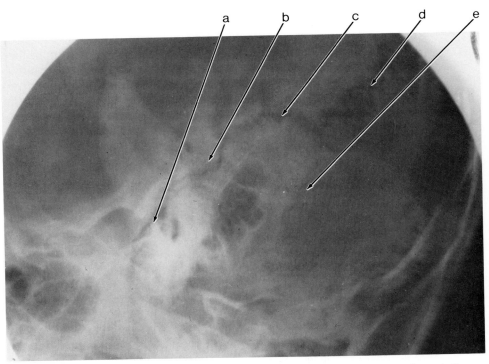

Fig. 14-52. Fracture of the temporal bone. Schüller's view shows (a) fracture through the anterior wall of the bony external canal; (b) linear fracture of the left mastoid extending into the squamosal portion of the temporal bone; (c) normal parietomastoid suture; (d) normal lambdoid suture; and (e) normal occipitomastoid suture.

may indicate a fracture through the internal auditory canal, the geniculate ganglion region, the horizontal portion of the nerve canal along the medial wall of the tympanic cavity, or distally, through the vertical portion of the canal. About 20% of fractures into the facial canal are associated with longitudinal fractures, 50% with transverse fractures.

All cases of trauma to the temporal bone require thin section tomography (polytomography) for optimal visualization of the affected area. AP, base, or Stenver's projections are preferable for transverse fractures; lateral and coronal views are adequate to show longitudinal fractures.

Temporal-bone fractures are often associated with various types of head injuries. CT scanning is the procedure of choice for the detection of intracranial bleeding. Fractures through the temporal bone may also be detected at the same time by a CT scan with the proper centering and window setting.

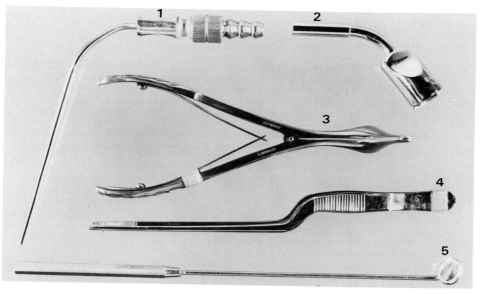

Fig. A-1. Nasal instruments. (*1*) Ferguson-Frazier nasal suction. (*2*) Transilluminator light for use with Welch-Allyn battery handle. (*3*) Nasal speculum, Vienna type. (*4*) Jansen-Gruenwald bayonet forceps. (*5*) Nasopharyngeal mirror.

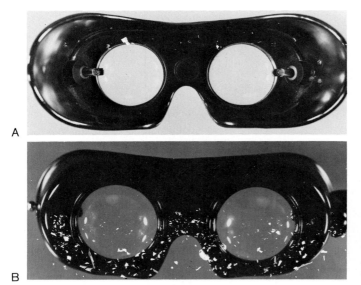

A

B

Fig. A-2. Frenzel's glasses. (*A*) Internal view with small lamp and 20 + diopter lenses. (*B*) External view.

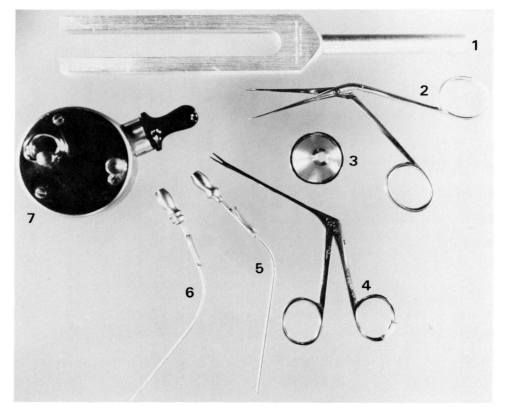

Fig. A-3. Ear instruments. (*1*) 512-Hz tuning fork. (*2*) Hartmann ear forceps. (*3*) Ear speculum. (*4*) Alligator forceps. (*5*) No.-5 ear suction. (*6*) No.-20 Schuknecht ear suction. (*7*) Bárány noise box.

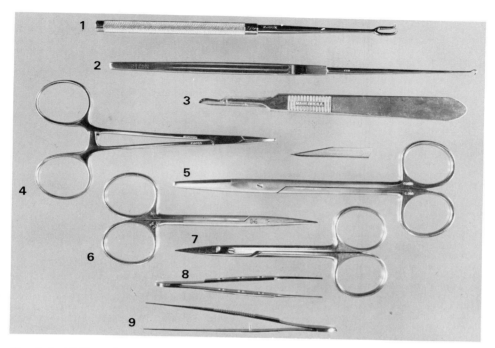

Fig. A-4. (*1*) Fine, double skin hook. (*2*) Fine, single skin hook. (*3*) Bard-Parker knife handle with No.-15 blade and No.-11 blade. (*4*) Fine mosquito hemostat. (*5*) Suture scissors. (*6*) Curved iris scissors. (*7*) Straight iris scissors. (*8*) Fine, toothed forceps. (*9*) Fine, smooth forceps.

Numerals followed by an "f" indicate a figure;
"t" following a page number indicates a table.

Abscesses
  brain
    frontal sinusitis and, 136-137
    otitis media and, 62-63
  mastoid, radiographic findings, 306-307,
    307f, 309f
  peritonsillar, 207
  retropharyngeal, radiographic findings in,
    295-296, 298f
  septal
    drainage of, 158, 158f
    septal hematoma and, 155
  sinusitis and, 136-137, 138
Acetaminophen, in viral rhinitis, 129
Acoustic neurinoma
  deafness with, 47-48
  and facial nerve weakness, 164f, 167
  radiographic findings in, 310-313, 310-312f
  and vertigo, 92, 96
Acoustic reflex decay, 21
Acoustic reflex threshold, 21
Acoustic trauma, 46, 106, 107f
Actinomycosis
  laryngeal, 218
  salivary gland infiltrates in, 192
Adenoidectomy, 33, 123
Adenoids
  hypertrophy of, 122-123
  in nasopharynx, 122
  radiologic evaluation of, lateral view, 260,
    261f, 262f
Adenovirus, and laryngitis, 229
Ageusia, 143-144
Aging. See Elderly patient
Air-conducting hearing aids, 41
Airway. See also Oropharyngeal disorders;
    Laryngeal disorders, Radiology, of lar-
    ynx
  laryngeal papillomatosis and, 214

  in lingual tonsillitis, 208
  upper respiratory tract anatomy, 116-118
Airway emergencies
  acute, 228-231
    angioneurotic edema, 234-235
    croup, 228-229
    epiglottitis, 230-231
    foreign body, laryngeal, 228
    foreign body, tracheobronchial, 231
    laryngeal edema, 234
  obstruction, respiratory, 231-235
    in child, 231-233
    in newborn, 234
Albers-Schonberg disease, deafness with, 44
Albinism, with amino acid metabolic errors,
    43
Alcohol, vestibular toxicity of, 91-92
Allergy
  allergic rhinitis, 119, 131-133
  and chronic nasal obstruction, 123
  and laryngeal edema, 234
  nasal mucus in, 118, 119
  and nasal obstruction, chronic, 122
Alternate binaural loudness balance test, 16
Amaurotic familial idiocy, 43
Amikacin, ototoxicity of, 92
Amino acid metabolic errors, deafness with,
    42-43
ε-Aminocaproic acid, in HANE, 235
Aminoglycosides, ototoxicity of, 45, 92
Amphotericin B in fungal infections, 143, 218
Ampicillin, 58
Amplification
  in presbycusis, 41-42
  in stapes fixation, 37
Amyotrophic lateral sclerosis
  and facial nerve weakness, 164f, 167
  and palatal dysfunction, 125
Anaerobes, in sinusitis, 135
Analgesia, in otitis externa, 54
Androgens, in HANE, 235
Anesthesia
  for laceration repair, 160
  for myringotomy, 32
  for nasal reduction, 156

Aneurysm
  and conductive hearing loss, 33
  intracranial, and epistaxis, 154
Angina pectoris
  atypical, 184
  and pharyngeal pain, 210
Angiofibroma, juvenile nasopharyngeal, 148,
    154
Angiography, in vascular tumors, neck, 252
Angioneurotic edema, hereditary, 234-235
Anosmia, 143-144
Anoxia
  airway obstruction and, 228
  and deafness, 45
Antibiotics
  in auricular infections, 99, 102
  and candidiasis, 203
  in external otitis, 53-54
  in external otitis, malignant, 55
  in lateral venous thrombosis, 68
  in mastoiditis, 59
  in Meniere's disease, 87-88
  with nasal balloon, 149
  in nasopharyngitis, chronic, 124
  in otitis media, suppurative, 57
  ototoxicity of, 45, 92
  in septal abscesses, 158
  in sialadenitis, bacterial, 191
  in sinusitis, 135
  in syphilis, 203-204
  in viral rhinitis, for secondary infection,
    129
Anticholinergics, in vasomotor rhinitis, 133
Antihistamines, 32
  in allergic rhinitis, 131-132
  in otitis media, suppurative, 57
  in serous otitis, 123
  in vasomotor rhinitis, 133-134
  in viral rhinitis, 129
Antral wash, in maxillary sinusitis, 138, 139-
    140
Antrotomy, anatomy for, 64, 65f
Aphthous stomatitis, 201
AP view, of larynx, 291, 293f, 296f
Arnold's nerve, 177
Arterial disease, deafness with, 48
Arterial epistaxis, 147-148
Arteriography, with embolization, in epi-
    staxis, 154
Arteritis, temporal, hearing loss with, 49
Arthritis
  gonorrhea and, 204
  laryngeal involvement, 219
Aryepiglottic folds
  in epiglottitis, 297f
  radiography of, 292-294f
Arytenoid area
  in epiglottitis, 297f
  radiography of, 292-294f

Arytenoidectomy, in laryngeal arthritis, 219
Aspergillosis, and nasal obstruction, 143
Aspergillus fumigatus, laryngeal infections
    with, 218
Aspirin, in epistaxis, 148
Aspirin triad syndrome, 134
Asthma, in aspirin triad syndrome, 134
Ataxia, vestibular, 92
Atelectasis, middle-ear, tympanograms in, 21
Atresia, external auditory canal, 29
Atrophic rhinitis
  mucus in, 119
  and olfaction, 144
Atticoantrotomy, 64, 65f
Atticotomy
  anatomy for, 66-67f
  in otitis media, 61
Audiometry. *See* Auditory function tests
Auditory artery disease, and vertigo, 95
Auditory evoked-response testing, 16-17, 18-
    19f
Auditory function, mastoid surgery and, 69
Auditory function tests, 58
  in acoustic neurinoma, 92
  in acoustic trauma, 106, 107f
  auditory evoked response testing, 16-17,
    18-19f
  behavioral audiometry, 12-13, 14-15f
  behavioral tests, 13
  in foreign body injury, to external auditory
    canal, 102
  impedance audiometry, 17, 19-21, 20f
  in inner-ear membrane rupture, 89
  tuning fork and whisper tests, 11-12
  tympanometry, 17, 19-21, 20f
Auditory ganglion, 5f
Auditory labyrinth. *See* Cochlea
Auditory nerve, skull fractures and, 108, 109
Auditory nerve pathology, tests of, 16, 86
Auricle
  anatomy of, 2-3, 2f
  deformities of, and hearing loss, 29
  emergencies, 98-102, 100-101f
  and external otitis, 52
Axonotmesis
  in Bell's palsy, 171
  defined, 169

Bacterial meningitis, deafness with, 45
Balloons, nasal, 149-150
Barbiturates, and vestibular system, 92
Barium swallow
  in cervical lymphadenomegaly, 249-250
  in laryngeal radiography, 291
    in cancer, 305
    with foreign body, 299-300

Barotrauma, 27
  emergency management, 105
  inner-ear damage, 106
  and vertigo, 89
Base view, of sinuses, 259-260, 260f
Basilar artery disease, and vertigo, 95
Basilar membrane, 6-7, 7f
Basilar skull fracture, 107-110, 108f
Beclomethasone, in allergic rhinitis, 133
Behavioral audiometry, 12-13, 14-15f
Behcet's syndrome, 202
Bekesy audiometry, 16
Bell's palsy
  diagnosis, 165-166, 165f
  surgery in, 171-173
  therapy for, 171
Benign paroxysmal positional vertigo, 91
Bezold's abscess, 59, 307
Biopsy
  in cervical lymphadenomegaly, 250
  in laryngitis, 215
  in neck masses, 252
  salivary gland, 192, 193, 194-195
  serous otitis media, 32
Birth trauma
  and deafness, 45
  and laryngeal paralysis, 233
Black hairy tongue, 199
Blastomycosis, laryngeal, 218
Blindness, ethmoidectomy and, 141
Blowout fracture, 276, 280-281f
Bondy-modified mastoidectomy, 69
Bone conduction, masked, 15
Bone-conduction hearing aid, 41
Bonine, in vertigo, 81
Brain abscess. *See* Abscesses, brain
Brain-stem disorders, and vertigo, 95-96
Brain-stem evoked-response audiometry, 16-17, 18-19f, 47
Branchial arch abnormalities, and hearing loss, 29
Branchial arches, 2, 3
Branchial arch syndromes, 4-5, 34
Branchial cleft cysts, 250
Bridge, nasal, 114, 115f
Bronchitis, laryngotracheal, 230, 295, 296f
Bullous myringitis, 55
Burning-tongue syndrome, 199-200
Burns, pharyngeal, 208

C-1-Esterase inhibitor, 234, 235
Caffeine, vestibular toxicity of, 91-92
Calculi, salivary gland, 191, radiographic findings in, 285-286, 285-287f, 289-290
Caldwell-Luc procedure, 138
  in maxillary sinusitis, 139-140
  radiography after, 265

Caldwell view
  in acute sinusitis, 264, 265f
  in ethmoid sinus osteoma, 270f
  of orbit and facial bones, 278-279f
  of sinuses, 256, 257f, 258, 259f
Caloric test, 21, 77, 78, 80
  in cerebellopontine-angle tumors, 47
  in Meniere's disease, 86
  in vestibular neuritis, benign, 91
Candidiasis
  laryngeal, 218
  oropharyngeal, 203
Carbohydrate metabolic disorders, deafness with, 43
Carcinoma
  and facial nerve paralysis, 164f, 165, 167-168
  and hoarseness, 220
  laryngeal, 220-223
    radiographic findings in, 303-305, 303-304f
    subglottic, 223-226
    supraglottic, 221-223
    surgery for, 223-226
  nasopharyngeal. *See* Nasopharyngeal carcinoma
  salivary gland, 290, 291f
  of sinuses, radiographic findings in, 272, 273f
  vocal cord, 221
Carotid artery
  and conductive hearing loss, 33
  ligation of, in epistaxis, 154
Carotid body tumors, 252
Carotid triangle
  anatomy of, 238-239, 239f
  contents of, 240f, 241
Carotidynia, and ear pain, referred, 182
Cartilage, nasal, 114, 115f
Cartilaginous tumors, of neck, 253
Cavernous sinus thrombosis
  nasal furunculosis and, 128
  in sphenoid sinusitis, 137-138
Cawthorne-Cooksey exercises
  for Meniere's disease, 86
  in vertigo, 83-84
Cellulitis, orbital, 138
Central nervous system disorders, and facial nerve paralysis, 167
Cephalexin, with nasal balloon, 149
Cerebellar artery disease, and vertigo, 95, 96
Cerebellar artery syndrome, and vertigo, 96
Cerebellopontine angle tumors
  deafness with, 47-48
  and facial nerve paralysis, 164f, 167-168
Cerebral aneurysm, and epistaxis, 154
Cerebral edema, septic thrombosis and, 63
Cerebral ischemia, deafness with, 48

Cerebrospinal fluid leak
    ethmoidectomy and, 141
    nasal fractures and, 155-156
    skull fractures and, 103
    temporal bone fractures and, 107
Cerebrospinal fluid otorrhea, traumatic, 110
Cerumen, 2, 9
    and external otitis, 52
    and hearing loss, 28
Cervical lymph nodes, 244f, 246
Cervical osteophytes, 210
Cervical spine
    referred pain from, 180, 183
    skull fractures and, 109
Cervical triangles
    anatomy of, 238-240, 239f
    contents of, 239, 241-246, 244f
    examination of, 247
Cheilosis, 200
Chemicals, and laryngeal irritation, 216
Chemotherapeutic agents, deafness with, 45
Chlorpheniramine, in viral rhinitis, 129
Choanae, nasal
    adenoid hypertrophy and, 122
    anatomy of, 121, 122f
Choanal atresia
    and airway obstruction, 234
    and nasal obstruction, 130
Choanal polyps
    in polypoid rhinosinusitis, 135
    sinuses in, 267
Cholesteatoma, 22, 30
    diagnosis and treatment, 61
    and facial nerve paralysis, 167
    and facial nerve weakness, 164f
    in mastoiditis, 309-310, 310-311f
    otitis media with
        complications, 61-68, 64-67f
        surgery in, 68-69
Chondritis, auricular, 99, 102
Chondromas, of neck, 253
Chorda tympani, 23
Chorda tympani nerve, 9
Claudius' cells, 7f
Cleft palate, 32, 125
Coagulopathy, epistaxis in, 147
Coated tongue, 199
Cocaine, for nasal packing, 148
Coccidiomycosis, laryngeal, 218-219
Cochlea
    anatomy of, 5, 5f, 6-7, 6-7f
    drug toxicity, 91-92
    electrocochleography of, 17
    in temporal bone fractures, 313
    tests of, 16
Cochlear artery disease, and vertigo, 95
Cochlear duct, 6f
Cochlear hydrops, 74, 84-85
Cockayne's syndrome, deafness with, 44

Cogan's syndrome
    hearing loss with, 49
    vertigo in, 94
Collagen vascular diseases, hearing loss with,
    49
Columella, nasal, 114, 115f
Coma, airway obstruction and, 228
Compazine, in vertigo, 83
Computed-tomography scan. *See also* Radiol-
    ogy
    in acoustic neurinoma, 312-313
    in cerebellopontine-angle tumors, 47
    in laryngeal cancer, 305
    in nasal fracture, 156
    of neck, 295
    in otitic hydrocephalus, 63
    with sialography, 285
    in temporal bone fractures, 314
Conduction-latency tests, in facial nerve pa-
    ralysis, 170
Congenital anomalies
    and nasal obstruction, 129-130
    and respiratory obstruction, in newborn,
        234
Congenital anosmia, 144
Congenital cholesteatoma, and facial nerve
    paralysis, 167
Congenital cysts, neck, 248, 250-251
Congenital heart disease, deafness with,
    44
Congenital laryngeal webs, 232
Connective tissue disorders, with Sjogren's
    syndrome, 192
Contact ulcers, laryngeal, 213-214
Contralateral-routing-of-signals aid, 41
Contrast medium, for sialography, 283, 285,
    287-288, 289-290
Cortical evoked response, 17
Cortisone. *See* Steroids
Corti's organ, anatomy of, 6-7, 7f
Cortisporin, in external otitis, 53
Cough, allergic rhinitis and, 132
Coxsackie virus infections, pediatric, 205
Cranial nerve(s). *See also* Facial nerve, Inner-
    vation; *specific nerves*
    cerebellopontine angle lesions, 164f
    in cervical triangles, 239f, 240f, 241, 242,
        243
    ear innervation, 176-177
    electrocochleography of, 17
    in malignant external otitis, 54
    neuralgia of, and ear pain, 180-181
    in sphenoid sinusitis, 137-138
    tumors of, 252
Cribriform plate, nasal fractures and, 155
Cricoarytenoid arthritis, in lupus erythemato-
    sus, 220
Cricoarytenoid joint, arthritic involvement of,
    219

Cricoid cartilage
  chondromas, 253
  examination of, 247
Crista falciformis, 312
Cristae ampullares, anatomy of, 5, 7
Cromolyn sodium, in allergic rhinitis, 133
Croup, 300
  acute spasmodic, 228-229
  radiographic findings in, 295, 296f
Crouzon's disease, 5
Cryosurgery
  in epistaxis, 148
  in lingual tonsillitis, 208
  in rhinitis medicamentosa, 134
  in vasomotor rhinitis, 134
Cryoturbinectomy, 134
Cryptococcal infections, laryngeal, 218
Cupula, 6f
Cupulolithiasis, 77, 89-91, 90f
Cystic fibrosis, and mucoceles, sinus, 268
Cystic hygroma, 234, 251
Cysts
  congenital, neck, 248, 250-251
  frontal sinus, 139
  laryngeal, 214, 233
    radiologic findings in, 301, 301f
  nasopharyngeal, 124
  sebaceous, neck, 251
  sinus, radiographic findings in, 266, 267f, 269

Debris, in external otitis, 52, 53
Debrox, 28
Decongestants, in otitis media, suppurative, 57
Deiters' cells, 7f
Dental disorders. *See* Teeth
Dermoplasty, septal, 147
Developmental defects
  cysts, neck, 248, 250-251
  and hearing loss, 29
Dexamethasone, in allergic rhinitis, 133
Diabetes mellitus
  deafness with, 48
  and fungal infections, 143
  and hearing loss, sudden idiopathic, 111
  otitis externa in, 54, 167
Diagnostic tests, in facial nerve paralysis, 169-171. *See also* Auditory function tests; Electronystagmography
Diazepam, in vertigo, 81
Digastric triangle. *See* Submandibular triangle
Diphtheria, 216-217
Diploic veins, frontal sinusitis and, 136-137
Diverticulum, hypopharyngeal, 210, 253

Diving, and frontal sinusitis, 137
Dizziness. *See* Vertigo
Dorsum, nasal, 114, 115f
Drainage
  paranasal sinuses, 121
  septal, 157-158, 158f
  sinuses, 120, 135-140
Dramamine, in vertigo, 81
Drop attacks of Tumarkin, 73
Drugs
  deafness with, 45
  and dry mouth, 200
  and Stevens-Johnson syndrome, 201
  in vertigo, 81
  vestibulotoxic, 91-92
Ductus reuniens, 6, 6f
Dyskeratosis. *See* Leukoplakia
Dysostosies, deafness with, 43

Eagle's syndrome, 181-182, 209
Ear
  anatomy and physiology, 2-9, 2-3f, 5-8f
  auditory function tests, 11-21
    auditory evoked response testing, 16-17, 18-19f
    behavioral audiometry, 12-13, 14-15f
    tuning fork and whisper tests, 11-12
    tympanometry, 17, 19-21, 20f
  examination of, 9-11, 10f
  facial nerve tests, 22-23
  and headache, referred, 183
  infected, surgery with, 68-69. *See also* Otitis
  vestibular testing, 21-22
Ear emergencies
  auricle, 98-102, 100-101f
  external auditory canal, 102-103
  inner ear and temporal bone, 106-111, 107-108f
  tympanic membrane and middle ear, 103-105
Ear instruments, 316f
Ear pain, referred, 176-182
Eaton agent, and laryngitis, 229
Ectodermal defects, and deafness, 43
Edema
  in frontal sinusitis, 137
  in Melkersson-Rosenthal syndrome, 166
  in sphenoid sinusitis, 138
Effusions, and hearing loss, 31-33
Elderly patient. *See also* Presbycusis
  arterial epistaxis in, 147-148
  dysequilibrium in, 92-93
  external otitis in, 54
  ototoxic drugs in, 92

Electrocautery
  in rhinitis medicamentosa, 134
  turbinate, in chronic nasal obstruction, 123
  in vasomotor rhinitis, 134
Electrocochleography, 17
Electrodiagnostic testing, in facial nerve pa-
    ralysis, 169-171
Electrogustometer, 23
Electromyography, 23, 170-171
Electroneurography, 23
Electronystagmography, 21, 80-87
  in cerebellopontine-angle tumors, 47
  in vestibular neuritis, benign, 91
Electrosurgery
  in lingual tonsillitis, 208
  in subglottic hemangioma, 232-233
Embolism, septic, otitis media and, 63, 68
Embolization, arterial, in epistaxis, 154
Emergencies
  airway. *See* Airway emergencies
  nasal and facial
    epistaxis, 146-154, 151-153f
    facial nerve disorders, 163-173, 164-165f.
      See also Facial nerve degeneration
    nasal fractures, 154-157
    septal drainage, 157-158
    soft-tissue lacerations, 158-163, 161-162f
  septic thrombosis, venous sinus, 68
Endocochlear shunt, in Meniere's disease, 87
Endocrine abnormalities, deafness with, 44
Endolymph, 6
Endolymphatic duct, anatomy of, 5f, 6f
Endolymphatic fluid, in vertigo, 74
Endolymphatic space, anatomy of, 5f, 6
Endotracheal intubation. *See* Intubation
Epidural abscess, frontal sinusitis and, 136-
    137
Epiglottis
  examination of, 211
  radiography of, 292-294f, 301, 301f
Epiglottitis, 230-231
  radiographic findings in, 295, 297f
Epinephrine, in croup, 229
Epiphora, ethmoidectomy and, 141
Epistaxis
  anterior septal bleeding, 146-147, 147f
  arterial, 147-148
  rare disorders causing, 147
  treatment of, 148-154, 151-153f
    balloons, 148-150
    packing, 150-151, 151-153f
    surgical options, 151, 154
    tampons, 149
Epsilon aminocaproic acid, 235
Epstein-Barr virus, and nasopharyngeal carci-
    noma, 123
Erythromycin, 58
  with nasal balloon, 149
  in otitis media, suppurative, 57

Escherichia coli, in otitis media, 60
Esophageal disorders
  and ear pain, referred, 179-180
  neoplasms, 249, 253
  reflux esophagitis, 210
Esophageal speech, 225
Ethiodol, for sialography, 283, 285, 290, 290f
Ethmoid artery
  ligation of, in epistaxis, 154
  nasal blood supply, 119
Ethmoid bone, nasal fractures and, 155
Ethmoidectomy, 140-141
  in polypoid rhinosinusitis, 135
Ethmoiditis
  chronic, 140
  and olfaction, 144
Ethmoid sinus. *See also* Sinuses, paranasal
  anatomy of, 115-116
  Caldwell view, 259f
  mucoceles, 269
  osteoma of, 270
  in polypoid rhinosinusitis, 135
  polyps of, 266-267
  in Water's view, 256, 258f
Eustachian tube, 32-33
  anatomy of, 4, 121, 122f
  blockage, tympanometry patterns in, 20,
    21
  evaluation of, 10
  and serous otitis media, 58
Exercises
  for Meniere's disease, 86
  in vertigo, 83-84
Exophthalmos, in sphenoid sinusitis, 137-138
Exostoses, and hearing loss, 29
External auditory canal
  anatomy of, 2-3, 2f
  emergencies, 102-103
  examination of, in vertigo, 74-75
  external otitis, 52-59
  innervation of, 9
  obstruction, and hearing loss, 28-29
  octoscopy, 10
Eye abnormalities, deafness with, 44

Facial lacerations
  and facial nerve paralysis, 168
  repair of, 161-162, 161-162f
Facial lymph nodes, 244f, 245,
Facial nerve, 8-9, 8f
  auditory canal foreign bodies and, 102
  in cerebellopontine-angle tumors, 48
  mastoid surgery and, 69
  neoplasms, 252
  otitis media and, 60, 62

in salivary gland surgery, 194-195
skull fractures and, 108, 109
in temporal bone fractures, 313-314
tests of, 22
Facial nerve decompression, 171-172
Facial nerve degeneration
Bell's palsy
diagnosis of, 165-166
surgical, 171-173
therapy, 171
diagnosis, 163-168, 164-165f
central causes, 167-168
infectious causes, 166-167
inflammatory causes, 165-166
salivary gland disorders and, 189-190
stages of, 169-171
surgery, 171-173
Facial pain, referred, sources of, 182-184
Facial paresis, in otitis media, suppurative,
59
Facial trauma, radiology in. *See* Radiology, in
facial trauma
Falling attacks, vestibular, 73
Fallopian canal, 165, 165f
Familial hereditary telangiectasia, and epistaxis, 147
Fever, ototoxic drugs in, 92
Fibrosing external otitis, chronic, 56
Fibrous dysplasia, sinus, 271, 271f
Fick operation, in Meniere's disease, 87
Fissured tongue, 198-199
Fistula
cholesteatoma and, 310
labyrinthine, otitis media and, 61-62
Fistula test, 22, 74
Fluid, in sinuses, 266-267, 266f
Fluoroscopy, of larynx, 291
Foreign body
in auditory canal, 102-103
and epistaxis, 147
in external auditory canal, 28-29
laryngeal, 228
radiographic findings in, 296, 298-300,
299f
and nasal obstruction, 130
pharyngeal, 208-209
tracheobronchial, 231
Fossa of Rosenmuller. *See* Rosenmuller,
fossa of
Fractures. *See* Emergencies; Trauma; *specific
fracture sites*
Frenulum, tongue, 198
Frenzel's glasses, 21, 22, 74, 75, 316f
in cupulolithiasis, 90
with Hallpike positional tests, 90
in Meniere's disease, 86
Friedreich's ataxia, deafness with, 44
Frontal sinus
and mucoceles, sinus, 268-269, 269f

osteoma of, 270
radiography of, lateral sinus view, 261f
Frontal sinus, anatomy of, 116
Frontal sinusitis. *See also* Sinuses, paranasal
acute, 136-137
chronic, 139
Frontal sinus obliteration, osteoplastic, 141
FTA-ABS, in vertigo diagnosis, 94
Fungal infections
laryngeal, 218-219
and nasal obstruction, 143
oropharyngeal, 203
Furunculosis, nasal, 128

Gargoylism, 43
Gastroesophageal reflux, 210, 216
Genetic disorders
familial hereditary telangiectasia, 147
with hearing loss, 42-45
hereditary angioneurotic edema, 234-235
Geniculate ganglion, 8f
Geniculate neuralgia, and ear pain, referred,
181
Gentamicin
deafness with, 45
in Meniere's disease, 87-88
ototoxicity of, 92
Geographic tongue, 198
Gingivitis, acute necrotizing ulcerative, 202
Gingivostomatitis, herpetic, 204-205
Glabella, 115f
Glands, in cervical triangles, 239f, 240f, 241,
242, 243
Globus hystericus, 209-210
Glomus jugulare
and conductive hearing loss, 33
and facial nerve paralysis, 165, 168
Glomus tympanicum tumors, 252
Glossitis, 198, 199, 200
Glossopharyngeal nerve, neoplasms, 252
Glossopharyngeal neuralgia, 180-181, 209
Glottic region, defined, 221
Glottis, carcinoma of, 221
Goiter, deafness with, 44
Gonococcal infections, pharyngitis, 204
Granulation, in malignant external otitis, 54-
55
Granuloma
and epistaxis, 147
and nasal obstruction, 142-143
Granulomatous infiltration, of salivary gland,
192-193
Guillain-Barré syndrome
and facial nerve paralysis, 167
and facial nerve weakness, 164f

Habituation, 83
Hair cells, 6-7, 7f
Hallpike maneuvers, 76-77, 76f, 78, 90
Hand-foot-and-mouth disease, 205
Headache
  allergic rhinitis and, 132
  in polypoid rhinosinusitis, 134-135
  referred, sources of, 182-184
  sinus, 135-140
Head and neck, lymph nodes of, 243-246,
    244f
Hearing. *See also* Auditory function tests
  anatomy and physiology, 2-9, 2-3f, 5-8f
  mastoid surgery and, 69
  vertigo and, 73-74
Hearing aids
  hearing loss level for, 14f
  in presbycusis, 41-42
Hearing loss. *See also* Auditory function tests
  conductive, 27-37
    branchial arch syndromes and, 4-5
    middle ear disorders, 31-37, 34-35f
    obstructive, 28-29
    tympanic membrane, 30-31
  definitions and history taking, 26-27
  in external otitis, 53
  foreign bodies and, 102
  functional, tests for, 21
  in Meniere's disease, 85-86
  sensorineural, 15
    bilateral, 35-45, 36-39f
    with metabolic disorders, 48, 49
    presbycusis, 35, 38-42, 38-39f
    sudden idiopathic, 49, 110-111, 171
    unilateral, 45-48
    of unknown cause, 49
  sudden idiopathic, 49, 110-111, 171
  tympanic membrane perforation and, 104
  vertigo and, 74
Hemangioma
  cervical, 251
  subglottic, radiographic findings in, 300
Hematoma
  auricular, 98, 100-101f
  septal. *See* Septal hematoma
  subglottic, 232-233
Hemophilus influenzae
  in epiglottitis, 230
  in septal abscesses, 158
  in sinusitis, 135
  in suppurative otitis media, 56
  in tonsillitis, 205
  in viral rhinitis, 129
Hemorrhage
  intracranial, with temporal bone fracture,
    314
  laryngeal
    in lupus erythematosus, 219
    submucosal, 213

Hemotympanum
  emergency management, 105
  skull fractures and, 108
Hennebert's sign, 22
Hensen's cells, 7f
Hereditary angioneurotic edema, 234-235
Hereditary disorders, deafness with, 48
Hereditary nerve deafness, 42-45
Hermann's syndrome, 43
Hernia, hiatus, 210
Herpangina, 205
Herpes zoster infections
  varicella, 204
  and vertigo, 88
Herpes zoster oticus, 56, 74
  and deafness, 171
  and ear pain, referred, 180
  and facial nerve paralysis, 165, 166
  and vertigo, 88
Herpetic stomatitis, 201, 204-205
Hiatus hernia, 210
Histiocytosis X, and facial nerve paralysis, 168
Histoplasmosis, laryngeal, 218
Hoarseness, 211-216, 212f
Hormones, in HANE, 235
Humidification, nasal mucosa and, 117
Huntington's chorea, 43
Hurler's syndrome, 43
Hutchinson's incisors, in syphilis, congenital,
    204
Hyalinization, and hearing loss, 30
Hydrocephalus, otic, septic thrombosis and, 63
Hydrops, cochlear. *See* Cochlear hydrops
Hyoid bone
  in epiglottitis, 297f
  radiography of, 292-294f
Hyoid cartilage, examination of, 247
Hypaque Sodium 50%, for sialography, 285
Hyperkeratosis, of vocal cords, 212-213
Hyperlipidemia, and hearing loss, sudden
    idiopathic, 111
Hypernasal speech, palatal dysfunction and,
    125
Hyperventilation, and vestibular symptoms,
    72
Hypogeusia, 143-144
Hypoglossal nerve, neoplasms, 252
Hypoglossal nerve transplant, in facial nerve
    disorders, 172
Hyponasal speech, 117, 125
Hypopharynx
  examination of, 211
  Zenker's diverticulum, 210, 253
Hyposmia, 143-144
Hypothyroidism, laryngeal involvement, 219
Hypoxia, airway obstruction and, 228
Hysteria
  globus hystericus, 209-210
  and olfaction, 144

Immune response, pemphigus vs. pemphigoid, 202
Immunoglobulins
  in allergic rhinitis, 132
  in mucus, nasal, 117-118
  in viral rhinitis, 128
Incus. *See also* Ossicular chain
  anatomy of, 4
  resorption of, 33-36, 34-35f
Indomethacin, in aspirin triad syndrome, 134
Infections. *See also* Abscesses
  auricular chondritis, 99, 102
  and cervical lymphadenomegaly, 248, 249-250
  deafness with, 45
  ear. *See* Otitis
  laryngitis, acute viral, 229-230
  nasal mucus in, 19
  nasopharyngeal, 122
  olfactory disorders, 130-135, 141-143
  oropharyngeal, 201, 202-204
  palatal dysfunction and, 128-129
  in polypoid rhinosinusitis, 135
  salivary gland, 190-191
  sinus, 135-140
  upper respiratory. *See* Respiratory tract infections, upper
Infectious mononucleosis
  and facial nerve paralysis, 166
  oropharyngeal lesions in, 202-203
Infiltrative disorders, of salivary gland, 192-193
Inner ear
  anatomy of, 2f, 5-7, 5-7f
  in presbycusis, 39f
  trauma
    emergency management of, 106-111
    and vertigo, 89
Inner-ear disease, ototoxic drugs in, 92. *See also* Vertigo
Innervation
  of cervical triangles, 239f, 240f, 241, 242, 243
  ear and referred pain, 176-177
  inner ear, 5f, 6, 7, 7f, 8-9, 8f
  nasal, 118
  salivary glands, 186, 187, 188
Instrumentation, 315-317f
Intermittent positive pressure breathing, in croup, 229
Internal auditory canal
  anatomy of, 2f, 5-7, 5-7f,
  disorders of, with facial nerve involvement, 165f
  radiography of, 311, 312f
  in temporal bone fractures, 314
Intracranial aneurysm, and epistaxis, 154
Intracranial bleeding, in temporal bone fractures, 314

Intracranial lesions, and olfaction, 144
Intracranial pressure, increased, referred pain in, 182
Intraocular pressure, increased, 183-184
Intubation
  in croup, 229
  in epiglottitis, 230
  and laryngeal edema, 234-235
  in viral laryngitis, acute, 230
Ischemia
  deafness with, 48
  and vertigo, 95, 96

Jerk nystagmus. *See* Nystagmus
Jervell syndrome, deafness with, 44
Jugular bulb, and conductive hearing loss, 33
Jugular vein, internal, septic thrombosis of, 68
Juvenile nasopharyngeal angiofibroma, 148, 154

Kanamycin, ototoxicity of, 92
Kiesselbach's plexus, bleeding from, 146, 147f
Klippel-Feil syndrome, deafness with, 44
Kobrak test, 21

Labial artery, nasal blood supply, 119
Laboratory studies
  in laryngitis, 215
  in lupus erythematosus, 220
  in syphilis, 203
Labyrinth. *See* Vestibular labyrinth
Labyrinthectomy, in Meniere's disease, 87
Labyrinthitis
  otitis media and, 45
  and vertigo, 88-89
  viral, 88-89
Labyrinthotomy, in Meniere's disease, 87
Lacerations, head and neck
  auricular, 99
  closure, 160
  evaluation of, 159-160
  facial, 160-162, 161-162f
  and facial nerve paralysis, 168
  lip, 163
  mucosal, 163
Lacrimal glands
  nervus intermedius and, 163, 164f
  in Sjogren's syndrome, 200
  tumors of, radiologic findings, 262, 263f

Lacrimation, 23
Lange-Nielsen syndrome, deafness with, 44
Laryngeal atresia, congenital, of newborn,
    234
Laryngeal cysts, 233
Laryngeal disorders
    carcinoma, 220-223, 249, 253
    generalized diseases and, 219-220
    hoarseness, 211-216
    infection
        mycotic, 218-219
        subacute and chronic, 216-217
    surgery, 223-226
    vocal cord paralysis, 220
Laryngeal edema, allergic, 234
Laryngeal hemorrhage, submucosal, 213
Laryngeal neoplasms, 220-223, 249, 253
Laryngeal papillomatosis, 214
Laryngeal paralysis, in pediatric patient, 233
Laryngeal stenosis, 215
Laryngeal trichinosis, 217
Laryngeal web(s), congenital, 232, 234
Laryngectomy, 222f, 224-226, 224f
    rehabilitation after, 225
    supraglottic, 222f, 226
    total, 224-225, 224f
    vertical, 222f, 226
Laryngitis
    acute viral, 229-230
    lupus erythematosus and, 220
    subacute or chronic, 215-216
Laryngoceles, 233
    radiographic findings in, 302-303, 302f
Laryngomalacia, 231
Laryngopharyngeal disorders, and ear pain,
    referred, 179-180
Laryngopharyngitis, reflux, 216
Laryngoscopy, 211, 212f, 223
Laryngotracheal bronchitis, 216
    radiographic findings in, 295, 296f
Larynx
    examination of, 211
    foreign body in, 228
    nerve lesions, 233
    paralysis of, 48, 233
    radiology of. *See* Radiology, of larynx
Laser surgery
    for laryngeal papillomatosis, 214
    of larynx, 223
    in lingual tonsillitis, 208
    in subglottic hemangioma, 233
Lateral medullary syndrome, deafness with,
    48
Lateral view
    of nasal bones, 282-283f
    of neck, 290-291, 292f
        in epiglottitis, 297f
        with foreign body, laryngeal, 299f

in laryngeal cysts, 301f
in retropharyngeal abscess, 298f
of sinuses, 260, 261f, 262f
Le Fort fractures, radiographic findings in,
    274, 276, 276f
Leprosy, laryngeal involvement, 217
Lermoyez's syndrome, 86
Leukemic infiltrates, and facial nerve paraly-
    sis, 168
Leukoplakia
    laryngeal, 223
    and laryngitis, 215-216
    oropharyngeal, 199
    of vocal cords, 212-213
Lidocaine, for nasal packing, 148
Light reflex, 3, 3f
Lingual tonsillitis, 207-208
Lip
    cheilosis, 200
    herpetic lesions, 201
    laceration repair, 163
Lipid metabolic errors, deafness with, 43-44
Lipomas, neck, 251
Liver disease, epistaxis in, 147
Loop diuretics, deafness with, 45
Luetic otitis. *See* Syphilitic otitis
Lupus erythematosus, laryngeal involvement
    in, 219-220
Lymphadenomegaly, neck, 248, 249-250
Lymph nodes
    of cervical triangles, 239f, 240f, 241, 242,
        243
    of head and neck, 243-246, 244f, 248, 249-
        250
    neck, CT scans of, 295
Lymphoma
    nasopharyngeal, 124
    sinus, 272
Lymphomatous infiltration, of salivary gland,
    192
Lysozymes, in mucus, nasal, 117

Maculae, 7
Malar fractures, radiographic findings in,
    273, 274f, 275f
Malignancy. *See* Carcinoma; Neoplasms
Malleus. *See also* Ossicular chain
    anatomy of, 4
    otoscopic view of, 3
Malleus fixation, 33
Mandible, fractures of, radiographic findings
    in, 280-282, 284f
Manubrium, 3
Masking, 15
Masseter muscle, transposition of, 172-173

Mass lesions. *See also* Neoplasms
  middle ear, 33
  neck. *See* Neck masses
Mastoid
  cell system of, 4
  otitis media and, 60, 61-69, 65-67f
  temporal bone fractures and, 107
Mastoidectomy, 68-69
  anatomy for, 64-67f
  in otitis media, suppurative, 59
Mastoid films, in temporal bone fractures, 313, 314f
Mastoiditis
  in otitis media, suppurative, 59
  radiographic findings in, 305-309, 307-309f
Mastoid lymph nodes, 244-245, 244f
Mastoid surgery
  procedures, 65-67f
  temporal bone anatomy, 64f
Mastoid tip, in malignant external otitis, 54
Mastoid tympanoplasty, in otitis media, 61
Maxilla, in polypoid rhinosinusitis, 135
Maxillary antrum
  radiographic assessment, 265
  in Water's view, 256, 257f, 258
Maxillary artery ligation, in epistaxis, 154
Maxillary sinus, anatomy of, 116
Maxillary sinusitis. *See also* Sinuses, paranasal
  acute, 138
  chronic, 139-140
  drainage in, 136
Maxillofacial trauma. *See* Facial trauma; Radiology, in facial trauma
Measles
  deafness with, 45
  and laryngitis, 229
Meatus, anatomy of, 114-115
Mechanical presbycusis, 38f, 40
Meclizine, in vertigo, 81
Melkersson-Rosenthal syndrome, and facial nerve paralysis, 165, 166
Membrane ruptures, and vertigo, 89
Membranous labyrinth, anatomy of, 6, 6f
Meniere's disease, 22, 84-88
  and cochlear hydrops, 74
  hearing loss with, 49
  syphilis vs., 94
Meningioma
  and facial nerve paralysis, 167
  and facial nerve weakness, 164f
Meningiomas, deafness with, 47-48
Meningitis
  and congenital deafness, 46
  otitis media and, 62-63
Meningoencephalocele, and nasal obstruction, 130
Meningomyocele, and laryngeal paralysis, 233

Metabolic disorders. *See also* Systemic disease
  with hearing loss
    genetic, 42-43
    sudden idiopathic, 111
  salivary glands in, 193
Metabolic presbycusis, 38f, 40
Metastatic disease
  and facial nerve weakness, 164f, 167-168
  neck masses in, 248
  and vertigo, 96
Middle ear
  anatomy of, 2f, 4
  branchial arch syndromes, 4-5
  conductive hearing loss, 31-37
  emergencies, 103-105
  tomography of, 312f
Middle-ear space, 4
Mikulicz's disease, 192
Minimal caloric test, 21
Moniliasis
  laryngeal, 218
  oropharyngeal, 203
Mononucleosis. *See* Infectious mononucleosis
Morquio's disease, 43
Motor fibers, facial nerve, 8, 8f, 9
Mouth, lymphatic drainage of, 244f, 245
Mouth breathing, and dry mouth, 200
Mouth care, with nasal balloon, 149-150
Mouth disorders. *See also* Oropharyngeal disorders
  examination in, 198-199
  nonulcerative, 199-200
  ulcerative, 201-204
Mucoceles
  in frontal sinusitis, 139
  sinus, radiographic findings in, 267-269, 269f
Mucormycosis, and nasal obstruction, 143
Mucosa. *See also* Oropharyngeal disorders
  laceration repair, 163
  lymphatic drainage of, 244f, 245
  nasal, 116
    in allergic rhinitis, 133
    examination of, 119
    nerve section and, 118
  in pemphigus, 202
  sinus, radiologic assessment, 265, 265f
Mucosal injury, and olfaction, 144
Mucus
  composition of, 117-118
  in viral rhinitis, 128, 129
Mulberry incisors, in syphilis, congenital, 204
Multiple sclerosis
  and facial nerve paralysis, 167
  vertigo in, 93
Mumps, 45, 190
Muscle disorders, neck, 248

Muscles
  auricular, 2
  of cervical triangles, 239f, 240f, 241, 242, 243
  facial nerve innervation, 8-9, 8f
  middle ear, 5
  of palate, 125
  tensor veli palatini, 4
Muscle transposition, in facial nerve disorders, 172-173
Muscular triangle
  anatomy of, 239, 239f
  contents of, 240f, 242
Myasthenia gravis, and palatal dysfunction, 125
Mycobacterium tuberculosis. See Tuberculosis
Mycoplasma pneumoniae, and laryngitis, acute, 229, 230
Mycotic infections. *See* Fungal infections
Myringitis, bullous, 55
Myringostapediopexy, 34
Myringotomy, 32-33, 123
Myxedema, laryngeal involvement, 219

Nafcillin, in septal abscesses, 158
Nares, 114, 115f
Nasal anatomy and physiology
  examination, 119-120
  external, 114, 115f
  internal and paranasal sinuses, 114-116
  nasopharynx, 121-124, 122f
  palate, 124-125
  radiographic studies, 120-121, 121f
  upper respiratory tract, 116-118
  vasculature, 118-119
Nasal bleeding. *See* Epistaxis
Nasal cavity, fibroma of, 271
Nasal choanae, anatomy of, 121
Nasal congestion, and sinus infection, 135
Nasal cycle, 116-117
Nasal disorders
  and ear pain, referred, 178
  referred pain in, 183
Nasal fractures
  management of, 154-157
  and olfaction, 144
  radiographic findings in, 277, 279f, 280, 282-283f
Nasal furunculosis, 128
Nasal glands, nervus intermedius and, 163, 164f
Nasal infections, olfactory disorders, 143-144
Nasal instruments, 315f
Nasal obstruction
  bilateral, 130-135

  chronic, 122-123
  and dry mouth, 200
  in newborn, 234
  and olfaction, 144
  olfactory disorders, 143-144
  unilateral, 129-130
  unusual causes of, 141-143
Nasal polyps
  allergic rhinitis and, 133
  radiographic findings in, 266-267, 267f, 268f
Nasal septum. *See also specific septal disorders and procedures*
  anatomy of, 121, 122f
  in base view, 260f
  trauma to, and nasal obstruction, 130
Nasal spray, and rhinitis medicamentosa, 134
Nasal stenosis, and airway obstruction, 234
Nasal ulcerations, and epistaxis, 146-147
Nasal vestibulitis, recurrent, 128
Nasion, 115f
Nasofrontal duct, 121f, 136
Nasofrontal suture, 115f
Nasopharyngeal angiofibroma, juvenile, 154
Nasopharyngeal carcinoma, 121-122, 123-124
  and ear pain, referred, 178-179
  in fossa of Rosenmuller, 121-122
  serous otitis media, 32, 58
  tomography in, 262, 263
Nasopharyngitis, chronic, 124
Nasopharynx
  adenoidal hypertrophy and nasal obstruction, 122-123
  anatomy, 121-122, 122f
  carcinoma, 123-124. *See also* Nasopharyngeal carcinoma
  choanal polyps in, 267
  cysts, 124
  eustachian tube termination in, 4
  examination of, 120
  in lateral sinus view, 261f
  lymphatic drainage of, 244f, 245
  masses, radiologic evaluation of, 260, 261f, 262f
  nasopharyngitis, 124
  of newborn, 234
  palatal dysfunction, 124-125
  referred pain from, 178-179
Nasotracheal intubation. *See* Intubation
Nausea
  in Meniere's disease, 85
  in vertigo, 83
Neck disorders
  and ear pain, referred, 180
  referred pain in, 183
Neck injury, vertigo in, 94-95
Neck masses. *See also* Carcinoma; Neoplasm
  anatomical considerations
    lymph nodes of, 243-246, 243f

skeletal landmarks, 243
triangles, contents of, 241-246, 239f, 244f
triangles of neck, 238-240, 239-240f
congenital or developmental lesions, 251-252
diagnostic strategy, 247-253
lymphadenomegaly, 249-250
normal structures, masses attached to, 251-253
physical examination, 246-247
Neoplasm. *See also* Acoustic neurinoma; Carcinoma; Nasopharyngeal carcinoma
airway, in newborn, 234
cerebellopontine angle, 167-168
deafness with, 47-48
and ear pain, referred, 178-179
and epistaxis, 154
and facial nerve paralysis, 164f, 165, 167-168,
middle ear, 33
mucoceles, benign, 269-271, 270-271f
nasopharyngeal radiographic findings, 260, 261f, 262, 262f, 263
neck, 248, 251, 252, 253. *See also* Neck masses
and olfaction, 144
salivary gland, 193-195
radiographic findings in, 287, 290, 290f, 291f
in serous otitis media, 31, 32
and sialadenitis, 191
sinuses, radiographic findings in, 272, 273f
and vertigo, 96
Nephropathies, and deafness, 43
Nerve degeneration, 23
Nerve excitability testing, in facial nerve paralysis, 170
Nerve grafts, in facial nerve disorders, 172, 173
Nerve injury. *See also specific cranial nerves*
nasal, 118
skull fractures and, 108, 109
Nerve lesions, of larynx, 233
Nerve–muscle pedicle transfer, in facial nerve disorders, 173
Nerves, in sphenoid sinusitis, 137-138
Nerve sectioning
and nasal mucosa, 118
in vasomotor rhinitis, 134
vestibular, 87, 91
vidian, 118, 134
Nervus intermedius, 8f, 9, 163-165, 164f
Neuralgia. *See also* Cranial nerves; *specific nerves*
and ear pain, referred, 180-182
glossopharyngeal, 209
Neural presbycusis, 38f, 40
Neural tumors, neck, 248, 252

Neurapraxia
defined, 169
facial nerve decompression with, 171
Neuritis, viral vestibular, 91
Neurofibroma, cranial nerve, 252
Neurological evaluation, in Meniere's disease, 86
Neurologic disorders, and deafness, 43, 44, 46, 48
Neuroma, and facial nerve paralysis, 164f, 165, 168
Neuromuscular disorders
and deafness, 48
and facial nerve paralysis, 164f, 165, 168
and palatal dysfunction, 125
Neuro-ocular system, nystagmus, 75
Neuropraxia, 22, 23
Neurotmesis, 22
in Bell's palsy, 171
defined, 169
Newborn, respiratory obstruction in, 234
Nicotine, vestibular toxicity of, 91-92
Nicotine stomatitis, 210
Nocardiosis, laryngeal, 218
Nodules, 223
Nose drops, in otitis media, suppurative, 57
Nystagmus
with amino acid metabolic errors, 43
assessment, 74-84
caloric tests, 77, 78, 80
electronystagmography, 80-81
positional tests, 76-77
spontaneous, 75
in cupulolithiasis, 90-91
in inner-ear membrane rupture, 89
in Meniere's disease, 86
in multiple sclerosis, 93
perilymph leak and, 104
positional, 74
tests of, 21-22
types of, 74, 75
vestibular, 74-75
Nystatin, in candidiasis, 203

Obstruction, salivary gland, 191. *See also* Foreign body
Occipital lymph nodes, 244, 244f
Occipital triangle, contents of, 239f, 240, 242-243
Olfaction
allergic rhinitis and, 132
disorders of, 143-144
in ethmoiditis, 138
Olfactory epithelium, location of, 115
Omoclavicular triangle. *See* Subclavian triangle

Onychodystrophy, 43
Ophthalmoplegia, ethmoidectomy and, 141
Oral care, with nasal balloon, 149-150
Orbit
    in ethmoiditis, 138
    fibroma of, 271
    radiography of
        base view, 259, 260f
        Caldwell's view, 258, 259f
        Water's view, 256, 258, 258f
    referred pain from, 183-184
    sinus malignancy and, 272
    trauma of, 276-277, 278-281f
Organ of Corti. *See* Corti's organ
Ornade, in vasomotor rhinitis, 133
Oropharyngeal disorders
    congenital, in newborn, 234
    and ear pain, referred, 179
    examination of mouth and throat, 198-199
    fibroma, 271
    hoarseness, 211-216
    pediatric, 204-208
    pharyngeal pain, deep, 208-210
    respiratory tract infections, 216-217
    sore mouth, 199-205
        nonulcerative, 199-200
        pediatric, 204-205
        ulcerative, 200-204
Oropharynx
    lymphatic drainage of, 244f, 245
    radiography of, lateral sinus view, 261f
Osler-Weber-Randu disease, and epistaxis,
        147
Osseus spiral lamina, 7f
Ossicular chain. *See also* Incus; Malleus;
        Stapes
    anatomy of, 4-5
    cholesteatoma and, 310
    in conductive hearing loss, 33-37, 36-37f
    emergencies, 104-105
    skull fractures and, 109
    temporal bone fractures and, 107
Ossiculoplasty, 35, 36-37f
    in otitis media, 61
Ossifying fibroma, sinus, 271, 271f
Osteochondrodystrophy, 43
Osteomas, sinus, radiographic findings in,
        270, 270f
Osteomyelitis
    in malignant external otitis, 54
    in sphenoid sinusitis, 137
Osteophytes, cervical, 210
Osteoplastic frontal sinus obliteration, 139,
        141
Otic capsule
    otitis media and, 61
    perilymph and, 5
Otitic hydrocephalus, 63
Otitis, syphilitic, and cochlear hydrops, 74

Otitis externa
    auricular chondritis, 55
    bullous myringitis, 55-56
    chronic fibrosing, 57
    diagnosis, 52
    and hearing loss, 29
    herpes zoster oticus, 56
    malignant, 54-55, 167
    treatment of, 53-54
Otitis media
    acute suppurative
        complications, 58-59
        diagnosis and treatment, 57
        follow-up, 57-58
    chronic
        with cholesteatoma, 61
        without cholesteatoma, 60-61
        complications of, 64-67f, 64-68
        and facial nerve paralysis, 165
    deafness with, 45
    with external otitis, 52-53
    and facial nerve paralysis, 166-167
    nasopharyngeal carcinoma and, 124
    serous, 58
        adenoids and, 123
        and hearing loss, 31-33
        tympanometry patterns, 20
    surgery with, 68-69
    tympanometry patterns in, 20
Otoconia, in cupulolithiasis, 89-90, 90f
Otolithic membrane, 7
Otorrhea, cerebrospinal fluid, 110
Otosclerosis, 20, 34-35
Otoscopy, 3, 4, 8-11, 9f
Ototoxic drugs
    deafness with, 45
    in Meniere's disease, 87-88
Oval window
    anatomy of, 5f
    rupture of, 106
    tympanic membrane and, 4
Oxycel, in epistaxis, 147
Oxygen therapy
    in croup, 229
    in viral laryngitis, acute, 230
Oxymetazoline. *See* Vasoconstrictors

Packing
    in epistaxis, 147, 148, 150-151, 151-153f
    in nasal fracture, 156
Pain
    pharyngeal, 208-210
    in salivary gland disorders, 189
Pain, referred
    to ear, 176-182
    to head and face, 182-184

Pain syndromes, sinus, 135-140
Palate
    abnormalities of, and serous otitis media, 32
    anatomy of, 121, 122f
    dysfunctional, 124-125
    radiography of
        lateral sinus view, 261f
        tomography, 262, 263f
    syphilitic lesions of, 204
Palatine artery, nasal blood supply, 119
Panophthalmoplegia, in sphenoid sinusitis, 137-138
Pantopaque cisternography, in acoustic neuroma, 313
Papilledema
    septic thrombosis and, 63
    in sphenoid sinusitis, 138
Papillomatosis, laryngeal, 214, 223, 300
Paracentesis, in otitis media, suppurative, 57
Parainfluenza virus infections, laryngitis, 229
Paralysis, laryngeal, 233
Paresis, facial nerve, otitis media and, 62
Parotid gland
    anatomy of, 186-187, 187f
    sialography of, 285-286, 285f, 288-291f
Parotid gland tumor, and facial nerve paralysis, 168
Parotid lymph nodes, 244f, 245
Paroxysmal positional vertigo, 91
Pars flaccida, 3, 3f
Pars tensa, 3, 3f
Pediatric patients
    airway emergencies
        acute, 228-231
        chronic respiratory obstruction, 231-235
        newborn, 234
    airway foreign body, 300
    auditory canal foreign bodies, 102, 102-103
    epistaxis, 146, 147f
    nasopharynx of, 122
    oropharyngeal disorders, 204-208
    otitis media, serous, 31, 32-33
    paranasal sinus development, 116
Pedicle transfer, nerve-muscle, 173
Pemphigus and pemphigoid, 201-202
Pendred's syndrome, deafness with, 44, 48
Penicillin
    with nasal balloon, 149
    in otitis media, suppurative, 57
    in septal abscesses, 158
    in syphilis, 93, 203-204
Penrose drains, for septal drainage, 157, 158f
Perforation, of tympanic membrane, 30-31
Periarteritis nodosa, hearing loss with, 49
Perichondritis, auricular, 99, 102
Perilymph, 5, 6
    leakage of, trauma and, 104
Perilymphatic space, anatomy of, 5-6

Pes anserinus, 8-9
Petrositis, otitis media and, 62
Petrous bone, cholesteatoma and, 310
pH, mucous, 117
Pharyngeal disorders. *See* Oropharyngeal disorders
Pharyngeal pain, 208-210
Pharyngeal pouch, 4
Pharyngitis
    chronic, 210
    gonococcal, 204
    in mononucleosis, 103
Pharynx
    disorders of, 208-210
    in epiglottitis, 297f
    paralysis of, 48
Phenylephrine hydrochloride. *See* Vasoconstrictors
Phlebitis
    frontal sinusitis and, 136-137
    otitis media and, 63, 68
Photophobia, with amino acid metabolic errors, 43
Pierre Robin syndrome, 234
Pituitary tumors, sphenoid sinus involvement in, 270
Pneumococcus, in suppurative otitis media, 56
Politzer bag, 22
Polychondritis
    hearing loss with, 49
    relapsing, vertigo in, 94
Polypoid mass, in orbital fractures, 277, 281f
Polyps
    allergic rhinitis and, 133
    laryngeal, 223
    sinus, 134-135
        radiographic findings in, 266-267, 267f, 268f
    vocal cord, 212-213
        radiographic findings in, 303
Polytomography, in temporal bone fractures, 314
Pontine brain stem, facial nerve origination, 8, 8f
Positional nystagmus. *See* Nystagmus
Positional tests, 21-22, 76-77, 76f
Potassium, in endolymph, 6
Preauricular lymph nodes, 244, 245f
Presbycusis, 35, 38-42, 38-39f
PRIST, in allergic rhinitis, 132
Promethazine, in vertigo, 81
Pseudomonas aeruginosa
    in auricular chondritis, 55
    in external otitis, 53
    in malignant external otitis, 54, 167
    in otitis media, 60
Pseudomonas aeruginosa, in auricular infections, 99

Pyocidin, in external otitis, 53
Pyriform sinus, radiology of, 293f
Pyriform sinuses, examination of, 211

Quinine
  deafness with, 45
  vestibular toxicity of, 91-92

Radiology
  in acoustic neurinoma, 92
  in cerebellopontine-angle tumors, 47
  in cervical lymphadenomegaly, 249-250
  in ear pain, referred, 178, 180
  in facial trauma, 272-282, 274-284f
    Le Fort fractures, 274, 276f, 277-278f
    mandibular fractures, 280-282, 284f
    nasal fractures, 277, 280, 282-283f
    orbital trauma, 276-277, 280-281f
    trimalar fractures, 273, 274-275f
  of larynx, 290-305, 292-294f, 296-299f, 301-304f
    benign lesions, 295-303, 296-302f
    malignant lesions, 303-304f, 303-305
  in malignant external otitis, 55
  in mastoiditis, 59
  in maxillary sinusitis, 136, 138
  in nasal fractures, 155, 156
  of nasopharynx and paranasal sinuses, 120, 121, 179
  in neck masses, 252, 253
  in otitis media, 60
  in salivary gland disorders, 192, 193-194
  of salivary glands, 282-283, 285-289, 285-291f
    complications of, 288
    contraindications, 287-288
    findings, 289-290, 289-291f
  in serous otitis media, 31-32
  sinuses, 120, 121, 135, 136, 138
    benign tumors, 269-271, 270-271f
    interpretation of, 264-269, 265-269f
    malignant lesions, 272, 273f
    tomography, 261-263, 263f, 266f
    x-ray series, 256-261, 257-262f
  of temporal bone, 59, 305-314, 306-312f, 314f
    in acoustic neuroma, 310-313, 312f
    in cholesteatoma, 309-310, 311f
    in mastoiditis, 305-307, 309-310f
    in trauma, 313-314, 314f
Ramsay-Hunt syndrome. *See* Herpes zoster oticus

Rathke's pouch, cysts in, 124
Raynaud's phenomenon, sympathectomy effects, 118
Receptors, of nasal mucosa, 116
Recklinghausen's disease, 47, 92
Recruitment
  assessment of, 13, 16
  in Meniere's disease, 85-86
Referred pain, in sphenoid sinusitis, 137
Reflux esophagitis, 210
Reflux laryngopharyngitis, 216
Rehabilitation, after laryngectomy, 225
Reissner's membrane, 7f, 89
Renal disease
  epistaxis in, 147
  and hearing loss, sudden idiopathic, 111
Renal failure, and ototoxic drugs, 92
Renografin 60, for sialography, 285
Respiratory obstruction, in newborn, 234. *See also* Airway emergencies
Respiratory syncytial virus, and laryngitis, 229
Respiratory tract, upper, anatomy of, 116-118
Respiratory tract infections, subacute and chronic, 216-217
Respiratory tract infections, upper. *See also* Oropharyngeal disorders; Laryngeal disorders and ethmoiditis, 138
  mucus in, 119
  nasopharyngitis, chronic, 124
  and olfaction, 144
  and otitis media, 31
Retention cysts, sinus, 266, 267f
Retinitis pigmentosa, deafness with, 44
Retroauricular lymph nodes, 244-245, 244f
Retropharyngeal abscess, radiographic findings in, 295-296, 298f
Rhabdomyosarcoma, and facial nerve paralysis, 168
Rhagades, in syphilis, congenital, 204
Rhinitis
  allergic, 131-133
  mucus in, 119
  vasomotor, 133-134
  viral, 128-129
Rhinitis medicamentosa, 132, 134
Rhinoplasty, after septal abscess, 158
Rhinosinusitis, polypoid, 134-135
Rhizopus, and nasal obstruction, 143
Rinne test, 11
Rosenmuller, fossa of, anatomy, 121-122, 122f
Round window
  anatomy of, 5, 5f, 6f
  in conductive hearing loss, 34
  membrane rupture, 106
    and hearing loss, sudden idiopathic, 111
    skull fractures and, 109
  in temporal bone fractures, 313
  tympanic membrane and, 4

Rubella
  deafness with, 45
  and facial nerve paralysis, 166

Saccule, anatomy of, 5, 5f
Sac operation, in Meniere's disease, 87
Saddle deformity, septal abscess and, 158
Salicylates, deafness with, 45
Salivary flow test, 23
Salivary gland disorders
  anatomy, 186-188, 187f
  categories of, 190-195
    inflammatory, acute, 190-191
    inflammatory, chronic progressive, 192-
      193
    neoplastic, 193-195
  diagnosis, 188-190
  and ear pain, referred, 178
Salivary glands
  in cervical triangles, 239f, 240f, 241
  innervation, 9
  nervus intermedius and, 163, 164f
  radiology of. *See* Radiology, of salivary
    glands
  in Sjögren's syndrome, 200
Salivary glands, minor
  anatomy of, 188
  surgery of, 195
Sarcoidosis
  and nasal obstruction, 142
  salivary gland infiltrates in, 192
Sarcoma
  and facial nerve paralysis, 168
  sinus, 272
Scala media, 7f
Scala tympani, 6f, 7f
Scala vestibuli, 6f, 7f
Scarpa's ganglion, 5f
Schilder's disease, deafness with, 44
Schiller's view
  in mastoiditis, 305, 306-307f
  in temporal bone fractures, 313, 314f
Schirmer's test, 23
Schwannoma
  brain stem evoked response, 19
  deafness with, 47-48
Screamer's nodules, 213
Scrotal tongue, 198-199
Semicircular canals, anatomy of, 5, 5f, 6f, 7
Sensorineural disturbances, in Wallenberg's
    disease, 95-96
Sensory fibers, facial nerve, 8, 8f, 9
Sensory presbycusis, 38f, 40
Septal bleeding, surgery, 146-147, 147f
Septal dermoplasty, 147
Septal deviations, and epistaxis, 146-147

Septal drainage procedures, 157-158
Septal hematoma, 130, 131f
  drainage of, 157, 158
  nasal fractures and, 155
Septal spurs, and epistaxis, 146-147
Septic emboli, otitis media and, 68
Septic thrombosis, 63
Septum, anatomy of, 114, 115, 115f, 121, 122f
Shrapnell's membrane, 3
Sialadenitis, acute bacterial, 190-191, 192
Sialography, 192, 193-194
  in cervical lymphadenomegaly, 250
  technique and findings, 282-283, 285-290,
    285-291f
Sigmoid sinus, in malignant external otitis,
    54
Singer's nodules, 213
Singular nerve, sectioning of, 91
Sinuses, paranasal
  allergic rhinitis and, 133
  anatomy of, 114-116, 121f
  examination of, 120, 121f
  radiology of, 256-261, 257-262f
    base view, 259-260, 260f
    Caldwell view, 256, 257f, 258, 259f
    interpretation of, 264-269, 265-269f
    lateral view, 260, 261f, 262f
    tomography, 261-263, 263f
    Water's view, 256, 257f, 258f
  referred pain from, 178, 183
Sinusitis
  chronic, 139-140
  mucus in, 119
  with nasal balloon, 149
  and nasopharyngitis, chronic, 124
  polypoid rhinosinusitis, 134-135
  with viral rhinitis, 129
SISI, in Meniere's disease, 86
Sjögren's syndrome
  oral symptoms of, 200
  salivary gland swelling in, 189
  and sialadenitis, 191
  sialography in, 286-287, 288f
  triad of, 192
Skeletal defects, and deafness, 43
Skin, neck, masses within, 251
Skin tests, in allergic rhinitis, 132
Skull
  fibroma of, 271
  in malignant external otitis, 54
Skull fracture. *See also* Temporal bone, frac-
    tures of
  basilar, 107-110, 108f
  and CSF leakage, 103
Sleep preparations, vestibular toxicity of, 92
Smoking
  and laryngitis, 215
  and leukoplakia, 212
Sore throat, irritated, 210

Sound, transmission of, 4-7
Speech. *See also* Hoarseness; Voice
  esophageal, 225
  nasal obstruction and, 117
  palatal dysfunction and, 125
Speech-reception threshold, 12
Sphenoethmoidal recess, 115
Sphenoid sinus. *See also* Sinuses, paranasal
  anatomy of, 116
  pituitary adenomas and, 270
  in polypoid rhinosinusitis, 135
  radiography of
    base view, 259, 260, 260f
    lateral view, 260, 261, 261-262f
    tomography, 263, 263f, 266f
    Water's view, 256
Sphenoid sinusitis
  acute, 137-138
  chronic, 139
Sphenopalatine artery, nasal blood supply, 118-119
Sphenopalatine neuralgia, and ear pain, referred, 181
Spinal accessory nerve, neoplasms of, 252. *See also* Cranial nerves
Spinal disorders, referred pain in, 180, 183
Spiral ganglion, 5f, 7f
Spiral ligament, 7f
Spiral limbus, 7f
Stapedectomy, 35, 37f
Stapedial reflex, 23
Stapedius muscle, 5
Stapes. *See also* Ossicular chain
  anatomy of, 4
  fixation of, 34-35, 37f
  skull fractures and, 109
Staphylococcus aureus
  in auricular chondritis, 55
  in auricular infections, 99
  in external otitis, 53
  in herpes zoster oticus, 56
  in nasal furunculosis, 128
  in otitis media, 60
  in otitis media, suppurative, 58
  in septal abscesses, 158
  and sialadenitis, 191
  in sinusitis, 135
  in suppurative otitis media, 56
  in tonsillitis, 205
  in viral rhinitis, 129
Stenosis
  airway, in newborn, 234
  external auditory canal, 29
  laryngeal, 215
  subglottic, 232
Stensen's duct, 186, 187f
  obstruction of, 191
  in sialography, 283, 285, 285f
Stenting, in laryngeal stenosis, 215

Stenver's projection, in temporal bone fractures, 313, 314
Steroids
  in allergic rhinitis, 133
  in carotidynia, 182
  in external otitis, 53
  in hearing loss, sudden idiopathic, 111
  in idiopathic sensorineural hearing loss, 49
  for labyrinthitis, 88
  in mononucleosis, 103
  in rhinitis medicamentosa, 134
  in Stevens-Johnson syndrome, 201
  in syphilis, advanced, 93
  therapy for, 171
Stevens-Johnson syndrome, 201
Stiffness lesion, 39f
Stomatitis
  aphthous, 201
  herpetic, 201
  nicotine, 210
Strength–duration tests, in facial nerve paralysis, 170
Streptococcal infections
  otitis media, 56, 60
  sinusitis, 135
  tonsillitis, 205, 206
Streptococcus pneumoniae
  in septal abscesses, 158
  in sinusitis, 135
  in viral rhinitis, 129
Streptomycin
  deafness with, 45
  in Meniere's disease, 87-88
  ototoxicity of, 92
Stria vascularis, 6, 7f
  atrophy of, 39f
Strictures, salivary gland, 191
Stroke, and facial nerve weakness, 164f, 167
Styloid process, in Eagle's syndrome, 181, 209
Stylomastoid foramen, 8
Subclavian steal syndrome, and vertigo, 96
Subclavian triangle, anatomy of, 239, 240
Subdural abscess, frontal sinusitis and, 136-137
Subglottic area
  carcinoma of, 223
  defined, 221
  examination of, 211
  radiography of, 292-294f
Subglottic hemangioma, radiologic findings in, 300
Subglottic hematoma, 232-233
Subglottic stenosis, 232
Sublingual gland, anatomy of, 188
Submandibular ganglion, 9, 164f
Submandibular gland
  anatomy of, 187, 187f
  sialography of, 285-286, 286f, 287f

Submandibular lymph nodes, 244f, 245,
Submandibular triangle
  anatomy of, 238, 239f
  examination of, 247
Submental lymph nodes, 244f, 245
Submental triangle
  anatomy of, 239, 239f
  contents of, 240f, 242
  examination of, 247
Submentovertical view. *See* Base view
Submucous resection, in epistaxis, 147
Sulfisoxazole, 57, 58
Superficial petrosal nerve, 9
Superior orbital fissure syndrome, in sphen-
    oid sinusitis, 137-138
Supporting cells, of Corti's organ, 7f
Supraglottic area
  carcinoma of, 221, 223
  defined, 221
Supraglottic laryngectomy, 222f, 226
Supraglottitis, acute. *See* Croup
Suprahyoid triangle. *See* Submental triangle
Surgery
  in acute sinusitis, 136, 137, 138
  in airway obstruction, 232-233
  in chronic nasal obstruction, 123
  in chronic sinusitis, 139-140
  in epistaxis, 147, 151, 154
  in facial nerve disorders, 171-173
  and facial nerve paralysis, 168
  with infected ear, 68-69
  laceration repair, 158-163, 161-162f
  in lingual tonsillitis, 208
  for Meniere's disease, 86-87
  for nasopharyngeal cysts, 124
  in polypoid rhinosinusitis, 134-135
  in rhinitis medicamentosa, 134
  salivary gland, 191, 194-195
  sinus, 140-141
  tonsillectomy, 206
  in vasomotor rhinitis, 134
Surgical, in epistaxis, 147, 148
Suturing, facial lacerations, 160-162, 161-
    162f
Swallowing
  globus hystericus, 209-210
  after laryngectomy, 226
Swimmer's ear. *See* Otitis externa
Syphilis
  and cochlear hydrops, 74
  deafness with, 46
  larynx in, 217
  in Meniere's disease, 86
  and nasal obstruction, 142
  oropharyngeal, 203-204
  and vertigo, 93-94
Systemic disease. *See also* Metabolic disorders
  and hearing loss, sudden idiopathic, 111
  with laryngeal involvement, 219-220

Tack operation, in Meniere's disease, 87
Tampons, nasal, 149
Tarsorrhaphy, in Bell's palsy, 171-172
Tartrazene, in aspirin triad syndrome, 134
Taste, test of, 23
Tattoo, traumatic, 160
Tay-Sachs disease, 43
Technetium scan, in Warthin's tumor, 194
Teeth
  lymphatic drainage of, 244f, 245
  in maxillary sinusitis, 138
  referred pain from, 177-178, 183
  in syphilis, congenital, 204
Telangiectasia, familial hereditary, and epi-
    staxis, 147
Temporal arteritis, hearing loss with, 49
Temporal bone
  anatomy, 64f
  fractures of, 106-111, 107f, 108f. *See also* Ra-
      diology, of temporal bone
    and CSF leakage, 103
    and facial nerve paralysis, 165, 168
    radiographic findings in, 313-314, 314f
  mastoid surgery, 65-67f
  nervus intermedius and, 164f, 165
Temporal bone tumors, and facial nerve pa-
    ralysis, 167-168
Temporalis muscle, transposition of, 172-173
Temporomandibular joint syndrome, and ear
    pain, referred, 177-178
Tensor tympani, 5
Tensor veli palatini, 4
Tetanus immunization, with lacerations, 160
Thayer-Martin medium, for gonococcal cul-
    ture, 204
Threshold shift, in acoustic trauma, 106, 107f
Throat. *See* Oropharyngeal disorders; Laryn-
    geal disorders; Nasopharynx
Thrombosis
  cavernous sinus. *See* Cavernous sinus
      thrombosis
  lateral venous, 68
  nasal furunculosis and, 128
  otitis media and, 63
Thyroglossal duct cysts, 251
Thyroid cartilage, chondromas, 253
Thyroid disease
  deafness with, 48
  and hearing loss, sudden idiopathic, 111
Thyroid gland
  examination of, 247
  neoplasms, 249, 252
Tietze's syndrome, 42
Tigan, in vertigo, 83
Tinnitus, 26
  in Meniere's disease, 85
  vertigo and, 74
Tobey-Ayer test, in lateral venous thrombo-
    sis, 63

Tobramycin, ototoxicity of, 92
Tomography
  in facial trauma, 272
  of internal auditory canal, 311, 312f
  of larynx, 294, 294f
  in mastoiditis, 307
  in nasal fractures, 280
  in orbital fractures, 279f
  salivary gland, 290
  of sinuses, 261-263, 262-263f, 266f
  in temporal bone fractures, 313, 314
Tone-decay test, 16, 86
Tongue. *See also* Oropharyngeal disorders
  base of, examination of, 211
  burning, 199-200
  examination of, 198-199
  lymphatic drainage of, 244f, 245
  vitamin deficiencies and, 200
Tonsil, in nasopharynx, 122
Tonsillectomy, 206-207, 208
Tonsillitis
  in mononucleosis, 202
  pediatric, 205-208
Torticollis, 248
Towne view, in mastoiditis, 305, 306f, 308-309f
Toynbee tube, 26
Trachea
  in epiglottitis, 297f
  radiology of, 292-294f
  vascular compression of, in pediatric patient, 233
Tracheal rings, examination of, 247
Tracheobronchial foreign bodies, 231
Tracheoesophageal fistula, in newborn, 234
Tracheostomy, 223-224
Tracheotomy, 223-224
  in airway obstruction, 232
  in laryngeal arthritis, 219
  for newborn, 234
  in viral laryngitis, acute, 230
Tractus solitarius, 9
Tranquilizers, vestibular toxicity of, 92
Transgrow bottles, for gonococcal culture, 204
Transorbital view, in mastoiditis, 305, 306f, 308f
Trauma. *See also* Emergencies; *specific fracture site*
  to auditory canal, 103
  deafness with, 45-46
  and facial nerve paralysis, 168
  in HANE, 234
  inner ear and temporal bone, 106-111, 107f
  middle ear and temporal bone, 103-104
  and nasal obstruction, 130, 131f
  and olfaction, 144
  and vertigo, 94-95

Treacher-Collins syndrome, 5
Trendelenburg position, in airway obstruction, 228
Treponema pallidum. See Syphilis
Triangles, cervical. *See* Cervical triangles
Trichinosis, laryngeal, 217
Trigeminal nerve, neoplasms, 252
Trigeminal neuralgia, and ear pain, referred, 180-181
Trimalar fractures, radiographic findings in, 273, 274f, 275f
Trisomies, deafness with, 44
Tuberculosis, 217
  and nasal obstruction, 141
  and otitis media, 60
  salivary gland infiltrates in, 192
Tumarkin, drop attacks of, 73
Tuning-fork test, 11-12
  in Meniere's disease, 86
Turbinates
  anatomy of, 114, 121, 122f
  electrocautery of, 123
  in vasomotor rhinitis, 134
Tympanic membrane
  anatomy of, 3-4, 3f
  auditory canal foreign bodies and, 102-103
  barotrauma, 105
  disorders of, and hearing loss, 30-31
  emergencies, 103-105
  examination of, in vertigo, 74-75
  in hearing loss. *See* Hearing loss
  in otitis media
    serous, 123
    suppurative, 56-57, 58
    tuberculous, 60
  otoscopy, 10
  skull fractures and, 108
  temporal bone fractures and, 107
Tympanic neuralgia, and ear pain, referred, 180-181
Tympanomastoidectomy, 68
Tympanometry, 17, 19-21, 21f
Tympanoplasty
  anatomy for, 66, 67f
  with mastoidectomy, 68-69
  in otitis media, 61
Tympanosclerosis, and hearing loss, 30

Ulcers
  laryngeal
    contact, 213-214
    in lupus erythematosus, 219
  of mouth, 201-204
  nasal, and epistaxis, 146-147
Ultrasound ablation, in Meniere's disease, 87

Unverricht's epilepsy, deafness with, 44
Usher's syndrome, 44
Utricle, anatomy of, 5, 5f, 6f, 7

Vagus nerve, neoplasms, 252
Valsalva maneuver, 10, 11
Varicella, 204
Varicosities, oropharyngeal, 199
Vascular anomalies, and tracheal compression, in pediatric patient, 233
Vascular disease
    deafness with, 48
    and epistaxis, 154
    otitis media and, 63
    septic thrombosis, 68
    and vertigo, 95, 96
Vascular tumors
    and epistaxis, 154
    neck, 248, 251, 252
    sinus, radiographic findings, 270
Vasculature
    of cervical triangles, 239f, 240f, 241, 242, 243
    frontal sinusitis and, 136-137
    nasal, 118-119
Vasoconstrictors
    in allergic rhinitis, 131-132
    in epistaxis, 146, 147, 148, 149
    for nasal examinations, 119
    in serous otitis, 123
    in sinusitis, 135-136
    in vasomotor rhinitis, 133-134
    in viral rhinitis, 129
Vasomotor rhinitis, 118, 119, 133-134
Venous sinus thrombosis, otitis media and, 63, 68
Vertebrobasilar ischemia, deafness with, 48
Vertical laryngectomy, 222f, 226
Vertigo
    benign paroxysmal positional, 91
    of brain-stem origin, 95-96
    evaluation of, 72-81
        caloric tests, 77, 80
        ear canal and tympanic membrane, 74-75
        electronystagmography, 80-81
        history, 72-74
        positional tests, 76-77, 78-79
        spontaneous nystagmus, 75
    with inner ear and vestibular nerve involvement, 89-91
        cupulolithiasis, 89-91
        vestibular neuritis, viral, 91
    labyrinthitis, acute viral, 88-89
    Meniere's disease, 84-88
    neck injury and, 94-95

    positional, 72-73
    stapedectomy and, 37
    systemic disorders and, 91-95
        acoustic neurinoma, 92
        aging, 92-93
        multiple sclerosis, 93
        rare disorders, 94-95
        syphilis, 93-94
        vestibular toxicity, 91-92
    treatment of, 81-84
Vestibular artery disease, and vertigo, 95
Vestibular end-organ ablation, in Meniere's disease, 87
Vestibular function
    aging and, 92-93
    mastoid surgery and, 69
    testing, 21-22
Vestibular ganglion, 5f
Vestibular labyrinth. *See also* Labyrinthitis
    anatomy of, 5-7, 5-7f
    drug toxicity, 91-92
    otitis media and, 61-62
    skull fractures and, 109, 313
Vestibular nerve
    schwannoma, deafness with, 47-48
    sectioning of
        in BPPV, 91
        in Meniere's disease, 87
    skull fractures and, 108
    viral neuritis, 91
Vestibular symptoms, 72. *See also* Vertigo
    in cerebellopontine-angle tumors, 47
    perilymph leak and, 104
Vestibule, tomographic view, 312f
Vidian nerve, sectioning of, 118, 134
Vincent's angina, 202
Viral infections
    and Bell's palsy, 166
    and ethmoiditis, 138
    and facial nerve paralysis, 166
    and hearing loss, sudden idiopathic, 111
    infectious mononucleosis, 202-203. *See also* Infectious mononucleosis
    labyrinthitis, and vertigo, 88-89
    laryngitis, acute, 229-230
    and nasopharyngeal carcinoma, 123
    pediatric, 204-205
    respiratory tract, 216-217
    rhinitis, 119, 128-129
    and sinus infection, 135
    vestibular neuritis, 91
Vision
    ethmoidectomy and, 141
    nystagmus and, 75
    in sphenoid sinusitis, 138
    in Wallenberg's disease, 95-96
Visual fixation, and nystagmus, 75
Vitamin deficiencies, and glossitis, 200

Vocal cords
    carcinoma of, 221
    cysts of, radiologic findings in, 301, 301f
    examination of, 211, 212f
    hyperkeratosis of, 212-213
    lupus erythematosus and, 220
    paralysis of, 220
        and hoarseness, 220
        in pediatric patients, 233
    polyps of, 212-213
        radiographic findings in, 303
    radiography of, 292-294f
    singer's nodules, 213
    submucosal hemorrhage, 213
Voice, in lingual tonsillitis, 208. *See also*
        Hoarseness; Speech
Vomiting
    in Meniere's disease, 85
    in vertigo, 83
von Recklinghausen's disease, 47, 92
Vosol, in external otitis, 53

Waardenburg's syndrome, 42
Waldenstrom's macroglobulinemia, vertigo
        in, 94
Wallenberg's syndrome
    deafness with, 48
    and vertigo, 95-96
Warthin's tumor, technetium incorporation
        in, 194
Water's view
    in acute sinusitis, 264, 265f
    in ethmoid sinus osteoma, 271, 271f
    in maxillary antrum carcinoma, 273f
    in nasal fractures, 277, 280
    in orbital fractures, 276, 277, 278f, 281f
    of sinuses, 256, 257f, 258f
Weber test, 11-12
Wegener's granulomatosis, 60
    hearing loss with, 49
    and nasal obstruction, 142
Wharton's duct, 187, 187f
    obstruction of, 191
    in sialography, 283
Whiplash, and vertigo, 94-95
Whisper test, 11-12, 86
Wicks', ear, in external otitis, 53-54
Wilson's disease, deafness with, 44
Word-discrimination test, 13
Wound closure, in laceration repair, 160
Wrisberg, nervus intermedius of, 163-165,
        164f

Xeroradiogram, laryngeal, 291
Xylometasoline hydrochloride, in sinusitis,
        136. *See also* Vasoconstrictors

Zenker's diverticulum, 210, 253
Zygomatic arch, fractures of, 273, 274, 275f